Mental Disorders

Mental Disorders

Edited by **John Dalvi**

FOSTER ACADEMICS

New Jersey

Published by Foster Academics,
61 Van Reypen Street,
Jersey City, NJ 07306, USA
www.fosteracademics.com

Mental Disorders
Edited by John Dalvi

International Standard Book Number: 978-1-63242-273-6 (Hardback)

Printed in China.

Contents

	Preface	**VII**
Chapter 1	**Cognitive Behavioral Therapy Approach for Suicidal Thinking and Behaviors in Depression** John D. Matthews	**1**
Chapter 2	**Cognitive Behaviour Therapy in the Management of Conduct Disorder Among Adolescents** Afusat Olanike Busari	**22**
Chapter 3	**Treatment-Resistant Schizophrenia: Prevalence and Risk Factors** Mohamed Dammak	**41**
Chapter 4	**Anxiolytics Use in the Families with (Non)dependent Member: Relation to Dependence Indicators, Self and Family Perceptions Including Social Neuroscience Perspective** Maja Rus-Makovec, Karin Sernec and Velko S. Rus	**63**
Chapter 5	**Management of Delirium** Narong Maneeton and Benchalak Maneeton	**82**
Chapter 6	**Rethinking Dissociation in an Age of Virtual Worlds** Gregory Patrick Garvey	**116**
Chapter 7	**Racism and Mental Illness in the UK** Apu Chakraborty, Lance Patrick and Maria Lambri	**132**
Chapter 8	**Somatic Symptom Disorder** Lesley A. Allen and Robert L. Woolfolk	**169**

Chapter 9	**The Bond We Share: Experiences of Caring for a Person with Mental and Physical Health Conditions** Sharon Lawn, Jeannette Walsh, Anne Barbara, Margaret Springgay and Patricia Sutton	**194**
Chapter 10	**Parent-Child Attachment, Parental Depression, and Perception of Child Behavioural/Emotional Problems** Lawrence T. Lam	**225**
Chapter 11	**Working on Adolescent's Motivation to Improve the Outcome Within a Multimodal Treatment** Gatta Michela, Testa C. Paolo, Del Col Lara, Spoto Andrea, Dal Zotto Lara, De Sauma Maxim and Battistella Pier Antonio	**238**
Chapter 12	**Current Advances in the Treatment of Major Depression: Shift Towards Receptor Specific Drugs** Ashok Kumar Jainer, Rajkumar Kamatchi, Marek Marzanski and Bettahalasoor Somashekar	**262**
Chapter 13	**The Association Between Tinnitus and Mental Illnesses** Adeyi A. Adoga and Taiwo J. Obindo	**282**
Chapter 14	**The Characteristics of Nicotine Addiction Among Patients with Schizophrenia** Ewa Wojtyna and Agnieszka Wiszniewicz	**303**
Chapter 15	**Post Traumatic Eco-Stress Disorder (PTESD): A Qualitative Study from Sundarban Delta, India** Arabinda N. Chowdhury, Ranajit Mondal, Mrinal K Biswas and Arabinda Brahma	**322**
Chapter 16	**Attention - Deficit Hyperactivity Disorder (ADHD) in Psychiatry and Psychoanalysis** Crístia Rosineiri Gonçalves Lopes Corrêa	**361**
Chapter 17	**Quality in Delivery of Mental Health Services** Mary Ditton	**378**
	Permissions	
	List of Contributors	

Preface

This book is the result of collaboration of reputed experts from various countries around the world. Mental disorders are a domain undergoing continuous studies with times and still seem to be incomprehensible with discoveries of new challenges and cases emerging every new day. It is an up-to-date document that discusses issues of critical importance in psychopathology whose understanding has been limited so far. This book will serve as a valuable addition to any library available for reference to scholars and clinicians.

All of the data presented henceforth, was collaborated in the wake of recent advancements in the field. The aim of this book is to present the diversified developments from across the globe in a comprehensible manner. The opinions expressed in each chapter belong solely to the contributing authors. Their interpretations of the topics are the integral part of this book, which I have carefully compiled for a better understanding of the readers.

At the end, I would like to thank all those who dedicated their time and efforts for the successful completion of this book. I also wish to convey my gratitude towards my friends and family who supported me at every step.

Editor

Chapter 1

Cognitive Behavioral Therapy Approach for Suicidal Thinking and Behaviors in Depression

John D. Matthews

Additional information is available at the end of the chapter

1. Introduction

1.1. Overview of cognitive behavioral therapy

Cognitive therapy is based on cognitive theory, which is an information processing model. Cognitive refers to how an individual interprets and assigns meaning to his or her experiences. We as humans are continually trying to make sense of our internal and external experiences for the purposes of survival and attachment. How we scan our environment and choose stimuli to attribute meanings is variable from person to person and based on past learning and beliefs. Over the course of our development, we acquire beliefs about ourselves, others, our environment, and our future. A.T. Beck et al. (1979) refers to these beliefs that have durability and rigidity over time as core beliefs [1]. J.S. Beck (2005) categorizes core beliefs based on individuals sense of their lovability, worth, and control [2]. These categories of core beliefs can be adaptive or maladaptive depending on our long-term experiences with significant people and situations. Thus, maladaptive core beliefs would be associated with beliefs of unlovability, worthlessness, and helplessness. New information is processed in the moment based on the balance between adaptive and maladaptive core beliefs among these three categories. Individuals who grow up in a mostly negative environment will likely develop more maladaptive than adaptive core beliefs. These core beliefs, when activated by associated events in the moment, influence objectivity and thus color how we interpret our experience in the present. Thus, the thoughts or interpretations in the present do not equal fact, but are subject to change with new information. When we are functioning well in the present moment, our adaptive core beliefs are prominent in conscious awareness and determine, in a positive manner, how we scan our environment and attribute meanings to new information. However, under stress, a crisis, or an acute onset or recurrence of a psychiatric disorder, our maladaptive core beliefs surface to conscious awareness and have a negative impact on how we scan our environment and process new information. When activated, maladaptive core beliefs mold new information to fit the current maladaptive core belief, thus making it stronger. Persistent maladaptive core beliefs are the basis, in part, of most psychopathology; however, CBT acknowledges the impact of biological and genetic factors, particularly in the case of major mental illnesses.

Cognitive theory teaches that our emotions, physiological responses, and behaviors are a product of our thinking in the present moment. The spontaneous, unpremeditated interpretations associated with specific events in the present are referred to as automatic thoughts [1]. When the automatic thoughts are misinterpretations of current events, Beck refers to then as dysfunctional automatic thoughts [1]. If in a given situation an individual has the dysfunctional automatic thought, "I'm a loser", this interpretation is likely due to the activation of the maladaptive core belief "I'm incompetent". The products of the dysfunctional automatic thought, "I'm a loser", might include sadness, anxiety, increased autonomic system activity, and a desire to avoid people. Cognitive theory also teaches that our emotions, physiological responses, and behavior influence our thinking and beliefs as well. Studies have shown that people who are depressed have difficulty accessing positive memories of past experiences and past successes [3,4]. Because depressed patients tend to withdraw and isolate, they miss opportunities to obtain information that might provide a more balanced view of themselves. Thus, there are multiple interactions among thoughts, feelings, physiological reactions, and behaviors as shown in Figure 1.

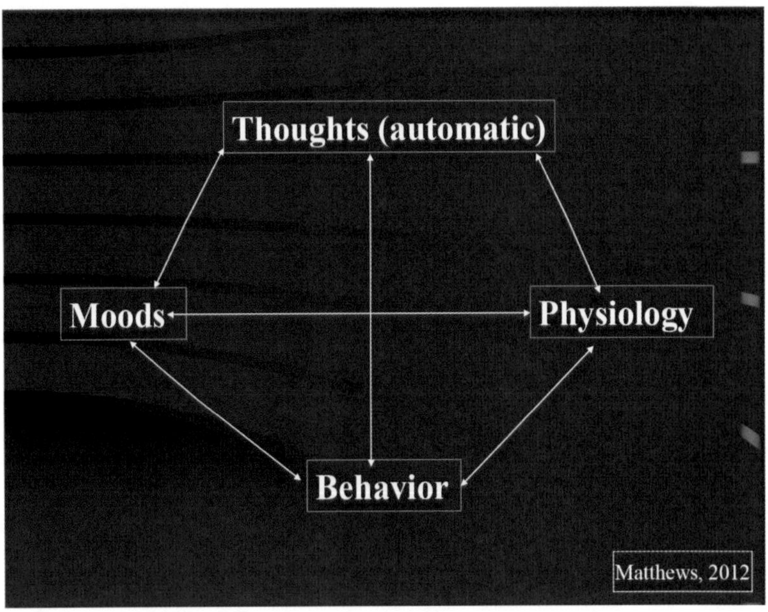

Figure 1.

The function of cognitive therapy is to reduce negative emotional reactions, distressing physiological responses, and self-defeating behaviors by modifying dysfunctional automatic thoughts, initially, followed by modifying maladaptive core beliefs. Dysfunctional automatic thoughts are challenged by having the patient look for evidence against the negative thoughts and/or by having the patient identify alternative explanations in a given situation. Maladaptive core beliefs are modified through a process called "belief work" [5], which will be reviewed later in the chapter. The underlying maladaptive core beliefs are revealed by observing patterns of dysfunctional automatic thoughts across multiple situations in the present. Although the primary focus of CBT is on targeting dysfunctional automatic thoughts and maladaptive core beliefs, negative emotions, distressing physiological responses, and self-defeating behaviors also become targets for treatment. In the case of a depressed patient, who was avoiding others out of fear of being criticized, behavioral activation strategies enabled him to discover that there were several supportive people available to him, which resulted in a marked decrease in his fear and anxiety. Thus, the behavioral intervention had a positive impact on both his negative thinking and negative emotions. According to A.T. Beck et al. (1979), in order to achieve lasting change of our emotional distress and self-defeating behaviors, cognitive and behavioral interventions are required to change the underlying maladaptive core beliefs [1].

In addition to dysfunctional automatic thoughts and maladaptive core beliefs, there are two other problematic aspects of cognition, maladaptive intermediate beliefs and errors in logic [5]. In view of the fact that awareness of one's maladaptive core beliefs creates emotional distress, the individual develops and implements cognitive compensatory strategies or maladaptive intermediate beliefs in order to prevent maladaptive core beliefs from being activated. Maladaptive intermediate beliefs consist of rules or assumptions that guide interactions with others and one's environment. These rules or assumptions take on a form of "if…then…" statements that take on either a positive or negative valence. For example, a patient with a core belief, "I am incompetent" may develop a maladaptive intermediate belief, "If I avoid making mistakes, my weaknesses will not be seen by others" (positive form). Alternatively, "If I do not perform perfectly, I will fail" (negative form). In stressful situations, the negative forms are more prominent [5]. From a treatment perspective, it is important to identify a patient's maladaptive intermediate beliefs since they contribute to his or her self-defeating behaviors. Frequently, there are corresponding maladaptive behaviors associated with maladaptive intermediate beliefs. J.S. Beck (2011) refers to these behaviors as compensatory strategies [5]. Like maladaptive intermediate beliefs, compensatory strategies serve the function of preventing maladaptive core beliefs from being activated. In the above example, "If I avoid making mistakes, my weaknesses will not be seen by others", a typical behavioral compensatory strategy might be perfectionism. A patient would try to do his or her work perfectly in or to avoid the activation of his or her core belief "I'm incompetent". Although performing perfectly has value in many situations, when perfectionism becomes a way of life, it can limit one's experience and interfere with achieving value-based goals. Errors in logic are the final problematic aspects of cognition to be addressed. The most common errors in logic include: mind reading (assumption that others are reacting negatively without sufficient evidence); overgeneralization (specific events defines life in general); all-or-nothing thinking (events are seen in one of two mutually exclusive extreme categories); personalization (assuming responsibility for negative outcomes without considering other contributing factors); and catastrophic thinking (experiences or events are interpreted in terms of the worst possible outcomes). Errors in logic also contribute to faulty information processing and thus lead to misinterpretations of events and experiences in the present.

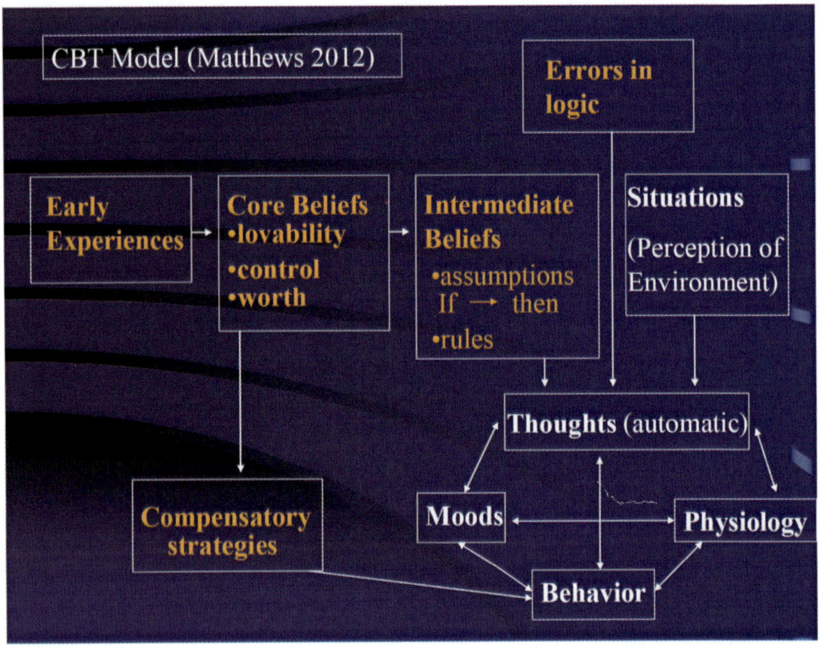

Figure 2.

Figure 2 summarizes what has been reviewed thus far. Cognitive therapy begins by helping patients see the relationships among thoughts, feelings, physiological responses, and behaviors in a variety of situations in the present (illustrated in white). As patterns of interpretations emerge, the therapist and patient develop a case formulation with the goal of identifying core beliefs, intermediate beliefs, and compensatory strategies based on an analysis of the interpretations from multiple situations in present, and based on a review of probable contributing negative experiences from the past (illustrated in yellow). Once the individual's core belief/s are identified, the focus of therapy is on modifying the underlying maladaptive core beliefs. J.S. Beck (2011) describes this process as "Belief Work" [5]. In the case of a patient with a core belief, "I'm a failure", the therapist would first have the patient reframe the maladaptive belief in less severe terms, "Having weaknesses does not mean I'm a total failure". The therapist next has the patient identify evidence against the maladaptive or old belief and supports the new belief, "My evaluations at work are good, but not perfect". Finally, the therapist has the patient identify evidence that supports the old belief, but with a reframe, "Although I have deficiencies, I am more than my weaknesses." To further enhance perspective building with regards to maladaptive core beliefs, the therapist has the patient perform a historical review in order to identify important events in his or her life that might have contributed to the development of the maladaptive core belief. The therapist then has the patient focus on specific relevant events and generate alternative explanations by taking on an observer role using cognitive restructuring (identifying evidence for and against the belief); in addition, the therapist assists the patient in collateral data collection by designing behavioral experiments [5].

2. Cognitive factors for suicidal thinking and behaviors

There are a number of cognitive factors that contribute to suicidal thinking and behaviors. These factors can be categorized as cognitive content deficits and cognitive information processing deficits.

2.1. Cognitive content deficits

Beck's cognitive triad: A. T. Beck's cognitive triad forms the foundation of the CBT model for suicidal thinking and behaviors. According to A.T. Beck, depressed suicidal patients view themselves as defective, inadequate, diseased, or deprived and thus worthless and undesirable; they view others as rejecting and unsupportive by making too many demands; and they view their future as hopeless since they do not believe that they have the internal and external resources to solve their problems [1].Their sense of defectiveness contributes to a passive approach to solving the problems that are creating their distress; they avoid making attempts at solving their problem/s and they may even hope for a spontaneous solution [6]. Because they believe that no one really cares about them and because their problem/s seem overwhelming to manage on their own, they give up. Without the personal skills and the support of others, they conclude that there can be no future.

Hopelessness: Hopelessness is a primary contributing factor in the development of suicidal thinking and behaviors and distinguishes depressed suicidal patients from depressed non-suicidal patients [7]. Hopeless is the consequence of seeing no solutions to problems and the activation of beliefs related to negative expectations: *"I can never be happy"; "I am a burden to my family and they will be better without me".* Hopelessness is more strongly related to suicide intent than depression or severity of symptoms [1,8]. More recent studies have demonstrated that hopelessness can be measured reliably and that it is a mediator between depression severity and suicidal thinking and behaviors [9]. Thus, hopelessness predicts current and future suicidal thinking and behaviors. Researchers have distinguished between state and trait hopelessness. State hopelessness is associated with the acute act of suicide; whereas, trait hopelessness is associated with long-term negative expectations for the future. A. T. Beck (1986) argues that with strong trait hopelessness, it takes less stress to trigger a suicidal crisis and state hopelessness [10]. Young et al. (1996) found that persistent levels of hopelessness, in depressed patients who had achieved remission, was more predictive of suicide attempts than high levels of hopelessness at a given time [11].

Psychological/Physical Pain: Shneidman was among the first to stress the importance of the experience of pain in contributing to suicidal thinking and behaviors. He referred to the pain of the suicidal patient as *psychache* and he strongly believed that *psychache* was the driving force for a patient attempting suicide. "Psychache is at the dark heart of suicide; no psychache, no suicide" (p.200) [12]. Chiles and Strosahl (2005) note that in a suicidal crisis, it is likely that an individual will experience emotional or physical pain that he or she believes is "Intolerable", "Inescapable", "Interminable" [13]. According to Chiles and Strosahl, pain is viewed as intolerable if it exceeds one's defined threshold; pain is viewed as inescapable if one does not see any solutions to the problem causing the pain; and pain is viewed as interminable if one believes that it will never change on its own accord. The authors also stress that much of the distress associated with pain is due to one's relationship to his or her pain. A patient gets into a struggle with his or her pain by resisting it and refusing to accept it in the context of there being no immediate solutions. Acceptance does not mean that a patient is giving-in, giving-up, or has to be satisfied with his or her situation. Acceptance reduces the distress of wanting to be elsewhere then where one is, thus putting him or her in a better attitude or frame of mind to work on the problem that is responsible for his or her pain.

2.2. Cognitive information processing deficits

Cognitive rigidity and dichotomous: Cognitive rigidity and dichotomous thinking are constructs that were proposed by Shneidman (1959) [14] and validated through research by Neuringer [15,16]. Cognitive rigidity refers to the inability to see options or alternative courses of actions in problematic situations; in addition, a patient also fails to anticipate the array of possible consequences. Dichotomous thinking ("all-or-nothing thinking") categorizes experiences into one of two extremes, "good/bad" or "success/failure". Thus a patient experiences difficulty in acknowledging nuances and subtleties in problem situations. These two cognitive processes contribute to the problem solving deficits seen in a depressed suicidal patient [17]. The steps to effective problem solving include: identify the possible solutions; review the pros and cons of each possible solution; choose the best solution from the pros and cons analysis; plan the implementation of the best solution; implement the plan; and evaluate the effectiveness of the plan [18, 19]. Problem solving deficits are a function of cognitive rigidity and dichotomous thinking. Cognitive rigidity contributes to a decreased ability to generate new ideas and anticipate various course outcomes; whereas, dichotomous thinking contributes to a tendency to focus on the negative consequences of potential courses of action.

Attentional bias: As previously discussed, cognitive theory teaches that an individual selectively scans his or her environment, makes interpretations of his or her observations, and recalls relevant information from the past in the process of trying to make sense of his or her internal experiences. The processes of selection and interpretation are determined by past experiences, memories, and beliefs. Suicidal patients will automatically focus and select information that is suicide-related, thus narrowing their perspective and awareness of other courses of action than suicide. Studies supporting this concept have shown that patients who have attempted suicide show an attentional bias towards words that are related to suicide on the Emotional Stroop Task compared to negative or neutral words [20, 21].

Attentional fixation: Wenzel et al. (2009) note that in suicidal patients that they have studied, patients report a mental state of confusion and disorientation immediately prior to their suicide attempt [22]. They are experiencing racing thoughts, agitation, "tunnel vision" as well as deep emotional pain. Suicide seems to be the only way out of their distress. Wenzel et al. (2009) compare this state of mind to what patients with panic disorder experience during a panic attack. Beck (1988) describes a "dissociation of higher-level reflective processes from automatic cognitive processing" [23]. Wenzel et al. (2009) believe that there is a similar process in operation just prior to a suicide attempt [22]. Higher-level processing is unavailable to broaden awareness and to assist in identifying options that could lead to solving those problems that are creating deep emotional pain. Attentional fixation interferes with rational information processing and makes it difficult to disengage from suicide-related information, thus interfering with problem solving and increasing as sense of hopelessness.

Overgeneralized memory: Overgeneralized memory is another information processing defect observed in depressed suicidal patients [24]. Studies have demonstrated that when patients who have made recent suicide attempts are cued to provide details about a past personal experience, they respond with vague recollections that summarize multiple experiences; these results were independent of processing speed [25, 21]. This finding is also seen when suicidal patients were provided further prompts, explanations, and practice items in an attempt to help clarify their responses [26]. This type of information processing interferes with effective problem solving, which relies on the recall of details from past problem solving successes.

3. A CBT model of suicide

Figure 3 summarizes the research that has been presented in the previous paragraphs. This model emphasizes that an individual considers suicide if he or she sees no solutions to the problem that is creating pain that is perceived as intolerable, inescapable, and interminable. Thus, the focus of CBT in the depressed suicidal patient is to: identify the perceived unsolvable problem; reduce cognitive distortions and errors in logic with regards to his or her views of self, others, and future; improve problem solving skills; increase motivation to problem solve; reduce perceived emotional pain; and encourage acceptance of emotional pain as part of everyday life.

4. Assessment

There are a number of predictors of suicidal thinking and behaviors that have been identified over the years including being elderly, male, divorced, widowed, separated, medically ill in the past 6 months, depressed, addicted to substances, and having made suicide attempts in the past to name a few [27]. However, from a CBT perspective, it is not solely the situation that determines suicidal thinking and behaviors, but, the meaning that an individual attributes to his or her situation. This is not to say that the above predictors do not have some contribution to an individual's decision to attempt suicide; rather, these predictors might indirectly contribute by increasing the individual's vulnerability to choose suicide.

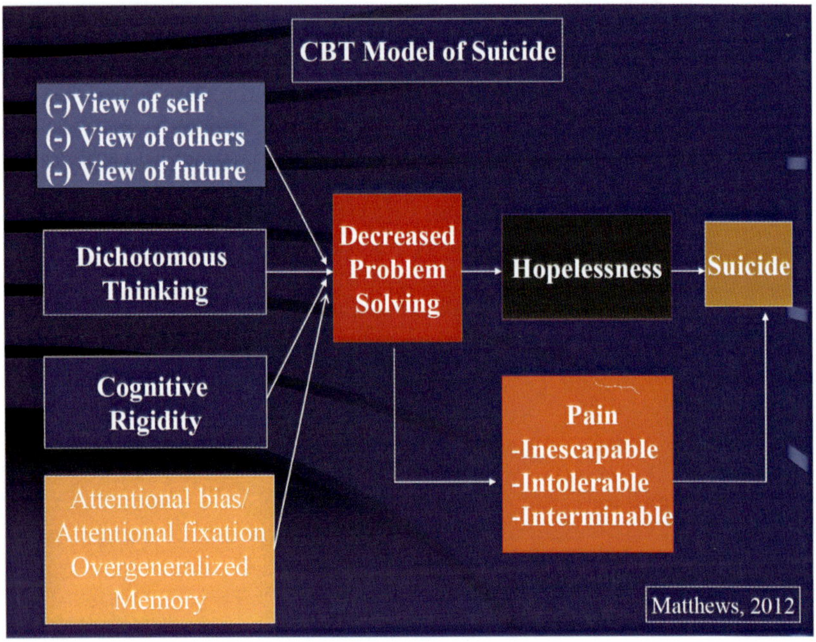

Figure 3.

4.1. Rating scales

Beck Hopelessness Scale (BHS) [8]: The Beck Hopelessness Scale is a twenty item, self-administered, true false questionnaire developed to assess the degree of positive and negative beliefs about the future during the previous week. It can be used in inpatient and outpatient settings and for both adults and adolescence. The score ranges from 0 to 20; patients who score above 8 are 11 times more likely to commit suicide than patients who score 8 or below [28]. In a study to predict suicide over a 10-year period in outpatients with mixed diagnoses (N=1,958), while using a total score of ≥9, Beck et al. (1990) found a false-positive rate of 59% (those with a score of ≥9 and who did not commit suicide) and a false-negative rate of 5.9% (those with a score of <9, but committed suicide) [29]. The test is an indirect indicator of suicide risk in depressed patients who have made suicide attempts and it is also useful for detecting hopelessness severity.

Beck Scale for Suicidal Ideation (BSS) [30]: The Beck Scale for Suicidal Ideation measures the intensity, pervasiveness, and characteristics of suicidal ideations in adults and adolescence and has been used in a variety settings including, inpatient, outpatient, emergency services, and medical services [30]. An earlier self-administered version, the Scale for Suicidal Ideation (SSI) used the same questions, but is no longer in print. The BSS is a 21-item, self-administered questionnaire that asks questions regarding suicidal ideations over the past week. It is scored on a 3-point Likert scale from 0=not present to 2=maximum severity of suicidal ideation. If items 4 ("Desire to make active suicide attempt") and 5 ("Passive suicidal desire") are rated as a 1 (weak) or 2 (moderate to strong), the patient rates the rest of the items. The severity of the suicidal ideations are calculated from the first 19-items and the range of scores is from 0-38. There is no cut-off score, but the severity of suicidal ideations are determined by increasing scores. Items on the scale can be re-examined over time in order to monitor for changes in the risk for suicide. The scale does not predict since there are no studies demonstrating that higher scores on the BSS predict immediate risk for a suicide attempt. Although most individuals who have suicidal ideations do not attempt suicide, high scores on the BSS can alert clinicians to perform a more comprehensive assessment of suicide risk.

Beck Suicide Intent Scale (SIS) is a clinician-administered measure of the intensity of the suicide attempter's desire to die at the time of the attempt [31, 32]. The scale consists of 20 items on a 0-2 Likert scale for each item. Items 1-8 focus on preparation and manner of execution of the attempt, the setting, likelihood of rescue. Items 9-15 focus on the attempter's perception of the lethality of the attempt, expectations of rescue, degree of premeditation, and the purpose of the attempt. Items 16-20 include the attempter's reaction to the attempt, number of previous attempts, and the use of substances at the time of the attempt; items 16-20 are not included in the total score. Studies have shown that items 1-8 distinguished fatal from non-fatal attempts. The total score differentiates repeat attempters from non-repeaters. One study found that the "Precautions against Discovery and/or Intervention was associated with increased risk of eventual suicide [28]. However, there is no data to suggest that the SIS can be used to predict suicide.

Columbia-Suicide Severity Rating Scale (CSSRS) The Columbia-Suicide Severity Rating Scale was developed as a single measure to assess severity of suicidal ideation and behavior and to track them as well. The CSSRS was designed to distinguish suicidal ideation and behavior. In the past, suicidal ideation and behavior were considered to be on a continuum [33]. The scale is divided into four subscales: severity subscale; intensity subscale; behavior subscale; and the lethality subscale. The severity subscale measure severity of suicidal ideations on a 5-point ordinal scale where 1=wish to be dead, 2=nonspecific active suicidal thoughts, 3=suicidal thoughts with methods, 4=suicidal intent, and 5=suicidal intent and plan. The intensity subscale consists of 5 items, each rated on a 5-point ordinal scale with measures on frequency, duration, controllability, deterrents, and reasons for ideations. The behavior subscale is rated on a nominal scale that includes actual, aborted, and interrupted suicide attempts as well as measures on preparatory behavior and non-suicidal self-injurious behavior. The lethality subscale, which assess actual attempts, is rated on a 6-point ordinal scale; an actual attempt is given a score of 0 and potential lethality of attempts is rated on a 3-point ordinal scale. The CSSRS uses different life-time assessment periods and studies have shown that the "worst-point ideation" was a stronger predictor of subsequent suicide than current ideation [34,35]. The inclusion of all of the items in the scale were based on previous research that demonstrated that these measures predicted risk for future suicidal behaviors. In a recent study, Posner et al. (2011) demonstrated that the CSSRS has good convergent and divergent validity with other suicidal ideation and behavior scales (e.g. Scale for Suicidal Ideation, Beck's Lethality Scale, Beck Depression Inventory, Columbia Suicide History Form) and high sensitivity and specificity for suicidal behavior compared to another behavior scale [33]. In addition, they found that the ideation and behavior subscales were sensitive to change over time.

4.2. Motivation for suicide

Identifying the motive for suicide is crucial for determining the treatment approach. There are two primary motives for suicide, to escape from life with its pain or to produce some interpersonal change or change in their environment [36]. In a study of 200 inpatients who had made a suicide attempt prior to admission, Kovacs, et al. (1975) found that 111 (56%) reported escape as their primary motive, whereas, 26 (13%) reported hope to effect a change in others or in their environment [36]. The reminder reported motives that were a combination of the two. The motive to escape was associated with more serious suicide attempts. Escape from life with its pain may be based on reality (poverty, medical problems, social isolation, chronic illness); thus, the focus of treatment is on appropriate biopsychosocial interventions. However, the motivation to end one's life may be based on distorted or pathological ways of viewing oneself, others, and the world, thus, the focus is directed on misperceptions and irrational belief systems. When the primary motivation is to create interpersonal or environmental change, the common reasons are for love and affection, revenge, or control. Under these circumstances, the focus of treatment is on improving social skills and learning more effective and adaptive ways of communicating.

4.3. Triggers for suicide

Rudd et al. (2001) stress the importance of identifying triggers of suicidal thinking and behaviors [6]. Triggers can be categorized as being internal and external experiences or themes. Internal triggers include thoughts, images, feelings and physical sensations. External triggers include people, places, circumstances, and situations. Thematic triggers include activation of abandonment concerns or fears of rejection. Tools that can assist in identifying triggers include dysfunctional thought records and chain analyses. A dysfunctional thought record is divided into five columns including: situation, emotions, dysfunctional automatic thoughts, rational response, and re-rating the belief in the original dysfunctional automatic thoughts. The Dysfunctional Thought Record provides a strategy to not only identify the trigger for the decision to choose suicide, but it identifies the misinterpretations associated with the trigger as well. The sequential links in the Chain Analysis strategy include: **vulnerabilities** (depression, stress, substance use, medical illness, loss etc.) → **prompting event** (the event outside of the person that was the "last straw") → **linked thoughts and feelings** → **suicide attempt** → **review consequences of suicide attempt** → **review alternatives to suicide attempt.**

5. Treatment

The goals of treatment for the depressed suicidal patient include: address specific cognitive biases and distortions; develop behavior skills (problem solving); acceptance and tolerance of emotional pain; improve communication skills (social skills, assertiveness training, conflict resolution skills); reduce environmental stress; and develop supports [13,27].

In order to engage a patient in the treatment of his or her suicidal thinking and behaviors, the clinician must convey an empathic approach. The patient enters therapy with concerns that he or she will be perceived as being irrational, trying to get attention, not being taken seriously, or potentially being punished. These are based on typical responses he or she has received from relatives and friends. It is important not to start psychotherapy by trying to talk him or her out of suicide. Such an approach convinces the patient that the therapist does not understand his or her situation and what he or she is experiencing. Rather, try to understand the patient's logic for choosing suicide. Ask the question, "Help me understand what got you to the point that suicide seemed to be the only solution". Through understanding his or her logic, the therapist may experience, to some degree, the patient's despair. The therapist might also help normalize the patient's decision by saying that "If I was in your situation, I might have also considered suicide". However, it is important to offer hope by informing the patient that, by working together, solutions or partial solutions to his or her problem will emerge, thus, providing alternatives suicide. It is also important for the therapist to be aware of his or her beliefs about the patient, such as "He is untreatable" or "He is just being manipulative". Awareness of these negative beliefs must be addressed by finding common ground from which to continue to work together.

5.1. Cognitive/behavioral targets for treatment

Hopelessness: The immediate goal in addressing hopelessness is to challenge the belief that the patient's situation cannot get better. The depressed suicidal patient overestimates the magnitude of his or her problem and underestimates the available resources. It is important to create a disequilibrium in the patient's distorted beliefs by introducing evidence that contradicts his or her belief. Teaching problem solving skills and identifying available family and community resources provide internal and external resources that can be used to solve his or her problems, thus, enhancing self-efficacy. For a patient who became suicidal because he believed that his musical career was over because of a single poor performance at a recent concert, his overestimation of the consequences and his belief he had no resources were challenged by having him market himself, which resulted in him successfully getting another performance. He had resisted marketing himself in the past; however, his success at marketing enhanced his self-efficacy.

Cognitive rigidity: With regards to cognitive rigidity, it is important to frame beliefs as testable hypotheses and not fixed rules and to generate alternative explanations and test them behaviorally. Strategies to accomplish this include role play and visual imagery. In the case of role play, the patient plays his or her critical voice and the therapist rationally responds; this is followed by reverse role play where the patient is played by the therapist and the patient responds to the critical voice. Visual imagery provides the patient an opportunity to imagine the various solutions and potential outcomes. Both strategies enhance self-efficacy and reduce his or her sense of helplessness and vulnerability. In the case of a patient who was convinced that his mother wanted him dead because she did not come to rescue him when he was feeling very depressed and suicidal, he discovered later that she had not come to see him because of her own insecurities about being a good mother and because of her fears that she might say the wrong thing and, thus, make him feel worse. This only became clear after the patient queried about why she did not come to visit him when he was at a very low point; he had not anticipated that this would have been his mother's response.

Dichotomous thinking: Challenge dichotomous thinking by developing a continuum between extremes. In the case of a suicidal patient who overdosed because he believed that he could never have another job as good as the one he lost, the therapist had the patient list the elements of the ideal job, The therapist then had the patient compare his previous jobs with each element of the ideal job; the patient discovered that many of his past jobs also had value and shared many of the listed ideal elements. When previous jobs were placed on a continuum, some of his previous jobs ranked higher, in some respects, than the job that he had just lost. The patient's all-or-nothing thinking interfered with being aware of the strengths of previous jobs. Another strategy is to have the patient keep track of all-or-nothing thinking and then practice thinking and speaking in less extreme terms; a less extreme response to the belief, "I'm a total failure" could be, "Although I am not perfect, I have made some accomplishments".

Problem solving: Schotte and Clum (1982) [37] were among the first to show that there is a significant relationship between poor problem solvers, who are experiencing high levels of stress, and the likelihood of developing suicidal thoughts. These researchers subsequently demonstrated that patients with suicidal ideations are less likely to come up with alternative solutions to their problems, they have little confidence in their problem solving ability, and they tend to focus on the potentially negative outcomes of their problem solving attempts. D'Zurilla et al. (2004) [38] conceptualize the problem solving deficits seen in suicidal patients into two categories, deficits in the skill of rational problem solving and deficits in motivation to engage in problem solving due to the lack of confidence and the tendency to expect negative outcomes. This distinction helps therapist to decide whether to focus treatment on building problem solving skills or working on the development of confidence while addressing unrealistic expectations or both. Reinecke et al. (2001) [39] demonstrated that the severity of depressed mood also interferes with problem solving by not only impacting motivation but by interfering with the encoding and retrieval of information. Studies by Teasdale and others have shown that the depressed state interferes with the acquisition of past positive experiences and successes [3,4].

Reinecke (2006) recommends the following approach to problem solving with the depressed suicidal patient [40]. Treatment begins by helping the patient identify the problem that suicide would solve and to provide psychoeducation and understanding of potential contributing factors. From a CBT perspective, suicide is one solution to the problem that is creating emotional distress. The therapist next assesses the patient's motivation and attitude about engaging in problem solving. According to Reinecke, ways to promote a more positive attitude about problem solving include helping the patient to accept that problems are a part of normal life, identifying possible contributing factors to his or her problem, identifying and correcting errors in logic (magnification, overgeneralization, personalization, etc.) that may interfere with problem solving, instilling a sense of self-efficacy and expectation that solutions will come, acknowledging that there may be only partial solutions, and that it might take time for the solutions to be realized [40]. With improvement in motivation, the focus of therapy turns to improving rational problem solving skills. Once the problem is clearly identified, the patient is encouraged to articulate his or her related concerns and understanding of what maintains the problem. The patient is then encouraged to identify realistic goals regarding the problem and then start working on steps to solve the problem. Skills in generating alternative solutions, than suicide, become the next focus of attention. With each alternative solution, the patient carries out a pros and cons analysis, determines the short- and long-term consequences, selects what appears to be the most effective solution, implements a plan, and assesses the outcome. Reinecke utilizes psychoeducation, Socratic dialogue, role plays, and modeling to effect this approach.

Acceptance of pain: One of the essential goals of therapy with the suicidal patient is to assist the patient in being able to have a life in spite of his or her pain. The suicidal patient is operating out of the belief that there is no reason to live if there is suffering. As a result, the patient's predominant focus of attention is to resist their pain and ruminate about how this could have happened to him or her and to worry about a future of suffering. As a result there is no room in the patient's experience for a purposeful and meaningful life. Unfortunately, for many of the problems that create suffering in suicidal patients, there are no immediate solutions. So the task is to make room in conscious awareness for suffering while carrying out one's responsibilities and working on solutions to the problem that is creating the suffering.

Chiles and Strosahl (2005) identify two strategies, recontextualization and comprehensive distancing, to assist the patient in accepting painful thoughts and feelings [13]. According to Chiles and Strosahl, "The objective of recontextualization is not to get rid of disturbing thoughts or feelings but to teach the patient to make room for them and do what needs to be done to get on with life. The objective is met when your patient learns that negative thoughts or feelings do not block adaptive behavior. The two can coexist". With recontextualization, our thoughts and feelings do not define our experience, but are just there to be observed as an opportunity to learn in the process of problem solving. Comprehensive distancing refers to the willingness of the suicidal patient to detach from his or her suicidal thoughts and emotional distress. Chiles and Strosahl recommend the dual-thermometer exercise which is carried out by the patient daily. The patient will keep a daily diary and make daily ratings on two 1-10 thermometer scales with regards to two dimensions of experience, willingness and suffering. The ratings on the Willingness Thermometer, measure willingness of being present without judgment, being mildly interested, and being just an observant of what is. Alternatively, the Suffering Thermometer rates how much distress the patient feels with his or her daily experiences as a result of ruminating and worrying about his or her condition. The patient makes daily notes on factors that either increase or decrease ratings on the two measures. The ratings tend to be reciprocal of each other. The purpose of this exercise is to point out the uselessness of attaching to our negative thoughts and feelings. During the course of therapy, suicidal thoughts can be used as a measure of non-acceptance of negative emotions since the purpose of suicidal thinking is to avoid experiencing negative emotions.

View of suicide as being a desirable solution: The desirability of suicide as a solution also needs to be a target of treatment. In the case where a patient's motive is to create a change in his or her relationships or environment, it is important to have the patient challenge the assumption that suicide will achieve his or her goal. Typical motives include revenge or to provide relief for family and friends. In the case of seeking revenge, the patient can be asked, "How certain are you that the person for whom you are seeking revenge will own the intended responsibility". Another patient may believe that the act of suicide will provide relief for his or her family. Pointing out evidence to the contrary may help the patient achieve a more realistic perspective. It is also important to have the patient consider the short- and long-term consequences of committing suicide. A patient in our clinic acknowledged that she would miss seeing her nephew's graduation from high school. Marsha Linehan (1993) stresses the importance of having the suicidal patient identify reasons for living in order to motivate him or her to consider alternatives to suicide [41]. The advantages and disadvantages of suicide and not suicide analysis is an effective technique to identify the positive and negative reinforcers of suicide. By identifying the positive reinforcers, the focus of treatment is directed towards identifying alternatives to suicide in order to achieve the desired results; it is also important to correct any cognitive distortions about the advantages of dying. Awareness of the negative reinforcers provides motivation not to suicide. In the case of a patient in our clinic, the **advantage of suicide** was that she would no longer be a burden to her family; the **disadvantage of not suicide** was that her pain would continue; the **advantage of not suicide** was that she could enjoy her children and grandchildren; and the **disadvantage of suicide** was that it would prove that she was a failure. The advantage of not suicide and the disadvantage of suicide were the negative reinforcers and helped motivate her not to act on her suicidal thoughts. The advantage of suicide and the disadvantage of not suicide were the positive reinforcers to suicide; however, these positive reinforcers were challenged in therapy and she realized that her children and grandchildren would be devastated if she ended her life and that there were alternative ways of managing her pain using Mindfulness techniques and psychopharmacological interventions.

6. Summary of a CBT approach to suicidal thinking and behavior in depression

In summary, I recommend the following approach to the acutely depressed patient with suicidal thoughts and behaviors. First, the therapist must determine what problem suicide would solve, followed by identifying the individual's motive for suicide; is suicide desired to escape from pain or to make a change in his or her relationships or environment or a combination of both. In order to engage the patient and to develop trust, the therapist should inquire as to what got him or her to the point that suicide seemed to be the only solution; the therapists asks for understanding. Once the therapist believes he or she understands the patient's logic, the therapist can acknowledge with the patient that he or she might have come to the same conclusion under similar circumstances; this response serves to help normalize the patient's experience. However, the therapist next provides hope by stressing that there are solutions or partial solutions that the patient might have overlooked and that together alternatives to suicide will become apparent. If the patient believes that the therapist understands his or her perspective and rationale without judgment, the patient will more likely engage in treatment. Once engaged, the task is to understand the internal, external, and or thematic triggers for suicidal thinking and behaviors, as well as the factors that maintain the desire to suicide, using thoughts records and/or chain analyses. Next, the therapist assists the patient in challenging the distortions and misconceptions, including core beliefs, that interfered with his or her motivation to initiate the process of problem solving; this is followed by promoting the development of problem solving skills, if needed. In addition, the therapist addresses the patient's view that he or she does not have the internal or external resources to solve his or her problem. An advantages and disadvantages analysis of suicide and not suicide should be performed early in the treatment in order to identify the positive and negative reinforcers for suicide. The negative reinforcers will help motivate the patient to think of reasons to live and not choose suicide; the positive reinforcers will be used to assist in identifying alternatives to suicide. Also, identifying alternatives to suicide helps to begin the task of problem solving. Once the alternatives have been identified, the patient continues with a pros and cons analysis for each alternative. The patient then develops an action plan once the best alternative is identified; this helps motivate the patient to implement the plan followed by an assessment of the outcome. Effective problem solving will be in the service of developing self-efficacy and to counter the patient's sense of helplessness and worthlessness. Simultaneously with problem solving, the therapist helps the patient reduce his or her level of distress by working on acceptance of emotional and/or physical pain. The mindfulness strategy of learning the skill to broaden one's awareness in the moment enables the patient to see that there is more to his or her reality than one's pain. Learning to refocus attention on purpose without judgment, especially when the pain is intense, or observing the pain in order to determine what makes it worse or better are mindfulness skills that can be empowering. As with all CBT treatments, the final phase of treatment focuses on relapse prevention. The relapse prevention phase gives the patient an opportunity to demonstrate his or her ability to make use of the skills learned during the treatment and it gives the therapist an opportunity to assess whether the patient is appropriately applying his or her new skills, and thus ready for termination. Wenzel et al., (2009) caution about the risk of having an unprepared patient destabilize while re-examining the events that lead to the suicide attempt, especially through imagery [22]. Careful collaboration with the patient about his or her readiness to review the suicide attempt in detail is essential along with close monitoring of his or her distress level in the review process. The patient may find it too overwhelming to use imagery, as if the events were occurring in the present. In this case, Wenzel et al. recommend using the past tense in summarizing the events and applying the newly learned techniques. I refer the reader to Wenzel et al. (2009) for the details regarding this exercise. Finally, relapse prevention focuses on having the patient imagine potential future suicide crises and review in detail how he or she would make use of cognitive and behavioral strategies to reduce the chance that he or she would engage in suicidal behaviors.

7. Evidence for CBT preventing suicide in depressed patients

There are very few randomized controlled trial (RCT) studies assessing the effectiveness of CBT in preventing suicide attempts in adult depressed patients. Earlier studies that focused on problem solving alone have failed to consistently demonstrate a reduction in future suicidal thinking and behaviors when compared to treatment as usual (TAU) [40]. These findings argue for a more comprehensive CBT approach including not only problem solving, but cognitive restructuring, behavioral strategies, stress reduction and mindfulness, and interpersonal skills training. To date, there is only one adequately powered (RCT) study that included many of these treatment elements [42]. Most other studies target changes in predictors of suicidal attempts rather than suicide attempts as the primary outcome measure. In the Brown et al., (2005) study, the researchers evaluated 350 adults and randomized 120 to 10 sessions of CBT or TAU, within 48 hours of admission to a university hospital emergency room after a suicide attempt [44]. Seventy-seven per cent of the patients met DSM-IV criteria (SCID interview) for major depressive disorder and 68% had a substance use disorder; 85% had more than one psychiatric disorder. Sixty per cent were African American, 35% Caucasian, and 5% were Hispanic. The elements of the CBT treatment included; identification of proximal thoughts, images, and core beliefs to the suicide attempt; cognitive and behavioral strategies to address the identified proximal thoughts and beliefs prior to the suicide attempt; development of adaptive ways of coping with stress; targeting hopelessness, poor problem solving, impaired impulse control, non-adherence to treatment, social isolation; and relapse prevention. From baseline to reassessment at 18 months, 24% of the CBT group and 41.6% of TAU group made at least one suicide attempt (asymptotic z score, 1.97; P=.049). Survival analysis (Kaplan-Meier) at month-18 showed a reattempt-free probability of 0.76(95% confidence interval [Cl], 0.62-0.85) in the CBT group and 0.58(95% Cl, 0.44-0.70) in the TAU group. Patients in the CBT group had a significantly lower reattempt rate (Wald X2/1=3.9; P=.049) and were 50% less likely to reattempt suicide than the TAU group (hazard ratio, 0.51;95% Cl, 0.26-0.997). With regards to the secondary analyses, the CBT group scored significantly lower than the TAU group on Beck Depression Inventory at 6 months (P=.02), 12 months (P=.009), and 18 months (P=.046). The CBT group scored significantly lower on the Beck Hopelessness Scale than the TAU group at 6 months (P=.045). There were no differences between the two groups in the Scale for Suicide Ideation. It is important to point out that Brown et al. adequately powered their study; the sample size of 120 provided at least 80% power to detect a hazard ratio of 0.44 with regards to a subsequent suicide attempt between the two groups [42]. Brown et al., point out that their results were consistent with an earlier small RCT study (n=20) by Salkovskis et al. (1990) [43]. Salkovskis et al. demonstrated that patients randomized to a CBT problem solving therapy were significantly (p=0.049) less likely to repeat a suicide attempt compared with the TAU group at six months after the index suicide attempt. The mean time to the next suicide attempt was 9.3 months for the CBT group compared to 3 months in the TAU group. Raj et al., (2001) [44] examined the effectiveness of CBT (n=20) versus treatment as usual (n=20) in ages between 16 and 50 in reducing deliberate self-harm. Patients were included with anxiety, depression, or adjustment disorder; psychotic patients were excluded. The 10 session CBT therapy consisted of cognitive and behavioral strategies, problem-solving skills, and behavioral counseling to significant others. The CBT group, compared to TAU, showed significant decreases on the Scale for Suicidal Ideations, Beck Hopelessness Scale, Problem Solving Inventory, and on the Hospital Anxiety and Depression Scale.

Tarrier et al. (2008) performed a meta-analysis on 28 select studies (based on quality) to investigate whether CBT reduced future suicidal behavior [45]. This is the first systematic review and meta-analysis of CBT and the prevention of suicidal behaviors. Suicidal behavior included completed suicides, suicide attempts, suicide intent or plans, and suicidal ideations. The diagnostic categories were broad across the 28 studies and not limited to depression. There were studies of patients with schizophrenia, first psychotic episodes, borderline personality, major depressive disorder, and personality disturbances. Thus their findings were not limited to a particular diagnostic disorder. Tarrier et al., concluded that CBT was highly effective in reducing suicidal behaviors within the 3 month period post treatment (combined Hedge's $g=-0.59$, $z=-5.26$, $p<.0001$, 95% CI=-0.811 to -0.371). Subgroup analysis of CBT demonstrated significant results with: controls of minimal treatment, treatment as usual, or active psychological treatments; adults only; treatment directed towards reducing suicidal behavior rather than associated symptoms like depression; and reductions in hopelessness. Also, CBT studies using an individual approach were effective whereas group CBT was ineffective. The authors are cautious in their conclusions because of publication biases. Small studies with large effect sizes had a disproportionately large impact on the overall effect size.

A recent study by Stewart et al. (2009) [46] was among the first to compare CBT and SPST (Social Problem Solving Therapy) with each other and against TAU. However, rather than measuring suicide attempts as their primary outcome measure, their outcome measures focused on predictors of suicide attempts including hopelessness (Beck Hopelessness scale), poor problems solving (Social Problem Solving Therapy), suicidal ideation (Beck Scale for Suicidal Ideation), and treatment dissatisfaction (Client Satisfaction Questionnaire-8). Subjects completed 8.73 treatment sessions in the CBT group (SD=1.04, range from 7-10 sessions), 4.75 sessions in the SPST group (SD=1.42, range 3-7 sessions), and.67 in the TAU group (SD=2.0, range from 0-6 session). Eleven subjects completed the CBT therapy, compared to 12 subjects in the SPST therapy, and 9 in the TAU intervention (334.4%, 37.5%, and 26.1% respectively). Over the course of treatment, subjects receiving CBT showed significant improvement in hopelessness (Beck Hopelessness Scale) ($z=-1.79$, $p<.05$, $r=.49$), suicidal ideations (Beck Scale for Suicidal Ideations) ($z=-2.32$, $p<.05$, $r=.49$), and patient satisfaction (Client Satisfaction Questionnaire-8) ($z=-2.81$, p<, $r=.60$); however, the CBT group did not show improvement in problem solving (Social Problem Solving Therapy) ($z=-1.02$, ns, $r=.21$). The TAU group did not show significant improvement in any of the predictors of suicidal behaviors. The authors suggest that treatment with CBT reduced hopelessness and suicidal ideations while improving treatment satisfaction. All three measures would presumably reduce the risk for future suicidal attempts. Also, the authors conclude that by empowering individuals to solve their problems, it follows that there was a reduction in hopelessness and suicidal ideations and an increase in patient satisfaction, all of which should help reduce the risk for future suicide attempts.

8. Conclusions

These limited studies provide cautious optimism that CBT is effective in reducing suicide attempts. However, there continues to be a great need for more studies, that are adequately powered and that not only examine the effectiveness of CBT in reducing predictors of suicide (e.g. hopelessness; decreased problem solving) but also measure the rates of suicide attempts as the primary outcome measure. As noted above, the Brown et al. (2005) protocol included several treatment components including cognitive restructuring, problem solving, treatment adherence, and identification of social supports [42]. It is unclear which elements are essential or most important for a positive outcome. Stress management and mindfulness training have not been consistently incorporated into CBT protocols for the suicidal patient; however, these elements should be considered for future studies. The duration, frequency, and intensity of CBT treatment for optimal outcomes is yet to be determined. Finally, future research needs to consider the value of CBT across clinical settings and various social economic groups.

Author details

John D. Matthews

Address all correspondence to: jmatthews@partners.org

Harvard Medical School, USA

References

[1] Beck, A. T, Rush, A. J, Shaw, B. F, & Emery, G. Cognitive Therapy of Depression. New York: The Guildford Press; (1979).

[2] Beck, J. Cognitive Therapy for Challenging Problems: What to do when the Basics don't Work. New York: The Guilford Press; (2005).

[3] Clark, D. M, & Teasdale, J. D. Diurnal Variation in Clinical Depression and Accessibility of Memories of Positive and Negative Experiences. Journal of Abnormal Psychology (1982). , 91-87.

[4] Teasdale, J. D, & Taylor, R. Induced Mood and Accessibility of Memories: An Effect of Mood State or of Induction Procedure? British Journal of Clinical Psychology (1981). , 20-39.

[5] Beck, J. S. Cognitive Behavior Therapy: Basics and Beyond (2nd edition). New York: The Guildford Press; (2011).

[6] Rudd, M. D, Joiner, T, & Rajab, M. H. Treating Suicidal Behavior: An Effective, Time-Limited Approach. New York: The Guildford Press; (2001).

[7] Beck, A. T, Kovacs, M, & Weissman, A. Hopelessness and Suicidal Behavior: An Overview. JAMA (1975). , 234-1146.

[8] Beck, A. T, Weissman, A, Lester, D, & Trexler, L. Beck Hopelessness Scale (BHS). In: Rush JA, First MB, Blacker D. (eds.) Handbook of Psychiatric Measures (2nd edition). Washington, DC: American Psychiatric Publishing, Inc; (2008). , 247-248.

[9] Beck, A. T, & Weishaar, M. E. Suicide Risk Assessment and Prediction. Crisis (1990). , 11(2), 22-30.

[10] Beck, A. T. Hopelessness as a Predictor of Eventual Suicide. In: Mann JJ, Stanley M. (eds.) Annals of the New York Academy of Sciences, Psychology and Suicidal Behavior. New York: New York Academy of Sciences; (1986). , 487, 90-96.

[11] Young, M, Fogg, L, Scheftner, W, Fawcett, J, Akiskal, H, & Maser, J. Stable Trait Components of Hopelessness: Baseline and Sensitivity of Depression. Journal of Abnormal Psychology (1996). , 105-105.

[12] Shneidman, E. S. Comprehending Suicide: Landmarks in 20th Century Suicidology. Washington, DC: American Psychological Association; (2001).

[13] Chiles, J. A, & Strosahl, K. D. Clinical Manual for Assessment and Treatment of Suicidal Patients. Washington, DC: American Psychiatric Publishing, Inc; (2005).

[14] Shneidman, E. S. The Logic of Suicide. In: Scheidman ES, Farberow N. (eds.) Clues to Suicide. New York: McGraw-Hill; (1959).

[15] Neuringer, C. Dichotomous Evaluations in Suicidal Individuals. Journal of Consulting Psychology (1961). , 25-445.

[16] Neuringer, C. Rigid Thinking in Suicidal Individuals. Journal of Consulting Psychology (1964). , 28-54.

[17] Shneidman, E. S. Suicide as Psychache: A Clinical Approach to Self-Destructive Behavior. Northvale, NJ: Aronson; (1993).

[18] Zurilla, D, Nezu, T, & Problem-solving, A. Therapy: A Social Competence Approach to Clinical Intervention (2nd edition). New York: Springer Publishing Company; (1999).

[19] Zurilla, D, Chang, T, Nottingham, E, & Faccini, E. L. Social Problem-Solving Deficits and Hopelessness, Depression, and Suicidal Risk in College Students and Psychiatric Inpatients. Journal of Clinical Psychology (1998). , 54-1091.

[20] Becker, E. S, Strohbach, D, & Rinck, M. A Specific Attentional Bias in Suicide Attempters. The Journal of Nervous and Mental Disease (1999). , 187-730.

[21] Williams JMGBroadbent K. Autobiographical Memory in Suicide Attempters. Journal of Abnormal Psychology (1986). , 95-144.

[22] Wenzel, A, Brown, G. K, & Beck, A. T. Cognitive Therapy for Suicidal Patients: Scientific and Clinical Applications. Washington, DC: American Psychological Association; (2009).

[23] Beck, A. T. Cognitive Approaches to Panic Disorder: Theory and Therapy. In: Rachman S, Maser JD. (eds.) Panic: Psychological Perspectives. Hillsdale, NJ: Erlbaum; (1988). , 91-109.

[24] Williams JMGBarnhofer T, Crane C, Duggan DS. The Role of Overgeneral Memory in Suicidality. In: Ellis ET. (ed.) Cognition and Suicide: Theory, Research, and Therapy. New York: American Psychological Association; (2006). , 173-192.

[25] Pollock, L. R. Williams JMG. Effective Problem Solving in Suicide Attempters Depends on Specific Autobiographical Recall. Suicide and Life-Threatening Behavior (2001). , 31-386.

[26] Williams JMGDritschel BH. Emotional Disturbance and the Specificity of Autobiographical Memory. Cognition & Emotion (1988). , 2-221.

[27] Reinecke, M. Suicide and Depression. In: Dattilio FM, Freeman A. (eds.) Cognitive-Behavioral Strategies in Crisis Intervention. New York: The Guilford Press; (1994). , 67-103.

[28] Beck, A. T, Brown, G, & Steer, R. A. Prediction of Eventual Suicide in Psychiatric Inpatients by Clinical Rating of Hopelessness. Journal of Consulting and Clinical Psychology (1989). , 57-309.

[29] Beck, A. T, Brown, G. K, Berchick, R. J, Stewart, B. L, & Steer, R. A. Relationship between Hopelessness and Ultimate Suicide: A Replication with Psychiatric Outpatients. American Journal of Psychiatry (1990). , 147-190.

[30] Beck, A, Kovacs, M, & Weissman, A. Beck Scale for Suicide Ideation (BSS); Scale for Suicide Ideation (SSI). In: Rush JA, First MB, Blacker D. (eds.) Handbook of Psychiatric Measures (2nd edition). Washington, DC: American Psychiatric Publishing, Inc; (2008). , 242-244.

[31] Beck, A, Schuyler, D, & Herman, I. Suicide Intent Scale (SIS). In: Rush JA, First MB, Blacker D. (eds.) Handbook of Psychiatric Measures (2nd edition). Washington, DC: American Psychiatric Publishing, Inc; (2008). , 244-245.

[32] Beck, A. T, Schuyler, D, & Herman, I. Development of Suicidal Intent Scales. In: Beck T, Resnik HLP, Lettier DJ. (eds.) The Prediction of Suicide. Bowie, MD: Charles Press; (1974).

[33] Posner, K, Brown, G. K, Stanley, B, Brent, D. A, Yershova, K. V, Oquendo, M. A, Currier, G. W, Greenhill, L, Shen, S, & Mann, J. J. The Columbia-Suicide Severity Rating Scale: Initial Validity and Internal Consistency Findings from Three Multisite Studies

with Adolescents and Adults. American Journal of Psychiatry (2011). , 168(12), 1266-1277.

[34] Joiner TE JrSteer RA, Brown G, Beck AT, Pettit JW, Rudd MD. Worst-Point Suicidal Plans: A Dimension of Suicidality Predictive of Past Suicide Attempts and Eventual Death by Suicide. Behav Res Ther (2003). , 41-1469.

[35] Beck, A. T, Brown, G. K, Steer, R. A, Dahlsgaard, K. K, & Grisham, J. R. Suicide Ideation at its Worst Point: A Predictor of Eventual Suicide in Psychiatric Outpatients. Suicide Life Threatening Behavior (1999). , 29-1.

[36] Kovacs, M, Beck, A, & Weissman, A. Hopelessness: An indicator of suicide risk. Suicide (1975). , 5-98.

[37] Schotte, D, & Clum, G. Suicide Ideation in a College Population: A Test of a Model. Journal of Consulting and Clinical Psychology (1982). , 50-690.

[38] Zurilla, D, Nezu, T, & Maydeu-olicares, A. A. Social Problem Solving : Theory and Assessment. In: Chang E, D'Zurilla T, Sanna C. (eds.) Social Problem Solving: Theory, Research, and Training. Washingtown, DC: American Psychological Association; (2004). , 11-27.

[39] Reinecke, M. DuBois D, Schultz T. Social Problem Solving, Mood, and Suicidality among Inpatient Adolescents. Cognitive Therapy and Resaerch (2001). , 25-743.

[40] Reinecke, M. A. Problem Solving: A Conceptual Approach to Suicidality and Psychotherapy. In: Ellis ET. (ed.) Cognition and Suicide: Theory, Research, and Therapy. Washington, DC: American Psychological Association; (2006). , 237-260.

[41] Linehan, M. M. Cognitive-Behavioral Treatment of Borderline Personality Disorder. New York: The Guildford Press; (1993).

[42] Brown, G. K. Ten Have T. Henriques GR, Xie SX, Hollander JE, Beck AT. Cognitive Therapy for the Prevention of Suicide Attempts: A Randomized Controlled Trial. JAMA (2005). , 294(5), 563-570.

[43] Salkovskis, P. M, Atha, C, & Strorer, D. Cognitive-Behavioural Problem Solving in the Treatment of Patients who Repeatedly Attempt Suicide: A Controlled Trial. British Journal of Psychiatry (1990). , 157-871.

[44] Raj, A. J, Kumaraiah, V, & Bhide, A. V. Cognitive-Behavioural Intervention in Deliberate Self-Harm. Acta Psychiatrica Scandinavica (2008). , 104-340.

[45] Tarrier, N, Taylor, K, & Gooding, P. Cognitive-Behavioral Interventions to Reduce Suicide Behavior: A Systematic Review and Meta-Analysis. Behavior Modification (2008). , 32(1), 77-108.

[46] Stewart, C. D, Quinn, A, Plever, S, & Emmerson, B. Comparing Cognitive Behavior Therapy, Problem Solving Therapy, and Treatment as Usual in a High Risk Population. Suicide and Life-Threatening Behavior (2010). , 39-538.

Chapter 2

Cognitive Behaviour Therapy in the Management of Conduct Disorder Among Adolescents

Afusat Olanike Busari

Additional information is available at the end of the chapter

1. Introduction

When asked what developmental stage is diagnosed with conduct disorder the primary answer would be adolescent. However, based on research the greatest damage to society is the result of actions by delinquent adolescents but conduct disorder begins below the age of 7 (Scott, 2007). The researcher hypothesis suggests conduct disorder has a multi-factorial causation which includes biologic, psychosocial and numerous facets of the family unit. The research reveals a negative combination of these factors may predispose young children to exhibit symptoms of conduct disorder. The following questions will hopefully be answered: (1) What causes conduct disorder? (2) Can conduct disorder be prevented or predicted? (3) Does parenting style promote symptoms of conduct disorder? and (4) What are the intervention programmes that can be used to manage conduct disorder in adolescents.

2. Definition of conduct disorder

According to Evans (2003) conduct disorder is a steady pattern of harming others or their property, lying, stealing, or breaking societal rules of behaviour. Remote instances of acute behaviour, running away, or vandalism is not enough to merit a diagnosis of conduct disorder. Most children exhibit instances of poor judgment and bad behaviour at least one time in their childhood. The distinction is children with conduct disorder break the rules over and over again, exhibit aggressive behaviour, and show no regard for others. The behaviour is not considered conduct disorder until the symptoms are displayed for one year or more. The disturbances in behaviour result in significant clinical impairment with social skills, academics and occupational functioning (American Psychiatric Association, 1994).

Conduct disorder is differentiated from other psychiatric disorders diagnosed in children by the following criteria: "persistent pattern of behavior in which the basic rights of others or major age-appropriate societal norms or rules are violated" American Psychiatric Association (as cited from Tehama, 2007). According to them conduct disorder is a psychiatric syndrome occurring in childhood and adolescence which characterized by a longstanding pattern of violations of rules and antisocial behaviors. They interpret conduct disorder as:

Conduct disorder is a common childhood psychiatric problem that has increased incidence in adolescence. The primary diagnostic features of conduct disorder include aggression, theft, vandalism, violation of rules and/or lying. For a diagnosis these behaviors must occur for a least a six-month period.

3. Causes conduct disorder

The conditions that contribute to the development of conduct disorder are considered to be multifactorial, with many factors (multifactorial) contributing to the cause. Neuropsychological testing has shown that children and adolescents with conduct disorders seem to have an impairment in the frontal lobe of the brain that interferes with their ability to plan, avoid harm, and learn from negative experiences. Childhood temperament is considered to have a genetic basis. Children or adolescents who are considered to have a difficult temperament are more likely to develop behaviour problems. Children or adolescents from disadvantaged, dysfunctional, and disorganized home environments are more likely to develop conduct disorders. Social problems and peer group rejection have been found to contribute to delinquency (Salaam 1992). Low socioeconomic status has been associated with conduct disorders (Busari & Adejumobi 2012). Children and adolescents exhibiting delinquent and aggressive behaviours have distinctive cognitive and psychological profiles when compared to children with other mental health problems and control groups (Aderanti 2006). All of the possible contributing factors influence how children and adolescents interact with other people.

The etiology of conduct disorder consists of the correlation of genetic, family and social factors. The child may inherit limited baseline autonomic nervous system activity, resulting in a need for greater stimulation to attain optimal arousal. This hereditary aspect may explain the high level of sensation-seeking activity associated with the disorder (Johnson et al., 2002). Several studies have revealed the role of autonomic under-arousal in conduct-disordered adolescents (Crowell et al., 2006). According to McBurnett&Lahey, 1994 & Scrapa & Raine, 1997 (as cited in Crowell et al., 2006) conduct disorder and antisocial behaviour in adulthood are marked by autonomic under-arousal which included reduced electro-dermal responding (EDR) and heart rate. Beauchaine, 2003 (as cited in Crowell et al., 2006) revealed both elementary children and adolescents have reduced sympathetic and parasympathetic linked cardiac activity when diagnosed with conduct disorder.

The importance of this research is evident when considering the critical period of preschool when noradrenergic, serotonergic, and dopaminergic systems which administer behavioural control are susceptible to long-term changes in functioning Bremner&Vermetten, 2001 (as cited in Crowell et al., 2006). Parasympathetic nervous system (PNS)-linked cardiac activity has been associated with emotional regulation capabilities Porges, 1995 (as cited in Crowell et al., 2006) in contrast to deficiencies in sympathetic nervous system (SNS)-linked cardiac activity have been linked with reward inconsiderateness.

During gestation the brain is vulnerable to the effects of environmental stressors; this statement applies to both prenatal and postnatal development Hulzink et al., 2004 (as cited in Van Goozen et al., 2007). Environmental factors which can affect brain development are:

- Poor nutrition
- Maternal psychopathology
- Atypical child interaction from a depressed mother

Baumrind (as cited in Marsiglia et al., 2007) classified three parenting styles: authoritarian, authoritative, and permissive. For the purpose of this research authoritarian parenting styles will be discussed. The characteristics of an authoritarian parent according to this researcher, are extremely restrictive and demanding rules. Parents who utilize this style tend to hamper children's autonomy and force them to follow stringent rules by threatening harsh punishment. This type of parenting may lead children to believe they are not responsible for their actions; by contrast, when actions are questions they assume it is not their fault. According to numerous psychological theories parent-child relationship can generate psychological disorders such as anxiety, identity confusion and conduct disorder (Dwairy, et al., 2006). Hoeve et al., (2008) concluded from their study a strong link between parenting styles and delinquency trajectories; therefore, they recommended future research include parenting styles in measuring serious behaviours which are classified as conduct disorders.

The link between exposure to violence in the home and community is a crucial risk factor for conduct disorder according to research by Elze et al., 1999; Fergusson &Horwood, 1998; ; Kaplan et al., 1998 (as cited in McCabe et al., 2005). Violence exposure can take place in many places within the child's environment including: (1) victimization and witnessing child abuse; (2) community violence; (3) parental abuse (McCabe et al., 2005).

Culture and societal norms make up the macro-system which is seen as the most distant factors; the eco-system is seen as a midlevel factor; and the micro-system is seen as the most proximal position to the child. Lynch &Cicchetti, 1998 (as cited in McCabe, et al., 2005) stress risk factors which have the most impact are the factors which are more proximal to the child. Family stresses: (1) substance abuse; (2) violence; and (3) social isolation etc. increase a child's risk of conduct disorder or other mental health disorders. Garrison et al., 1992 (as cited in Baker et al., 2007) reveals several studies have documented the relationship between childhood psychosocial issues and primary care visits. Pediatricians consistently under identify mental health problems in children. Behavioural problems have been linked to an increase in family stressors: (1) divorce; (2) relocation; and (3) financial issues Lavigne et al., 1998 (as cited in Baker et al., 2007). Pediatrician should be aware of these factors when addressing repetitive visits to the office or the emergency room for treatment.

Parental psychopathology and parenting behaviour may be potentially important risk or protective factors in developmental outcomes for these children with concurrent conduct problems. Parental stress and maladaptive parenting may foster the development of conduct disorder Johnson & Mash, 2001 (as cited by Chronis et al., 2007). The researchers propose maternal smoking is a significant factor in conduct disorder because nicotine may interrupt fetal brain development. According to them, "Our study suggests that cigarette smoking may be one of the first prenatal risk factors for this very serious disorder" (University of Chicago Medical Center, 1997).

According to the ecological-transactional model child abuse has the greatest impact on child functioning. Kaplan et al., 1998 states several studies have correlated child maltreatment to an increase risk of conduct disorder (as cited in McCabe et al., 2005). A study at University of Chicago Medical Center (1997) reveals a link between smoking during pregnancy and the likelihood of having a son with conduct disorder. The researchers analyzed records of 177, 7-12 year-old boys who were referred for outpatient treatment for behavioural problems. The study indicated 24 percent of the mothers who reported smoking more than a half-pack of cigarettes per day during pregnancy, 80% of their sons had conduct disorder. This was in contrast to conduct disorder in 50% of the boys whose mothers did not smoke (University of Chicago Medical Center, 1997). According to the researcher "Our study indicates that regardless of other factors, smoking during pregnancy can have serious behavioural outcomes in children" (University of Chicago Medical Center, 1997).

The longitudinal and experimental studies on children who are raised in orphanages, children's homes, and foster homes have established the adverse effects of long-term institutional care on children's personality development according to the American Academy of Child and Adolescent Psychiatry, 2005 (as cited in Chronis et al., 2007). Consistent research has shown a correlation between institutional child rearing and hyperactivity and inattention (Busari & Ojo 2011). Both of these symptoms are precursors of conduct disorder Roy et al., 2000 (as cited in Chronis et al., 2007).

The research repeatedly exposes children who are diagnosed with ADHD and conduct disorder are predisposed for (1) risky sexual behaviour; (2) substance abuse; (3) delinquency; and (4) driving risks Barkley et al., 1993 (as cited in Chronis et al., 2007). The most disturbing fact is children who are diagnosed with ADHD and conduct disorder are at a greater risk of chronic criminal offenses Lyman, 1998 (as cited in Chronis et al., 2007). They identified children with conduct disorder at a greater jeopardy for continual offending and explained their perseverance by the correlation of their behaviour, neuropsychological and physiological deficits are comparable to adult psychopaths.

Childhood conduct disorder is a major risk factor for adult disorders especially anti-social behaviour. The key to diagnosing these children is to identify the origin of antisocial behaviour which is found in (1) difficult temperament and (2) ineffective socialization (Van Goozen et al., 2007). Conduct disorder in childhood which persists through adolescence is associated with co-morbidity, recurrence and resistance to treatment Moffit(2005). The study shows children and adolescence who struggle with signs and symptoms of conduct disorder continue to struggle throughout adulthood with psychosocial problems. The trajectories of antisocial behaviour influence these children throughout adulthood and influence the child-rearing environment (Jafee et al., 2006).

The influences of individual factors are multifaceted and confusion. Family dysfunction is repetitively identified as one of the crucial factor for conduct disorder in adolescence. Poor parental supervision is the preeminent predictor of violence and vandalism committed by boys. Psychosocial disturbances in children and adolescence bring together a comprehensive range of research to shed light on these young people who become parents of tomorrow; these parents who were diagnosed with conduct disorder predispose their child to the same disorder (Pearce, 1996).

The public debate concerning the relationship between family characteristics and children with conduct disorder continues to raise questions which researchers hope to answer. A longitudinal survey of children suggests ineffective parenting style is the strongest predictor of delinquent behaviour in children between the ages of 8 and 11 years. In addition, aversion tactics, low socioeconomic status and the number of siblings in the home are associated with higher probability of children exhibiting delinquent behaviour and conduct disorder (Busari&Adejumobi 2012). Somerstein (2007) reveals the common family dynamic in many individuals' histories of male terrorist is authoritarian parents.

4. Symptoms of conduct disorder

The clinical features of Conduct Disorder are:

- aggression or serious threats of harm to people or animals;
- deliberate property damage or destruction (i.e. fire setting);
- repeated violation of household or school rules, laws or both; and
- persistent lying to avoid consequences or to obtain tangible goods or privileges

The American Psychiatric Association (1994) provides further symptoms which support the clinician in diagnosis of conduct disorder. The child will often bully, threaten or intimidate others. They may intentionally set fires with the objective of harming others. The violation of rules would include: (1) often staying out late at night regardless of parental prohibitions which can begin before the age of 13; (2) has run away from home more than two times; and (3) the child is often truant from school which usually begins before the age of 13.

Additional features of conduct disorder include an indifference to the welfare of others and little if any remorse about harming others. Adolescents often verbalize outward remorse to avoid punishment but do not exhibit any guilt. They do not require an objective basis to conclude others are a threat to them. Because of this demeanor they may lash out aggressively without being provoked (Scott., 2007). During normal child development aggression and fighting is pertinent for defensive issues which do not escalate into anti-social behaviours; but, persistent anti-social behaviour collectively handicaps during childhood and leads to deprived adjustment during adulthood. The child often endures negative responses by their peers and high levels of disapproval from their parents (Scott, 2007).

Children who are diagnosed with conduct disorder judge the world as an antagonistic and intimidating place. They may tattle on friends or blame others for the harm they have caused. They have few if any friends because of their limited interpersonal skills. Peers and family members may view them as irritating because of their indifference to their actions. They often have low self-esteem internally but externally they appear tough, cocky or self-assured (Evans, 2003).

5. Prevalence of conduct disorder among the adolescents

Conduct disorder has become a major health and social problem; it is the most common psychiatric problem diagnosed among children. Around the world the prevalence of conduct disorder is 5% (Scott, 2007). A study conducted by Sujit et al., (2006) reveals 4.58% of boys and 4.5% of girls are diagnosed with conduct disorder worldwide. In their study of 240 students in four schools in Kanke childhood conduct disorder was found in 73% and in adolescent 27%. Mild conduct disorder was found in 36%, moderate in 64% and severe conduct disorder in none. Lying, bullying and cruelty to animals were the primary symptoms (Sujit, 2006).

Conduct disorder affects 1 to 4 percent of 9- to 17-year olds in the United States. The disorder is more predominate in boys than girls and more common in cities than in rural areas (U.S. Department of Health and Human Services, 1999). Between 6 to 16 percent of boys and 2 to 9 percent of girls meet the criteria to be diagnosed with conduct disorder. It is estimated 40 percent of these children will grow up to be adults with antisocial personality disorder (Searight, 2001).

Epidemiological studies state approximately 2% of girls and 9% of boys are afflicted with this disorder. Adolescents with more external signs and symptoms would amplify the percentage to one third or one half of all children and adolescent clinic referrals Kazdin et al., 1992 (as cited by McCabe et at., 2005).

6. What are the symptoms of conduct disorder?

Most symptoms seen in children with conduct disorder also occur at times in children without this disorder. However, in children with conduct disorder, these symptoms occur more frequently and interfere with learning, school adjustment, and, sometimes, with the child's relationships with others.

The following are the most common symptoms of conduct disorder. However, each child may experience symptoms differently. The four main groups of behaviours include the following:

- **Aggressive conduct.** Aggressive conduct causes or threatens physical harm to others and may include the following:
  - Intimidating behaviour
  - Bullying
  - Physical fights
  - Cruelty to others or animals
  - Use of a weapon(s)
  - Forcing someone into sexual activity, rape, molestation
- **Destructive conduct.** Destructive conduct may include the following:
  - Vandalism; intentional destruction to property
  - Arson
- **Deceitfulness.** Deceitful behaviour may include the following:
  - Lying
  - Theft
  - Shoplifting
  - Delinquency
- **Violation of rules.** Violation of ordinary rules of conduct or age-appropriate norms may include the following:
  - Truancy (failure to attend school)
  - Running away
  - Pranks
  - Mischief
  - Very early sexual activity

The symptoms of conduct disorder may resemble other medical conditions or behavioural problems.

7. How is conduct disorder diagnosed?

A child psychiatrist or a qualified mental health professional usually diagnoses conduct disorders in children and adolescents. A detailed history of the child's behaviour from parents and teachers, observations of the child's behaviour, and, sometimes, psychological testing contribute to the diagnosis. Parents who note symptoms of conduct disorder in their child or teen can help by seeking an evaluation and treatment early. Early treatment can often prevent future problems. Further, conduct disorder often coexists with other mental health disorders, including mood disorders, anxiety disorders, posttraumatic stress disorder, substance abuse, attention-deficit/hyperactivity disorder, and learning disorders, increasing the need for early diagnosis and treatment. Parents should consult their child's doctor for more information.

8. Prevention of conduct disorder in childhood

As with oppositional defiant disorder (ODD), some experts believe that a developmental sequence of experiences occurs in the development of conduct disorder. This sequence may start with ineffective parenting practices, followed by academic failure, and poor peer interactions. These experiences then often lead to depressed mood and involvement in a deviant peer group. Other experts, however, believe that many factors, including child abuse, genetic susceptibility, history of academic failure, brain damage, and/or a traumatic experience influence the expression of conduct disorder. Early detection and intervention into negative family and social experiences may be helpful in disrupting the development of the sequence of experiences that lead to more disruptive and aggressive behaviour

9. Relationship between conduct disorder, depression and opposition disorder

Many studies have shown that conduct disorder (CD) and depression often co-occur in late childhood and adolescence and have historically been regarded as the primary point of comorbidity between internalizing and behavioral disorders. On the other hand, recent evidence suggests that oppositional defiant disorder (ODD), and not CD, may best explain the comorbidity between disruptive behaviour disorders and depression. ODD typically onsets before CD and depression, changes in ODD symptoms predict changes in symptoms of CD and depression from one year to the next, and ODD in childhood and adolescence predicts depression in adulthood. Emerging evidence suggests that there are affective and behavioural dimensions of ODD symptoms, and those affective ODD symptoms (and not the behavioural symptoms) best predict later depression.

These results are highly relevant not only for our understanding of the etiology of the disorders, but also for optimizing early interventions aimed at reducing irritability in some ODD children. The new findings also stimulate new questions to be addressed with future research. In this review, the comorbidity between disruptive behaviour disorders (oppositional defiant disorder [ODD] and conduct disorder [CD]) and depression will be considered. The term comorbidity is used to indicate the concurrent co-occurrence of two disorders, but like Angold, Costello, and Erkanli (1999), the researcher do not use concurrent to imply that the two disorders onset or terminate at exactly the same time. In addition, the researcher is primarily interested in the heterotypic comorbidity (e.g., Angold et al., 1999) involving the disruptive behaviour disorders and depression. The term heterotypic continuity is used to refer to the continuity of psychopathology in different forms over time, such as children with ODD being more likely to become depressed in adulthood (e.g., Copeland, Shanahan, Costello, &Angold, 2009). This is in contrast to homotypic continuity, which refers to the continuity of the same type of psychopathology over time, such as depression in adolescence showing continuity in the form of depression in adulthood.

10. What is cognitive therapy?

Cognitive therapy is an active, structured form of psychotherapy that is designed to rapidly and effectively reduce and eliminate psychological symptoms. Cognitive is simply a fancy word that means thoughts. Cognitive behaviour therapy, sometimes known as CBT is a form of psychological treatment that focuses on the thoughts and behaviours that accompany psychological distress.

Traditionally, CBT has been relatively brief treatment compared to other types of psychotherapy. CBT is focused on achieving defined and measurable treatment goals. Progress towards these goals is regularly assessed to ensure that treatment is progressing in an efficient and effective manner.

There is a significant amount of scientific evidence demonstrating that CBT is effective in treating a wide variety of psychological difficulties including depression, anxiety, panic attacks, phobias, obsessive compulsive disorder, social anxiety and shyness, and post- traumatic stress disorder. The evidence suggests that CBT is not only effective in helping people get better but it is also effective in minimizing relapse or helping people stay better. Cognitive behaviour therapists (CBT) emphasise the process of learning in improving and maintaining behaviour. The client is encouraged to identify connections between thoughts and their responses to social situations.

CBT often involves problem solving skills training. This type of training has been widely evaluated and there is evidence for its efficacy in the short term in treating aggression and conduct disorders in children. CBT is used for a range of problems for children and adults. It places emphasis on certain cognitive techniques that are designed to produce changes in thinking and therefore changes in behaviour or mood (Busari & Uwakwe 2001). CBT also emphasises the learning process and the ways in which external environments can change both cognition and behaviour. CBT for children and adolescents usually includes a range of behaviour performance-based procedures, and often involve the family or school in therapy. It may include individual work, group sessions, or both. The length of treatment varies considerably and depends on the severity of difficulties experienced.

For children with conduct disorder CBT usually has a strong focus on social cognitions and interpersonal problem-solving. Programmes are often quite long and may take up to 25 or 30 weekly sessions. The therapist is active and involved and tries to develop a collaborative relationship that stimulates the child to think for him or herself. The approach aims to give the child the opportunity to try things out and develop new skills

11. Problem solving skills training

A basic ingredient in CBT is to improve the problem-solving abilities of children and adolescents with conduct disorder. The training helps them to deal with external problems that may provoke behaviours. The child is first encouraged to generate potential solutions to a problem. The child and the therapist then decide on the best solution and identify steps in implementing it. The child practices these steps, and finally the whole process is evaluated.

There is some evidence that suggests that clients that develop new ways of thinking get better from psychological difficulties. When clients develop skills that enable them to identify, evaluate and change their thoughts they are likely to get better. In fact, there is proof, in the form of research studies that suggests that when clients develop these new thinking skills that they tend to get better and stay better, or have a lower chance of relapse (Busari 2012).

Cognitive behaviour therapy aims at changing clients' beliefs by treating beliefs as testable hypothesis to be examined through behavioural experiments jointly agreed upon by the clients and the therapists. The therapist does not tell the client that his belief is wrong but rather asks questions to elicit the meaning, function, usefulness, and consequences of clients' beliefs (Busari, 2000).

Cognitive behaviour therapy also challenges adolescents to make conscious choices and to accept full responsibility for their choices (Martye 2004). Cognitive behaviour therapy has been found to be very effective in the treatment of all forms of antisocial behaviours such as stealing (Obalowo, 2004), socially undesirable behavior, faulty thinking.frustration, recidivism and delinquent behaviour (Busari & Adejumo 2012). Cognitive Behaviour Therapy also involves self-management which explains the self- which believes that individuals have potential for self-actualization. The proponent of this theory believed that human beings have inherent tendency to develop their "self" in the process of interpersonal and social experiences, which they have in the environment (Chauman 2000). Since individual has the potential for self-actualization, self-management techniques will make the delinquent individual take part in the management of his own behaviour. Research work cited in Juvenile Justice Bulletin (1999), Gardner 2003), revealed that self-management is effective in modifying deviant behaviours. The present study therefore investigates the effectiveness of cognitive – behaviour programme in the management of adolescents conduct disorder.

12. Hypotheses

The following four null hypotheses were formulated and tested to guide this study at 0.05 level of significant.

Ho1: There is no significant difference in the level of reduction of conduct disorder of participants in the experimental and those in the control group

Ho2: There is no significant difference in the level of reduction of conduct disorder of participants based on gender after exposure to therapeutic treatment

Ho3: There is no significant difference in the level of reduction of conduct disorder of participants from separated and those from intact homes exposed to cognitive behaviour intervention

Ho4: There is no significant difference in the level of reduction of conduct disorder exhibited by participants form polygamous and those from monogamous home after therapeutic treatment

13. Methodology

13.1. Design

The design adopted for this study was a two group (experimental vs control) pretest-post - test design with dependent variable (conduct disorder) and independent variable (Cognitive Behaviour Therapy). Participants were assigned to either experimental or control group by randomly alternating sign-up at counter balanced times.

13.2. Participants

The participants of is study were 350 adolescents pre-selected using conduct disorder questionnaire. The participant's ages between 10-19 years from five secondary schools selected through stratified random sampling techniques in Ibadan metropolis of Oyo State, Nigeria. Out of 350 (72%) 252 were males while (28%) 98 were females 58% (203) were from monogamous home while (42%) 147 were from polygamous homes. (84%) 294 were from intact family while (16%) 56 were form separated family.

13.3. Instrument

The instrument used for collecting data was conduct disorder questionnaire (CDQ) designed by the researcher. It consists of two sections with section A consisting of Demographic data such as age, sex, religion, type of home, type of family, class, etc. while section B consists of 37 items eliciting information on conduct disorder of the participants. These items requires the participants to indicate their degree of agreement with each item on a five point likert type scale ranging from 1 (most unlike me) to 5 (very much like me). Total scores range thus from 37 to 185. High score indicate highest level of conduct disorder. These instrument (conduct disorder questionnaire) was cross-validated with two other instruments (Juvenile Delinquency Questionnaire and Anti-social Behaviour Scale) in a pilot study among randomly selected adolescents in the Junior secondary School, different form the participants (n= 150). The result when correlated with conduct disorder questionnaire was (.

763) at 0.01. A test-retest method was used to establish the reliability of the instrument. A reliability coefficient of 0.83 was obtained, thus indicating that the instrument was highly reliable. Some of the items in the instrument (conduct disorder questionnaire) include:

- Fighting is okay, so far you are not caught
- Running away from school to avoid punishment is okay
- Stealing is not bad so far you don't exceed what you need
- Rules are not meant to be strictly obeyed

13.4. Procedure

This study was carried out in three phases. In the first phase, the participants were screened through conduct disorder questionnaire (CDQ). In the second phase, the participants were randomly assigned to the treatment group (cognitive behaviour therapy) and the control group respectively. At phase three, the experimental group went through eight weeks (1 hour a week) of intensive training consisting of discussion/lecture, discussion of the previous assignment given to the participants, summary and given of assignment for the next session. Instructions and explanations on the task involved in the experimental group such as lectures, discussion and assignment were given to all participants.

In the first session, participants introduced themselves to one another and the therapist familiarized them with the entire programme, she also created a good climate for discussion sessions. Pre-test questionnaire was administered to the participants. A contract was then made between the therapist and the participants such as agreeing on the venue, and time of meeting for the next eight sessions. The participants were encouraged to participate actively in the discussions and to do hoe work/assignments.

The second session witnessed conceptualization of Cognitive Behaviour Therapy (CBT) which was discussed with participants as an active, structured form of psychotherapy designed to rapidly and effectively reduce and eliminate psychological symptoms. The participants were taught that CBT is a form of psychological treatment that focuses on the thoughts and behaviours that accompany psychological distress.

In the third session the participants and the therapist discussed negative effects of conduct disorder to include school drop- out, inferiority complex, low self-esteem, lack of ambition, lack of decision making skills, inability to set goals and make plans inability to clarify values, feelings of guilt, unhappiness etc.

During the fourth session participants were asked to write down various conduct disorder experienced. Among the conduct disorder experienced as mentioned by the participants include truancy, aggression, theft, violation of rules, stealing, disobedience to parents and teachers etc.

The fifth session witnessed, teaching of various personal skills needed by the adolescents to make life meaningful to them. Various personal skills taught the adolescents include decision making goal setting, values of honest, honour, respect, self-control, responsibility, equality, social justice etc. others include communication skills, assertiveness, negotiation. When asked why they engage in conduct disorder the participants mentioned cruelity by parents, teachers and other siblings, inadequate provision of needed materials, lack of love and affection by relations, etc.

In the sixth session participants were taught to replace negative conducts, behaviours and feelings with positive ones; for example they were asked to substitute statement like

- Rules are not meant to be strictly obeyed with
- To avoid punishment rules must be strictly obeyed. In this session the process of learning in improving and maintain behaviour was emphasized. The participants were encouraged to identify connections between thoughts and their responses to social situations.

During the seventh session the participants were taught that the various negative thoughts and behaviors were learned and therefore can be unlearned. They were therefore trained in the emphasis of certain cognitive techniques that are deigned to produce changes in thinking and therefore changes in behavior or mood. They were taught on how learning process and the ways in which external environments can change both cognition and behaviour. They were taught how to strongly focus on social cognitions and inter-personal problem-solving techniques.

Session eight witnessed review of previous session activities rehearsal, role play and administration of post-test instrument.

The control group were given a brief educational review in conduct disorder but no treatment was applied to them both the pre and post -test measures were also administered on them.

Follow-up: Six weeks after the treatment programme, conduct disorder questionnaire was administered on the participants. The results obtained from the data indicates that cognitive behaviour therapy was effective in the management of conduct disorder among adolescent.

Data analysis: The data obtained from this study was analysed using analysis of co-variance (ANCOVA).

14. Results

In order to estimate the effects of the independent variable in the observed differences in the pre- and post- treatment scores of the participants on the dependent measures,an Analysis of Covariance (ANCOVA) was ran, using the pre- test scores as covariates and the post- test scores a criterion. ANCOVA is used to adjust for the initial differences that existed between the groups, since they were randomly selected. Thus, this study adopted ANCOVA to test the hypotheses formulated.

Source of variation	DF	SS	MS	F-ratio Obs.	F-ratio Crit.	Test decision
Between group	7	6376.44	910.92			
				18.74	2.81	Reject Ho
Within group	342	17681.4	51.7			
Total	349	24057.84	962.62			
Critical value F (7,342 = 18.74; P>0.05						

Table 1. Post-treatment Comparison of Cognitive Behaviour Therapy (CBT) and the Control Group using ANCOVA.

With regard to between group differences, there was a significant main effect of treatment(Cognitive Behaviour Therapy) on participants' mean level of conduct disorder (Dependent Variable)scores, F(7,342=18.74;p>0.05.Treatment was found to have contributed significantly to variations in participants' conduct disorder scores.

As shown in table 1, the computed outcome of pre and post treatment evaluation revealed that the null hypothesis was not confirmed at 0.05 alpha level. The finding showed that the critical value F (7,342) = 18.74 has P>0.05 and thus simultaneously indicated that a statistical significant difference existed in the investigated conditions.

Source of variation	DF	SS	MS	F-ratio Obs.	F-ratio Crit.	Test decision
Between group	3	54948.3	18316.1			
				47.91	3.72	Reject Ho
Within group	346	156911.0	453.5			
Total	349	211859.3	18769.6			
Critical value F (7,346 = 47.91; P>0.05						

Table 2. Pre and post-treatment comparison of male and female participants using ANCOVA.

A significant main effect of treatment (Cognitive Behaviour Therapy) on participants' mean level of conduct disorder (Dependent Variable) was evident F(3, 346,=47.91;p>0.05.Post treatment comparison outcome of pre and post -test indicates treatment was found to have contributed significantly to variations in participants' conduct disorder scores.

As shown in table 2, the compared pre and post-treatment outcome with the critical value F (3,346) = 47.91 and P>0.05 showed that there was statistical significant difference between male and female participants exposed to cognitive behaviour therapy. The null hypothesis therefore was not supported.

Source of variation	**DF**	**SS**	**MS**	F-ratio Obs.	F-ratio Crit.	**Test decision**
Between group	5	156528.0	31305.6			
				194.57	2.72	Reject Ho
Within group	344	107293.6	311.9			
Total	349	263821.6	31617.5			
Critical value F(5,344 = 194.57; P>0.05						

Table 3. Pre and post-treatment comparison participants from intact and those form separate family using ANCOVA.

The between group differences, shows that a main significant effect of treatment (Cognitive Behaviour Therapy)on participants' mean level of conduct disorder (Dependent Variable) scores existed F(5,344=194.57;p>0.05. Treatment was found to have contributed significantly to variations in participants' conduct disorder scores.

As indicated in table 3, the outcome of pre and post treatment details among participants from intact and those form separated family showed that there was statistical significant difference in the results obtained contrary to the postulated null hypothesis. Consequently, therefore, the null hypothesis was rejected at 0.05 level of significance.

Source of variation	**DF**	**SS**	**MS**	F-ratio Obs.	F-ratio Crit.	**Test decision**
Between group	5	78299.5	15659.9			
				125.9	2.72	Reject Ho
Within group	344	1836157.6	5337.65			
Total	349	1914451.1	20997.55			
Critical value F(5,344 = 125.9; P>0.05						

Table 4. Pre and Post-treatment comparison of participants from Monogamous and those from Polygamous Homes using ANCOVA.

There was a significant main effect of treatment (Cognitive Behaviour Therapy) on participants' mean level of conduct disorder scores (Dependent Variable) F(5,344=125.9;p>0.05.Post treatment comparisons revealed its significant contribution to variations in participants' conduct disorder scores.

In table 4, the compared computed pre-and post –treatment outcome of participants from monogamous and polygamous homes showed that there was statistical significant difference following the alpha level of 0.05. The findings revealed that the critical value of F(5,344)=125.9; P>0.05 evidently failed to support the predicted null hypothesis.

15. Discussion of the findings

The result of the first hypothesis shows that there was a significant difference in the level of reduction of conduct disorder of participants in the experimental and those in the control group.

This result corroborates the findings of Wolinsky and Miller (2006) when they found that cognitive training would affect the cognitive ability targeted by that training and these effects would be maintained over time. It also indicates that maintained on improvements in cognitive ability would have a positive transfer effect on everyday function.

Gardner (2003) also confirms the effectiveness of cognitive behaviour therapy in treating rebelliousness, delinquency and conduct disorder. According to him, cognitive factors play an important and well documented roles in these undesirable behaviors since the way people think has a controlling effect on their action and that replacement of negative habits with positive ones and rethinking will help individual to generate more adaptive behaviour. Moreover, an individual cognition is important in the acquisition of a new behaviour.

Results emanated from hypothesis two indicates that there exists significant difference in the level of reduction of conduct disorder of male and female participants.

This finding agrees with that of Rathus (1996) who suggested that females who have become involved in criminality must somehow be more male-like than their law abiding counterparts. Some researchers have suggested that where the females have been involved in crime, they have typically played a more passive compliance role, their male counterparts are actually responsible for the planning and execution of the crime. Moreover, it was observed that females restricted their criminal activities to such female crimes as shoplifting, incorrigibility, sex offences or running away whereas males participates in offences like homicide, forcible rape, aggravated assault, robbery, burglary, and auto-theft.

The findings from the result of hypothesis three reveals that there exist significant difference in the response to treatment of participants form intact and those from separated homes. Parents are responsible for the upbringing and development of their children and make provision for their basic needs such as food, education, shelter, protection etc. the family integrates the child into the community. Families raise children to learn the cultural norms. They are the teacher of the rules which in most cases are not written down but may be passed from one generation to another through the process of socialization. In a situation where the two parents are not living together proper upbringing of the children might be impossible. Actions and behaviours which do not promote positive development and growth of the children are likely to be the end product of separated parents whereas the opposite is find in the intact homes (Busari & Adejumobi, 2012).

Results from the findings of the fourth and the last hypothesis indicates that there was significant difference in the level of education of conduct disorder of participants form monogamous and those from polygamous homes after exposure to treatment.

This findings is in line with the findings of Mathye (2004) which reveals that family size is a variable which makes major contribution to the explanation of degree of participation of children in anti-social behaviour such as delinquent acts, rebelliousness, conduct disorder etc. He further expantiate that large family is believed to be negatively related to high rate of anti-social behaviours and that as family increases a child's undesirable behaviour increases. The findings also appear to be consistent with the finding that poor living conditions may slow down growth and maturity among growing children and thrown them off their "programmed curve" that is off the curve that they normally follow under optimal conditions.

16. Conclusion / recommendation

The main objective of this study was to investigate the effects of cognitive behaviour therapy on the management of conduct disorder among adolescents. This study provided substantial evidence to support the fact that cognitive behaviour therapy was effective in the reduction of conduct disorder among the adolescents.

Clearly the research reveals the correlation of diverse factors which promote conduct disorder. Parenting styles play a key role in promoting an environment which is conductive to this disorder. It follows therefore that therapist need to educate their clients, public, parents, families etc. on the negative effects authoritarian parenting styles have on their children.

The research suggests that children with conduct disorder become adults with anti-social behaviour and other psychological problems. The disorder is more than a fussy child it is a serious issue which parents, teachers and the mental health professionals needs to address.

Another aspect to consider is the link between nicotine and conduct disorder. Pregnant women need to be warned against smoking during and after pregnancy. There are significant risks with cigarette smoking during pregnancy.

Author details

Afusat Olanike Busari

University of Ibadan, Ibadan, Nigeria

References

[1] Aderanti, R. A. (2006). Prevalent of adolescents' delinquent behavioral patterns: An issue in counseling psychology and implications for national development. A paper presented at the 1st National Conference of Colelge of Applied education and Vocaitoanl Technology. Tai Solarin University of Education, Ijagun (unpublished)

[2] American Psychiatric Association.(2000). Diagnostic and statistical manual of mental disorders (4th ed. Tex. t Revision). Washington D.C.: Author.

[3] Barton, A., et al. (2007). Functional Family Therapy: blueprint for violence Prevention.Institute of Behavioral Science. Retrieved June 19, 2011 from http:www.colorado.edu/cspv/blueprints/model/programs/FFT.html

[4] Functional Family Therapy Website. (2007). http://www.fftinc.om.

[5] Busari, A. O. (2000). Stress Inculcation Training and Self Statement Monitoring Techniques in the Reduction of Test Anxiety Among Adolescent Under Achievers in Ibadan Metropolis, Nigeria. An unpublished Ph.D Thesis, University of Ibadan , 309.

[6] Busari, A. O. ., & Uwakwe, C. B. U. (2001). The Effects of Stress Inoculation Training-Techniques in the Management of Worry as a self Handicapping Strategy in IntellectualPerformance. Nigerian Journal of Emotional Psychology and Sport Ethics 3:, 6-12.

[7] Busari, A. O., & Ojo, R. A. (2011). Empowering Youth in Remand Home Against Risk Taking Behaviours for Effective Transition to Independence. Ethno Medicine. 5(3)India, 217-222.

[8] Busari, A. O. (2012). Cognitive Training Intervention and Daily Functioning Improvement among the Retirees of University of Ibadan, Nigeria. European Journal of Globalization and Development Research.3(1) , 143-153.

[9] Busari & Adejumobi(2012). Cognitive Behaviour Therapy in the Management of Juvenile Delinquency; being a paper presented at the International Conference on Sustainable Development in Africa. Held at R.S. Amegashie Auditorium University of Ghana, Legon, Accra, Ghana between 25th- 27th July.

[10] Edelson, S. M. (2004). Self-management center for autism. Retrieved from the web November 22, 2011 http://www.ojdpncjrs.org

[11] Garner, J. R. (2003). Cognitive Rehabilitation. Retrieved from the web November 22, 2010

[12] Hoeve et al.(2008). Trajectories of delinquency and parenting styles.Journal of Abnormal Child Psychology, 36 (2), 223-235. Retrieved May 23, 2011 from http://www.pubmedcentral.nih.gov/

[13] Hoagwood, K., et al. (2007). Empirically-based school interventions targeted at academic and mental health functioning. *Journal of emotional and behavioral disorders*, 66 EOF-92 EOF.

[14] Marsiglia et al.(2007). Impact of parenting styles and locus of control on emerging psychosocial success. Journal of Education and Human Development, 1. Retrieved April 29, 2012 from: http://www.scientificjournals.org

[15] Mathye, L. V. (2004). Therapeutic techniques for treatment of adolescents with rebellious behavior.

[16] National Institute for Health & Clinical Excellence.(2007). Conduct disorder programs {Electronic Version}. Community Care, Retrieved June 22, 2012 http://www.nice.org.uk/page.aspx?0=529846, 1672(1672), 32-33.

[17] Obalowo, Y. O. (2004). Cognitive restructuring and contigency management in the treatment of stealing behavior among some Nigerian adolescents. Unpublished Ph.D Thesis, Olabisi Onabanjo University, Ago-Iwoye.

[18] Ray, D. (2007). Two counseling interventions to reduce teacher-child relationship Stress {Electronic version}. Professional School Counseling, 10(4), 428-440. http://www.goliath.ecnext.com/coms2.

[19] (1990). Screening for Signs and Symptoms of Juvenile Delinquency in Secondary School Students.In Kajola Local Government area of Oyo State.An Unpublished B.Ed Project, University of Ibadan , 127.

[20] Scott, S. (2007). Conduct disorder in children.BMJ 2007. Retrieved July 13, 2012 from http://www.bmj.com/cgi/content/full/334/7595/646

[21] Somerstein, L. (2007). I came with a sword on judgment day: a psychoanalytic look at terrorist enactments. Psychoanalytic Review, 94 (5).

[22] Stevenson, K. (1999). Family characteristics of problem kids.Canadian Social Trends.

[23] U.S.Department of Health and Human Services. ((1999). Mental Health: A report of the Surgeon General {Electronic Version}.Rockville, MD. Retrieved July 13, 2010 from http://mentalhealth.samsha.gov/publications

[24] U.S. Department of Justice.(2000). Juvenile Justice Bulletin. Washington, D.C.

[25] Van Goozen et al. (2007). The evidence for a neurobiological model of childhood anti-social behavior. *Psychological Bulletin*, 149-182.

Chapter 3

Treatment-Resistant Schizophrenia: Prevalence and Risk Factors

Mohamed Dammak

Additional information is available at the end of the chapter

1. Introduction

Despite significant progress in the treatment of schizophrenia in recent decades, the evolution of a large rate of patients suffering from this mental disorder is little influenced by treatment [1]. The management of these patients, so-called treatment resistant, constitutes a public health problem. Indeed, these very symptomatic patients often require long periods of hospitalization [2], and their care consumes a disproportionately large share of total cost management of schizophrenia [3].

Following the renewed interest in clozapine since 1988, thanks to the baseline study on the neuroleptic Kane and al [4], and the development in this period of several explicit criteria defining treatment-resistant schizophrenia (TRS), like those of Kane [4], Dencker and al [5] and Brenner and al [6], some studies have subsequently estimated its prevalence.

The large number and variety of risk factors associated with poor prognosis or poor response to treatment, reported in the literature, suggest that several pathophysiological mechanisms may contribute to the emergence of resistance.

In this work, we tried to shed light on the prevalence of this concept, as well as its risk factors, through a critical review of the literature.

2. Methodology

In our literature review, we conducted a literature search in two databases MEDLINE and PUBMED. We used the following keywords: treatment-resistant, refractory, schizophrenia, prevalence, Correlates, predictors, poor outcome, Treatment refractoriness, Treatment response, poor prognosis.

For studies estimating the prevalence of TRS, we selected the works that have considered the resistance as a categorical diagnosis, defining it by explicit criteria.

For risk factors of TRS, we selected studies that have specifically studied the risk factors of resistance, and the studies that studied the risk factors of poor prognosis or poor response to treatment.

3. Prevalence of treatment-resistant schizophrenia

3.1. Results

The prevalence of resistant schizophrenia ranged from 5 to 60% (Table 1) in the four studies in the literature. Vanelle only found a low rate of 5% resistance because of too restrictive criteria of resistance corresponding to stages 5 and 6 of Dencker and May defining TRS. The results of the other three studies suggest that an important rate of patients do not derive virtually any benefit of treatment and that the TRS is therefore a true public health problem [7]. Many authors agree on the fact that 1/5 to 1/3 of patients are resistant to treatment [1]. Methodological differences between these different studies concerning inclusion criteria and the TRS criteria were important, which explains the wide variation in the estimate of the prevalence of TRS: 5 to 60%. The study by Juarez-Reyes and al [8] illustrates this fact. Applying the criteria of the FDA (Food and Drugs Administration) for the prescription of Clozapine in the United States of America, Juarez-Reyes et al found in their sample a prevalence of 42.9% of resistant patients, but applying the more restrictive criteria of Kane on the same sample, the prevalence dropped to 12.9%.

These methodological differences reflect a lack of consensus on the concept of TRS, which seems to hamper research in this field, since the studies found were few, relatively old and only conducted between 1990 and 1996.

3.2. Discussion of methodological differences

The methodological differences were related to:

3.2.1. Inclusion criteria

Essock [11] required in his sample only inpatients that must have had a total hospitalization of at least 24 months for the preceding 5 years as inclusion criteria. It is clear that in such sample the prevalence of TRS will be overestimated. By applying FDA criteria for eligibility to Clozapine in this sample, Essock found the highest rate of TRS: 60%. Indeed, if outpatients were including in the sample, prevalence of TRS would be less elevated. Essock [11] justified such restrictive inclusion criteria by the fact "to ensure that Clozapine was most available for

Authors	Inclusion's criteria	Criteria of TRS				Prevalence of TRS
		Number of NLP trial	Minimal duration of NLP trial	Minimal dosage of CPZ or its equivalent	Assessment scales	
Terkelsen (1990) [9]	Retrospective estimates based on three large-scale surveys, of patients in New York State	unspecified	unspecified	unspecified	BPRS CGI	.58 % of inpatients and 24 % of outpatients
Vanelle (. 5995) [10]	566 SKZ or SAD inpatients since at least 6 months disease duration since 3 years	2	3 months	.5000 mg/a day	CGI level 5 and 6 of May and Dencker classification of treatment response	5%
Juarez-Reyes (. 5995) [8]	293 SKZ ou SAD	2	4 weeks	600 mg/a day	BPRS CGI GAF	42.9 +/- 5.9%
Essock (. 5996) [11]	803 SKZ or SAD inpatients since at least 4 months and at least 24 months of hospitalization during the last 5 years disease duration since 5 years	2	6 weeks	.5000 mg/a day	BPRS CGI FDA criteria for eligibility to Clozapine	60%

SKZ: schizophrenia; SAD: schizo-affective disorder; NLP: neuroleptic ; CPZ : Chlorpromazine; BPRS: Brief Psychiatric Rating Scale; CGI: clinical global impressions; GAF: global assessment of functioning.

Table 1. Prevalence of TRS in the literature.

those most in need", because of the high cost of this treatment, and thus he recognized that he did not screen TRS in all potentially patients in need to Clozapine, such as outpatients.

3.2.2. Criteria of TRS

3.2.2.1. Chronic hospitalization

In Vanelle's study [10], which is based on the Dencker and May criteria [5] to define the TRS, the need of continuous hospital stay was an essential criterion of resistance. Such highly restrictive criteria of resistance may underestimate TRS. This highly restrictive criterion seems explaining the low rate of TRS in Vanelle's study 5 % [10]. Currently, most authors agree that chronic hospitalization is not necessary for criteria of TRS [1].

3.2.2.2. *Duration criteria*

Persistence of illness for more than 5 years was taken as the duration criteria for TRS by Kane et al [4]. This was most probably the impact of serious side effects of clozapine (drug induced agranulocytosis), which made researchers so stringent about duration criteria. Essock [11] fixed this duration at 5 years and Vanelle [10] at 3 years. The other authors did not specify any duration. Currently, most authors agree that waiting such durations are not necessary and a clinical history of persistent psychosis for at least 2 years is sufficient for TRS [6,12]. Some researchers have mentioned that even one year of unresponsiveness to treatment may be an adequate time period [7].

3.2.2.3. *Criteria of adequate drug trial*

3.2.2.3.1. *Duration of adequate drug trial*

This duration ranged from 4 weeks to 3 months between the four studies (Table 1). Most authors agree with the fact a period of 4 to 8 weeks is sufficient to evaluate the efficacy of a therapeutic trial [13-17]. Conley [1] recommended in its definition of TRS established in 2001, a period of 4 to 6 weeks, while the NICE (national institute for clinical excellence) recommends a period of 6 to 8 weeks [18]. Nevertheless, some authors as Vannelle [10], Ciapparelli [19] and Lindenmayer [20] consider that a period less than three months is insufficient to assess the efficacy of a therapeutic trial.

This duration must vary according to symptoms taken into account when assessing the therapeutic trial, because the different symptomatic dimensions do not evolve synchronously. If the assessment of treatment response is based on the positive and negative symptoms, a relatively short period seems sufficient. If the dimensions, such as social functioning, occupational functioning, or quality of life, are included in the scope of the evaluation, a longer period of evaluation should be required. However, the functional dimension of schizophrenia is less specific to treatment response as positive or negative symptoms in a clinical trial, as it can be influenced by several factors other than treatment [21,22].

3.2.2.3.2. *Adequate dosage of neuroleptic*

Despite the variation of this dose (600 to 1000 mg per day of chlorpromazine equivalents) across studies, it was largely sufficient. Indeed, Kane set the minimum threshold dose, in its definition of resistance, to 1000 mg per day of chlorpromazine equivalent [4]. But the results of more recent studies, using the technique of positron emission tomography, showed that a dose of 400 mg of chlorpromazine daily can block 80-90% of dopamine D2 receptors in the nigrostriatal pathway, and an occupancy rate of 60 to 80% of these receptors is sufficient to obtain a response to neuroleptic treatment [23]. In addition It has been reported that higher doses produce no direct therapeutic benefit even in patients who are nonresponsive to therapy [24] and do not improve efficacy in acute treatment [25].This dopamine antagonism is considered the main mechanism of action of typical neuroleptics [23].Currently, most authors such as Barnes[13], McEvedy [13], Dixon [26], Kinon [24], Shalev [27] and Conley [1] consider that doses between 400 and 600 mg per day of chlorpromazine equivalents are sufficient.

3.2.2.4. Adequate number of trials

Terkelsen [9] could not assess the adequacy of previous trials in his study because he constructed retrospective estimation based on three large-scale surveys, conducted in 1987 and 1988, of patients in New York State. The remaining three authors (table 1) agree that the failure of two trials is a criterion of treatment resistance, and not three as Kane had proposed in the beginning in his initial definition of TRS. Indeed, the fact that there was only a 3% response rate to prospective haloperidol treatment and a 4% response rate to double blind chlorpromazine treatment in the Multicenter Clozapine Trial led to the belief that failure of two retrospective drug trials would be as effective as 3 in screening for treatment resistance [4]. Additionally, Kinon and al [24] mentioned that subjects who do not respond to 2 adequate antipsychotic trials (1 retrospective and 1 prospective) have less than 7% chance of responding to another trial. The FDA guidelines on clozapine use state that a patient before being treated with clozapine should have failed to respond to two separate trials of antipsychotics. Several guidelines such as APA (American Psychiatric Association) [28], NICE [18], IPAP (The International Psychopharmacology Algorithm Project) [29], and TMAP (the Texas Medication Algorithm Project) [30] also recommended that the number of trials of other antipsychotics that should precede a clozapine trial is 2. Thus, two drug trial failures are now generally accepted as the criterion for treatment resistance.

3.2.2.5. Scales for evaluating response to treatment

With the exception of the Vanelle's study, all of the other studies have used the BPRS as the main tool for assessing the clinical response (Table 1). In this scale the positive psychotic symptoms are the most important. The response to neuroleptic treatment was considered adequate if the score in the BPRS reduction ranges from 20 to 30% as suggested in the literature data [31]. Cognition and subjective perspectives or other illness domains again have not been incorporated into definitions of treatment response in TRS in these studies.

However, according to some authors, the definition of resistant schizophrenia must be multidimensional, and the field to assess during a clinical trial should be extended and include, besides the conventional positive and negative symptoms of schizophrenia, cognitive deficits, quality of life, social reintegration, occupational impairments and behavioral problems [32-35]. But these positions are still controversial. This higher level of requirement is motivated by improving in therapeutic arsenal in the field of schizophrenia as the widespread prescription of Second Generation Antipsychotic (SGA), cognitive remediation and several types of psychotherapy that are effective on certain dimensions of schizophrenia.

3.2.2.6. The question of the type of antipsychotic

The four studies were consistent in the type of neuroleptic. During clinical trials of these studies, only conventional neuroleptics (also called first generation antipsychotics: FGA) are used. The results of these studies, therefore, reflect only the resistance of schizophrenia in this type of neuroleptic. Recently, the evidence that second generation antipsychotics (SGA) are somewhat more effective than traditional medications has opened the question of the type of the drug patient should fail [36]. Currently, most authors [37] and guidelines such as APA (American Psychiatric Association) [28], NICE [18], IPAP [29], TMAP (the Texas Medication Algorithm Project) [30] and Clinical Practice Guidelines for the Treatment of Schizophrenia in Adults of the Department of the COMMONWEALTH OF MASSACHUSETTS [38] agree that failure to respond to second generation antipsychotics should precede a clozapine trial. In the Schizophrenia Algorithm of the International Psychopharmacology Algorithm Project (IPAP) [29] patient is regarded to be refractory if he or she failed to respond to monotherapy with Two trials of Two Different SGA (or Two trials with a FGA, if SGAs are not available). Indeed, atypical antipsychotics cause fewer early and late extrapyramidal neurological side effects, improve adherence to treatment, would be more effective than conventional neuroleptics in negative symptoms, cognitive deficits and mood symptoms, and may be effective in some cases resistant to conventional neuroleptics, but without reaching the effectiveness of clozapine for this indication [39].

3.2.2.7. Recommendations for future studies

Since 1996, the last date of study estimating the prevalence of TRS, there have been changes in treatment practices in schizophrenia, such as the widespread prescription of atypical antipsychotics, or more intensive *deinstitutionalization* of psychiatric cares in schizophrenia, which could change the rate of resistance. There has also been a revision of the criteria of TRS [1] as shown in the comparison of TRS criteria adopted by the four studies estimating the prevalence of TRS to the recent data from the literature given above. New studies estimating the prevalence of TRS and adopting the revised criteria of resistance seem to be necessary. Pending the establishment of a broad consensus on the criteria of TRS, this will be precious for research and therapeutic practice, the criteria of TRS that are currently almost unanimously accepted in the literature are:

- A period of two years, during which the patient does not improve significantly, and has a poor psychosocial functioning, seems reasonable even without long hospital stay.
- During this period, two well-conducted clinical trials have failed. The characteristics of an adequate therapeutic trial would be:
- A period of 4 to 6 weeks each,
- A dose of 400 to 600 mg equivalent of chlorpromazine to classical neuroleptics
- Among the two trials that failed, one should include an atypical antipsychotic.

Even more restrictive criteria, such as Kane, should be reserved for experimental studies evaluating the efficacy of new drugs in resistant schizophrenia.

4. Risk factors of TRS

In this field, the literature is dominated by studies that have examined factors associated with good or poor prognosis or outcome in general, or factors associated with good or poor response to neuroleptic treatment in particular.

4.1. Risk factors related to the patient

The male gender is among the most documented risk factors of poor prognosis [40]. It was also identified specifically as a factor associated with a poor response to neuroleptic treatment for chronic patients and for patients seen during their first psychotic episode, by numerous studies [41]. This male gender predominance in patients with TRS is explained by a greater sensitivity of dopamine receptors to dopamine antagonism of neuroleptics in women, due to the antidopaminergic effect of natural estrogen [42].

The results of studies correlating the early age of onset and poor outcome are consistent [43,44]. This risk factor was associated with greater dysfunction in prospective studies [45], with poor response to neuroleptics [46-48], with an increased risk of re hospitalization [49] and specifically to the resistance [10]. Schizophrenia has a later onset in females than in males and the difference has been found to be about 5 years in most studies [50] suggesting that the association between early age of onset and poor prognosis, is biased by the variable male gender. However, the fact that the difference in age of onset between men and women disappears in patients with TRS in many studies [44] argues for a direct influence, and independently of gender, of age at onset on treatment response. The association between early age of onset and poor outcome reflects a greater neurodevelopmental insult [51] that can be intensified by environmental factors.

In terms of symptoms, severity of negative symptoms was associated with poor response to treatment in many studies [35,52]. Other clinical aspects of schizophrenia were associated with poor prognosis in the literature, as asociality [53] inappropriate or blunted affects [35,53], the low level of premorbid functioning [54], a high degree of minor neurological signs [55], the absence of affective symptoms [56,57], negative formal thought [52], excessive summertime (July) and clustering of birthdates [58], morbid polydypsia [59], and a less severe overall basic symptomatology (before starting treatment) [60].

In the psychological level, insight, poor coping, and some personality traits such as low social skills, a lack of impulse control, and an intolerance of frustration, alogia would be factors of poor response to psychosocial treatment [61-63].

4.2. Family and socio-environmental risk factors

The presence of family history of schizophrenia would be a poor prognostic factor [64]. A high emotional expressiveness in the family environment was related to higher risk of relapses [65]. A history of obstetric complications is more common in patients not responding to neuroleptic treatment [66]. The absence of precipitating factors [35] and a history of substance abuse [67-70] were associated with poor response to treatment.

4.3. Risk factors associated with cognitive deficits

Several literature reviews have summarized the evidence for associations between functional outcome and cognitive deficits [71-73]. These reviews have regarded ranks of functional outcome measures, including measures of skill acquisition in psychosocial rehabilitation treatment, demonstration of ability to solve simulated interpersonal problems, and community (social and occupational) functioning. The reviews indicated consistent and highly significant relationships between ranks of key cognitive constructs such as episodic memory, immediate / working memory, vigilance, and executive functions, and functional outcome in schizophrenia. The effect sizes of these relationships tended to be in the medium to wide range.

According to several studies, the severity of cognitive deficits is equally or more important than positive or negative symptoms to predict prognosis in schizophrenia [74].

4.4. Para clinical risk factors

4.4.1. The data of brain neuroimaging

The ventricular enlargement is the variable most studied in this field. Over the last three decades, earlier computerized tomography and then MRI, cross sectional studies including chronic patients have found an association between ventricular enlargement and poor outcome [75-77]. Several longitudinal studies conducted during periods of 1 to 5 years of chronic patients [78,79] or first psychotic episode patients [77,80] confirmed these structural changes in the brain and found that they were progressive over the course of illness.

For the gray matter, reduction in total volume or located reduction in certain regions such as the frontal, temporal and occipital cortex and ventral thalamus were identified [77]. In addition, volumes of the putamen, especially dorsal and in the right hemisphere, showed increases in patients with better outcomes, whereas putamen volumes in patients with poor outcome did not differ from those in healthy comparison subjects [81]. Expansion of the putamen is known to occur as a result of antipsychotic treatment, so that failure to expand in patients with poor outcome may be related to their resistance to treatment [77].

Abnormalities of white matter located especially at the frontal and temporal lobe of the right hemisphere were associated with poor outcome [77].

The results of longitudinal studies suggest that these brain volume changes seem to be progressive, and occurred at an early stage of the illness [82].

Dynamic neuroimaging data found that lower pre-treatment striatal metabolism predicted better clinical response to neuroleptic treatment and that drug responders showed a greater increase in striatal metabolism after haloperidol therapy [83-85].

4.4.2. The biology data

In the literature, a smaller increase in plasma levels of prolactin [86,87], and a smaller decrease in plasma homovanillic acid [88-91] following administration of neuroleptic, were associated with poor response treatment. A lower baseline plasma levels of homovanillic acid (before the administration of a neuroleptic), was also associated with poor response to treatment [35,92]. A lack of clinical change after administration of amphetamine (central dopamine agonist) was associated with decreased response to antipsychotics [93]. A blunted response of growth hormone after stimulation with apomorphine [94] has been associated with poor prognosis.

All these factors reflect a poorer response to central dopaminergic action of dopamine antagonist antipsychotics. The hyperactivity of central dopaminergic mesolimbic pathway remains the predominant mechanism that explains the positive symptoms of schizophrenia [39].

4.4.3. The data of electrophysiology

The MMN (mismatch negativity) is an early component of auditory evoked potential, recorded after a disruptive auditory stimulus. The peak of MMN occurs after 100 to 150 milliseconds after the stimulus. Abnormally increased MMN amplitude, as well as abnormal MMN topographical distribution, was associated with a poor functional outcome in schizophrenia [95]. These anomalies reflect pre-attentive deficit process (or automatic attention), related to neuropathological changes in the auditory cortex in schizophrenia [95].

4.4.4. The Electrodermal Activity (EDA)

Some studies have found that heightened electrodermal activity, as indicated by frequent orienting responses to innocuous stimuli, elevated skin conductance level (SCL) and frequent nonspecific skin conductance responses (NS-SCR), is associated with most often poor symptomatic, social and occupational outcome in schizophrenic patients [96].

4.5. Risk factors associated with treatment

The initial duration of untreated psychosis, namely the time gap between the onset of psychotic symptoms and first treatment, also called DUP, is among the most studied risk factors for poor outcome during the last 2 decades [97]. Evidence from both retrospective and prospective studies suggests that a longer duration of untreated psychosis in the early stage of schizophrenia is associated with a longer time to remission and a lower level of recovery, a greater likelihood of relapse and a worse overall outcome [98]. Perkins in a recent meta-analysis has retained a total of 43 publications from 28 sites. He found that shorter DUP was associated with greater response to antipsychotic treatment, as measured by severity of global psychopathology, positive symptoms, negative symptoms, and functional outcomes [97].These findings are frequently interpreted as a consequence of a more intense and rapid progression of a neurodegenerative process in the first years of untreated illness [99].

Response to treatment, at least in some cases, appears to decrease over psychotic relapses. As a result patients have lower rates of remission and longer duration to achieve it [100]. Lieberman and colleagues [101] measured time to remission over three successive psychotic episodes and found that the time to reach remission more than tripled between the first and third episode.

Moreover, the absence of a significant and rapid reduction of symptoms during the first days of neuroleptic treatment (3 to 7 days) [60], the dysphoric subjective response type at an initial dose of neuroleptic [60], a bad alliance with the therapist [63], the occurrence of neurological side effects such as parkinsonism [102], akathisia [10] or tardive dyskinesia [102], predict a poor response to treatment.

4.6. Methodological considerations

In our literature review we have considered the factors influencing the prognosis and response to treatment as factors that may explain the resistance. This choice can be criticized. On the one hand, a poor prognosis or a poor response to neuroleptic treatment is not synonymous with therapeutic resistance. On the other hand, the prognosis is a broader concept that the response to treatment and thus the factors influencing prognosis and those influencing treatment response can be inter-related but not necessarily identical [60]. Accordingly, it is important to consider these potential factors of resistance with caution.

Tools for evaluating the response to treatment or prognosis varied widely, limiting their comparability. Consensus specifying tools for assessing treatment response and prognosis in schizophrenia is therefore of great interest for research in this field [60]. The criteria for remission in schizophrenia proposed by Andreasen et al [103] can be a great help for future studies [104].

In this area of research, the results of longitudinal studies examining schizophrenic patients prospectively from their first psychotic episode are more reliable than cross-sectional studies retrospectively examining chronic patients [102]. Indeed, in samples of chronic patients examined retrospectively, there is firstly an overrepresentation of poor responders or patients with less favorable prognosis, and secondly, a greater heterogeneity because these chronic patients are at different stages of the disease and were exposed for varying periods at different neuroleptics. While in samples of patients followed from their first psychotic episode in longitudinal studies, there is a greater representation of the broad spectrum of response to treatment or prognosis, and a greater homogeneity because patients are at the same stages of the disease (the first months or years of illness) and the exposure to neuroleptics was controlled [102].

Some risk factors of TRS are known to be interrelated, like poor premorbid sociosexual functioning [77] and cognitive deficits that are related to severity of the negative symptoms. At end of design studies with methodological rigor use of statistical techniques such as multiple regression and the development of more complex predictive models is needed for future studies in this area.

4.7. The pathophysiology of TRS

The pathophysiology of TRS is still unclear. Some risk factors for TRS cited above as the low level of premorbid adjustment, male gender, severity of primary negative symptoms, the greater frequency of obstetric complications, the high degree of minor neurological signs, and the vulnerability to develop tardive dyskinesia, suggest a neurodevelopmental origin [98].

These neurodevelopmental factors are more frequently found in patients resistant to treatment from the first clinical trial. Moreover, these factors may have an additive effect, i.e. there should be coexistence of a critical number of such factors for there to be resistance [98]. According to some authors [59,105,106] these factors are the characteristics of a more severe subtype of schizophrenia (Kraepelinian schizophrenia) less influenced by neuroleptic treatment.

However, some patients worsen over the course of their illness either because of its progression or because they become less responsive to treatment [101]. Other TRS risk factors mentioned above as DUP, progressive changes in brain volumes in early stage of illness and the deterioration of treatment response over relapses, support the hypothesis that the resistance would be secondary to a neurodegenerative process, which alters the response to treatment in a progressive manner, and not to a static and finished neurodevelopmental process [99]. Candidate's neurons for the seat of this neurodegeneration include dopaminergic projections to the cortex, and glutamatergic cortico-cortical projections. This neurodegeneration is due to excessive glutamatergic excitation (excitotoxicity) triggered by the disease, involving the NMDA subtype of glutamate receptor that is coupled to an ion channel for calcium. This excessive excitation induces an excess of intracellular calcium, which activates certain intracellular enzymes which dangerously begin to produce free radicals that destroy the cell [39].

For other authors, these two hypotheses, neurodevelopmental and neurodegenerative, are not mutually exclusive, but in fact they are complementary [98]. Each comes at different stages of the disease in the genesis of resistance to treatment. However, the neurodegenerative hypothesis is more optimistic, because it suggests that treatment resistance is not inevitable, it does not follow the law of all or nothing, at least for some patients, and it would be possible to protect patients against the development of resistance to treatment by receiving early effective and continuous treatment.

4.8. The perspectives

Some risk factors for TRS cited in this literature review, are promising and interesting, and require a particular interest in future studies because they offer an more positive and optimistic approach of the concept of TRS.

4.8.1. The initial duration of untreated psychosis

It is a potentially modifiable risk factor, offering hope for effective therapeutic intervention to avoid resistance by shortening this duration. Indeed, some preliminary studies have found that shortening this period is possible by means of early detection programs [107], and that early intervention can favorably influence the prognosis of schizophrenia [108,109]. Additionally, evidence for a neuroprotective effect of some forms of early treatment such as atypical antipsychotics is beginning to emerge. Atypical antipsychotics may counteract some of the progressive deteriorative effects by enhancing synaptic plasticity and cellular resilience [99]. Finally, understanding the mechanism by which duration of untreated psychosis influences prognosis may lead to better understanding of the pathophysiology of schizophrenia and to improved current treatment strategies [97].

4.8.2. Cognitive deficits

Cognitive impairment has emerged as an important new target in schizophrenia therapeutics in light of evidence that cognitive deficits are critically related to the functional of disability that is characteristic of the illness. The cognitive impairment is a risk factor for TRS that is potentially accessible to efficient therapeutic interventions. Indeed, in addition to atypical antipsychotics that are more effective in improving cognitive deficits than classical antipsychotics [39], there is now enough evidence that some rehabilitation therapies such as cognitive remediation - a cognitive computerized training - can change and improve these deficits [110], and thus it is another promising way forward.

4.8.3. Some paraclinical tests

The mismatch negativity (MMN) is an electrophysiological recording that could predict poor outcome in patients with schizophrenia. It has the advantage of being harmless, quick and easy to made, with low cost, and can be coupled with functional neuroimaging (fMRI) to increase its spatial resolution [95,111]. Like the mismatch negativity, research can provide "biomarkers" associated with prognosis or response to treatment. Predicting precociously a poor outcome using such convenient test will give the therapist the opportunity to optimize treatment at the first trial.

4.8.4. The glutamate hypothesis for schizophrenia

The promising findings of researches on the glutamate hypothesis in pathophysiology and treatment of schizophrenia allow hope for having future drugs modulating glutamatergic neurotransmission (such as NMDA-receptor agonists) that seem to be promising in difficult-to-improve symptoms as cognitive impairments and negative symptoms [112,113]

4.8.5. The need for future studies

Setrn and al found in there review of the literature about predictors of response to neuroleptic treatment in schizophrenia, that predictive models explained less then 80 % and more frequently less than 40 % of the outcome variance. These findings suggest that there are other factors influencing the prognosis of schizophrenia, which are still unknown [60], hence there is an important need for further studies in this area.

5. Conclusion

TRS remains a challenge for clinical practice and research. It is an undeniable and frequent clinic reality and a real public health problem. For research, having a wide consensus defining the boundaries of TRS is important for comparability and reliability of future studies. TRS is a heterogeneous entity, and has a multifactorial determinism. It is not, at least for some patients, a fatality, but rather the culmination of several risk factors, some of which seem to be accessible to effective therapeutic interventions. According to this opinion, TRS would be partly preventable and reversible.

Nomenclature

TRS : treatment-resistant schizophrenia;

SKZ: schizophrenia;

SAD: schizo-affective disorder;

NLP: neuroleptic;

CPZ: Chlorpromazine;

BPRS: Brief Psychiatric Rating Scale;

CGI: Clinical global impressions;

GAF: Global assessment of functioning;

SGA: Second generation antipsychotics;

FGA: first generation antipsychotics;

APA: American Psychiatric Association;

NICE: National institute for clinical excellence;

IPAP: The International Psychopharmacology Algorithm Project;

TMAP: The Texas Medication Algorithm Project

Acknowledgements

I offer my thanks to Karim Tabbane, Hatem Dammak and Mohamed Triki for their valuable assistance in the elaboration of this work. There were no funding sources for this work.

Author details

Mohamed Dammak*

Address all correspondence to: dr.dammak@gmail.com

Sfax, Tunisia

References

[1] Conley, R. R, & Kelly, D. L. Management of treatment resistance in schizophrenia. Biological Psychiatry (2001). Dec 1;, 50(11), 898-911.

[2] Mcglashan, T. H. A selective review of recent North American long-term followup studies of schizophrénia. Schizophr Bull (1988). , 14(4), 515-42.

[3] Revicki, D. A, Luce, B. R, Weschler, J. M, Brown, R. E, & Adler, M. A. Cost-effectiveness of clozapine for treatment resistant schizophrenic patients. Hosp Community Psychiatry (1990). Aug;, 41(8), 850-4.

[4] Kane, J, Honigfeld, G, Singer, J, & Meltzer, H. Clozapine for the treatment-resistant schizophrenic. A double-blind comparison with chlorpromazine. Arch Gen Psychiatry. (1988). Sep; , 45(9), 789-96.

[5] Dencker, S. J, & Kulhanet, F. eds. Treatment Resistance in Schizophrenia. Braunschweig, Germany: Vieweg Verlag; (1988).

[6] Brenner, H. D, Dencker, S. J, Goldstein, M. J, et al. Defining treatment refractoriness in schizophrenia. Schizophr Bull (1990). , 16(4), 551-61.

[7] Peuskens, J. The evolving definition of treatment resistance. J Clin Psychiatry (1999). Suppl , 12, 4-8.

[8] Juarez-reyes, M. G, Shumway, M, Battle, C, Bacchetti, P, Hansen, M. S, & Hargreaves, W. A. Effects of stringent criteria on eligibility for clozapine among public mental health clients. Psychiatr Serv. (1995). Aug;, 46(8), 801-806.

[9] Terkelsen, K. G, & Grosser, R. C. Estimating clozapine's cost to the nation. Hosp Community Psychiatry (1990). Aug;, 41(8), 863-869.

[10] Vanelle, J. M. Notion de schizophrénie résistante. L'Encéphale (1995). NS3) 13-21.

[11] Essock, S. M, Hargreaves, W. A, Dohm, F. A, Goethe, J, Carver, L, & Hipshman, L. Clozapine eligibility among state hospital patients. Schizophr Bull. (1996). , 22(1), 15-25.

[12] Painuly, N, Gupta, N, & Avasthi, A. Concept and Management of Treatment Resistant Schizophrenia (TRS). Indian J Psychiatry. (2004). Apr-Jun; , 46(2), 125-134.

[13] Barnes, T. R, & Mcevedy, C. J. Pharmacological treatment strategies in the non respensive schizophrenic patient. Int Clin Psychopharmacol (1996). Suppl 2): 67-71.

[14] Kane, J. M, Potkin, S. G, Daniel, D. G, Buckley, P. F, & Double-blind, A. randomized study comparing the efficacy and safety of sertindole and risperidone in patients with treatment-resistant schizophrenia. J. Clin. Psychiatry (2011). , 72, 194-204.

[15] Sacchetti, E, Galluzzo, A, Valsecchi, P, Romeo, F, Gorini, B, & Warrington, L. MOZART Study Group, Ziprasidone vs clozapine in schizophrenia patients refractory to

multiple antipsychotic treatments: the MOZART study. Schizophr. Res. (2009). , 113, 112-121.

[16] Bitter, I, Dossenbach, M. R, Brook, S, Feldman, P. D, Metcalfe, S, Gagiano, C. A, Füredi, J, Bartko, G, Janka, Z, Banki, C. M, Kovacs, G, & Breier, A. Olanzapine HGCK Study Group,. Olanzapine versus clozapine in treatment-resistant or treatmentintolerant schizophrenia. Prog. Neuropsychopharmacol. Biol. Psychiatry (2004). , 28, 173-180.

[17] Semiz, U. B, Cetin, M, Basoglu, C, Ebrinc, S, Uzun, O, Herken, H, Balibey, H, Algul, A, & Ates, A. Clinical predictors of therapeutic response to clozapine in a sample of Turkish patients with treatment-resistant schizophrenia. Prog. Neuropsychopharmacol. Biol. Psychiatry (2007). , 31, 1330-1336.

[18] National Institute for Clinical ExcellenceTechnology appraisal Guidance Guidance on the use of newer (atypical) antipsychotic drugs for the treatment of schizophrenia. London: NICE, (2002). (43)

[19] Ciapparelli, A. Dell'Osso, L., Bandettini di Poggio, A., Carmassi, C., Cecconi, D., Fenzi, M., Chiavacci, M.C., Bottai, M., Ramacciotti, C.E., Cassano, G.B. Clozapine in treatment-resistant patients with schizophrenia, schizoaffective disorder, or psychotic bipolar disorder: a naturalistic 48-month follow-up study. J. Clin. Psychiatry (2003)., 64, 451-458.

[20] Lindenmayer, J. P, Czobor, P, Volavka, J, Lieberman, J. A, Citrome, L, Sheitman, B, Chakos, M, & Mcevoy, J. P. Olanzapine in refractory schizophrenia after failure of typical or atypical antipsychotic treatment: an open-label switch study. J. Clin. Psychiatry.(2002). , 63, 931-935.

[21] Van Os, J, Burns, T, Cavallaro, R, Leucht, S, Peuskens, J, Helldin, L, Bernardo, M, Arango, C, Fleischhacker, W, Lachaux, B, & Kane, J. M. Standardized remission criteria in schizophrenia. Acta Psychiatr Scand. (2006). Feb;, 113(2), 91-5.

[22] Andreasen, N. C. Carpenter WT Jr, Kane JM, Lasser RA, Marder SR, Weinberger DR. Remission in schizophrenia: proposed criteria and rationale for consensus. Am J Psychiatry. (2005). Mar;, 162(3), 441-9.

[23] Farde, L, Nordstrom, A. L, Wiessel, F. A, et al. Positron emission tomographic analysis of central D1 and D2 dopamine receptor occupancy in patients treated with classical neuroleptics and Clozapine: Relation to extrapyramidal side effects. Archives of General Psychiatry, (1992). , 49, 538-544.

[24] Kinon, B. J, Kane, J. M, & John, C. Treatment of neuroleptic resistant schizophrenia relapse. Psychopharmacology Bulletin (1993). , 29, 309-314.

[25] Van Putten, T, Marder, S. R, & Mintz, J. A controlled dose comparison of haloperidol in newly admitted schizophrenic patients. Archives of General Psychiatry (1990). , 47, 754-758.

[26] Dixon, L. B, Lehman, A. F, & Levine, J. Conventional antipsychotic medications for schizophrenia. Schizophr Bull. (1995). , 21, 567-577.

[27] Shalev, A, Hermesh, H, Rothberg, J, & Munitz, H. Poor neuroleptic response in acutely exacerbated schizophrenic patients. Acta Psychiatr Scand. (1993). , 87, 86-91.

[28] Lehman, A. F, Lieberman, J. A, Dixon, L. B, Mcglashan, T. H, Miller, A. L, & Perkins, D. O. Kreyenbuhl J; American Psychiatric Association; Steering Committee on Practice Guidelines. Practice guideline for the treatment of patients with schizophrenia, second edition. Am J Psychiatry. (2004). Feb;161(2 Suppl):, 1-56.

[29] http://wwwipap.org/algorithms.php

[30] Moore, T. A, Buchanan, R. W, Buckley, P. F, Chiles, J. A, Conley, R. R, Crismon, M. L, Essock, S. M, Finnerty, M, Marder, S. R, Miller, D. D, Mcevoy, J. P, Robinson, D. G, Schooler, N. R, Shon, S. P, Stroup, T. S, & Miller, A. L. The Texas Medication Algorithm Project antipsychotic algorithm for schizophrenia: 2006 update. J Clin Psychiatry. (2007). Nov;, 68(11), 1751-62.

[31] Suzuki, T, Remington, G, Mulsant, B. H, Rajji, T. K, Uchida, H, Graff-guerrero, A, & Mamo, D. C. Treatment resistant schizophrenia and response to antipsychotics: a review. Schizophr Res. (2011). Dec;133(1-3):54-62. Epub 2011 Oct 14.

[32] Brenner, H. D, Dencker, S. J, Goldstein, M. J, Hubbard, J. W, Keegan, D. L, Kruger, G, Kulhanek, F, Liberman, R. P, Malm, U, & Midha, K. K. Defining treatment refractoriness in schizophrenia. Schizophr Bull. (1990). , 16(4), 551-61.

[33] Kulhara, P. Management of schizophrenia: an update. Indian Journal of Psychiatry (1998). , 40, 120-134.

[34] Conley, R. R, & Buchanan, R. W. Evaluation of treatment-resistant schizophrenia. Schizophr Bull. (1997). , 23(4), 663-74.

[35] Lindenmayer, J. P. Treatment refractory schizophrenia. Psychiatr Q.(2000). , 71, 373-384.

[36] Marder, S. R. Management of treatment-resistant patients with schozphrenia. Journal of Clinical Psychiatry (1996). Suppl 11): 26-30.

[37] Smith, T. E, & Docherty, J. P. Standards of care and clinical algorithms for treating schizophrenia. Psychiatr Clin North Am (1998). , 21, 203-20.

[38] http://wwwmass.gov/eohhs/docs/dmh/publications/schizophrenia-guidelines-full.pdf

[39] Stephen, M, Stahl, M. D, & Ph, D. Essential Psychopharmacology: Neuroscientific Basis and Practical Applications, 2nd ed. Cambridge University Press, New York, N.Y., (2000). pages.

[40] Leung, A, & Chue, P. Sex differences in schizophrenia, a review of the literature. Acta Psychiatr Scand (2000)., 101, 3-38.

[41] Szymanski, S, Lieberman, J. A, Alvir, J. M, Mayerhoff, D, Loebel, A, Geisler, S, et al. Gender differences in onset of illness, treatment response, course and biologic indexes in first-episode schizophrenic patients. Am J Psychiatry (1995). , 152(5), 698-703.

[42] Buckman, M. T, & Peake, G. T. Estrogen potentiation of phenothiazine-induced prolactin secretion in man. J Clin Endocrinol Metabol (1973)., 37(6), 977-980.

[43] De Lisi LE: The significance of age of onset for schizophreniaSchizophr Bull (1992)., 18, 209-215.

[44] Meltzer, H. Y, Rabinowitz, J, Lee, M. A, Cola, P. A, Ranjan, R, Findling, R. L, & Thompson, P. A. Age at Onset and Gender of Schizophrenic Patients in Relation to Neuroleptic Resistance. Am J Psychiatry (1997). Apr;, 154(4), 475-482.

[45] Johnstone, E. C, Owens, D. G, Bydder, G. M, Colter, N, & Crow, T. J. Frith CD: The spectrum of structural brain changes in schizophrenia: age of onset as a predictor of cognitive and clinical impairments and their cerebral correlates. Psychol Med (1989)., 19, 91-103.

[46] [46]. Kolakowska, T, Williams, A. O, Ardern, M, Reveley, M. A, Jambor, K, & Gelder, M. G. Mandelbrote BM: Schizophrenia with good and poor outcome, I: early clinical features, response to neuroleptics and signs of organic dysfunction. Br J Psychiatry (1985)., 146, 229-239.

[47] Nimgaonkar, V. L, Wesseley, S, & Tune, L. E. Murray RM: Response to drugs in schizophrenia: the influence of family history, obstetric complications and ventricular enlargement. Psychol Med (1988)., 18, 583-592.

[48] Eaton, W. W, Mortensen, P. B, Herrman, H, Freeman, H, Bilker, W, & Burgess, P. Wooff K: Long-term course of hospitalization for schizophrenia, part I: risk for rehospitalization. Schizophr Bull (1992)., 18, 217-228.

[49] Loebel, A. D, & Lieberman, J. A. Alvir JMJ, Mayerhoff DI, Geisler SH, Szymanski SR: Duration of psychosis and outcome in first-episode schizophrenia. Am J Psychiatry (1992)., 149, 1183-1188.

[50] Castle, D. J, Abel, K, Takei, N, & Murray, R. M. Gender differences in schizophrenia: hormonal effect or subtypes? Schizophr Bull. (1995)., 21(1), 1-12.

[51] Mcdonell, M, & Mcclellan, J. (2007). Early-onset schizophrenia. In E. Mash & R. Barkley (Eds.), Assessment of childhood disorders (4th ed., New York: Guilford Press., 526-550.

[52] Brickman, A. M, Buchsbaum, M. S, Shihabuddin, L, Byne, W, Newmark, R. E, Brand, J, et al. Thalamus size and outcome in schizophrenia. Schizophrenia Research (2004). , 71, 473-484.

[53] Cuesta, M. J, Peralta, V, & De Leon, J. Schizophrenic syndromes associated with treatment response. Prog Neuro Psychopharmacol & Biol Psychiat. (1994). , 18, 87-99.

[54] Wiersma, D, Wanderling, J, Dragomirecka, E, et al. Social disability in schizophrenia: its development and prediction over 15 years in incidence cohorts in six European centres. Psychol Med. (2000). , 30, 1155-1167.

[55] Schulz, S. C, Conley, R. R, Kahn, E. M, et al. Nonresponders to neuroleptics: a distinct subtype. In: Tamminga CA, ed. Schizoprenia Scientific Progress. Oxford, UK: Oxford University Press; (1989). , 1989, 341-350.

[56] Rieckmann, N, Reichenberg, A, Bowie, C. R, Parrella, M, White, L, Friedman, J. I, et al. Depressed mood and its functional correlates in institutionalized schizophrenia patients. Schizophrenia Research (2005). , 77, 179-187.

[57] Kilzieh, N, Wood, A. E, Erdmann, J, Raskind, M, & Tapp, A. Depression in Kraepelinian schizophrenia. Comprehensive Psychiatry (2003). , 44, 1-6.

[58] Bralet, M. C, Loas, G, Yon, V, & Marechal, V. Clinical characteristics and risk factors for Kraepelinian subtypeof schizophrenia: Replication of previous findings and relation to summer birth. Psychiatry Research (2002). , 111, 147-154.

[59] Bralet, M. C, Ton, T, & Falissard, B. Schizophrenic patients with polydypsia and water intoxication more often have a form of schizophrenia first described by Kraepelin. Psychiatry Res. 2007 Aug 30;152(2-3):267-71. Epub (2007). Apr 18.

[60] Stern, R. G, Kahn, R. S, & Davidson, M. Predictors of response to neuroleptic treatment in schizophrenia. Psychiatric Clinics Of North America. June (1993). , 16(2), 313-338.

[61] Naeem, F, Kingdon, D, & Turkington, D. Predictors of response to cognitive behavior therapy in the treatment of schizophrenia: a comparison of brief and standard interventions. Cognit Ther Res. (2008). , 32, 651-656.

[62] Tarrier, N, Yusupoff, L, Kinney, C, et al. A randomised controlled trial of intensive cognitive behaviour therapy for chronic schizophrenia. Br Med J. (1998). , 317, 303-307.

[63] Fassino, S, Pierò, A, Mongelli, E, Caviglia, M. L, Delsedime, N, Busso, F, et al. Baseline personality functioning correlates with 6 month outcome in schizophrenia. European Psychiatry (2003). , 18, 93-100.

[64] Malaspina, D, Goetz, R. R, Yale, S, et al. Relation of familial schizophrenia to negative symptoms but not to the deficit syndrome. Am J Psychiatry (2000). , 157, 994-1003.

[65] Butzlaff, R. L, & Hooley, J. M. Expressed emotion and psychiatric relapse: A meta-analysis. Arch Gen Psychiatry. (1998)., 55, 547-52.

[66] Alvir, J. M, Woerner, M. G, Gunduz, H, Degreef, G, & Lieberman, J. A. Obstetric complications predict treatment response in first-episode schizophrenia. Psychol Med. (1999)., 29, 621-627.

[67] Carpenter, M. D, Mulligan, J. C, Bader, I. A, & Meinzer, A. E. Multiple admissions to an urban psychiatric center: a comparative study. Hosp Community Psychiatry. (1985)., 36, 1305-1308.

[68] Gupta, S, Hendricks, S, Kenkel, A. M, Bhatia, S. C, & Haffke, E. A. Relapse in schizophrenia: is there a relationship to substance abuse? Schizophr Res. (1996). , 20, 153-156.

[69] Sullivan, G, Wells, K. B, Morgenstern, H, & Leake, B. Identifying modifiable risk factors for rehospitalization: a case-control study of seriously mentally ill persons in Mississippi. Am J Psychiatry. (1995)., 152, 1749-1756.

[70] Bailey, L. G, Maxwell, S, & Brandabur, M. M. Substance abuse as a risk factor for tardive dyskinesia: a retrospective analysis of 1027 patients. Psychopharmacol Bull. (1997)., 33, 177-181.

[71] Green, M. F, Kern, R. S, & Heaton, R. K. Longitudinal studies of cognition and functional outcome in schizophrenia: implications for MATRICS.Schizophr Res. (2004). Dec 15;, 72(1), 41-51.

[72] Green, M. F. What are the functional consequences of neurocognitive deficits in schizophrenia? American Journal of Psychiatry (1996)., 153, 321-330.

[73] Green, M. F, Kern, R. S, Braff, D. L, & Mintz, J. Neurocognitive deficits and functional outcome in schizophrenia: are we measuring the bright stuffQ? Schizophrenia Bulletin (2000)., 26-119.

[74] Gold, J. M. Cognitive deficits as treatment targets in schizophrenia. Schizophrenia Research. (2004)., 72, 21-28.

[75] Friedman, L, Lys, C, & Schulz, S. C. The Relationship of Structural Brain Imaging Parameters to Antipsychotic Treatment Response: A Review. J Psychiatr Neurosci, (1992)., 17(2)

[76] Staal, W. G. Hulshoff Pol HE, Schnack HG, van Haren NEM, Seifert N, Kahn RS. Structural brain abnormalities in chronic schizophrenia at the extremes of the outcome spectrum. American Journal of Psychiatry (2001)., 158, 1140-1142.

[77] Mitelman, S. A, & Buchsbaum, M. S. Very poor outcome schizophrenia: clinical and neuroimaging aspects. Int Rev Psychiatry. (2007). Aug;, 19(4), 345-57.

[78] Davis, K. L, Buchsbaum, M. S, Shihabuddin, L, Spiegel-cohen, J, Metzger, M, Frecska, E, et al. Ventricular enlargement in poor-outcome schizophrenia. Biological Psychiatry (1998). , 43, 783-793.

[79] Ho, B. C, Andreasen, N. C, Nopoulos, P, Magnotta, V, Arndt, S, & Flaum, M. Progressive structural brain abnormalities and their significance on outcome: A longitudinal MRI study early in the course of schizophrenia. Archives of General Psychiatry (2003). , 60, 585-594.

[80] Lieberman, J. A, Chakos, M. H, Wu, H, Alvir, J. M, Hoffman, E, Robinson, D, et al. Longitudinal study of brain morphology in first episode schizophrenia. Biological Psychiatry (2001). , 49, 487-499.

[81] Buchsbaum, M. S, Shihabuddin, L, Brickman, A. M, Miozzo, R, Prikryl, R, Shaw, R, et al. Caudate and putamen volumes in good and poor outcome patients with schizophrenia. Schizophrenia Research (2003). , 64, 53-62.

[82] Cahn, W. Hulshoff Pol HE, Lems EB, van Haren NE, Schnack HG, van der Linden JA, Schothorst PF, van Engeland H, Kahn RS. Brain volume changes in first-episode schizophrenia: a 1-year follow-up study. Arch Gen Psychiatry. (2002). Nov;, 59(11), 1002-10.

[83] Bartlett, E J, Brodie, J. D, Simkowitz, P, Schlösser, R, & Dewey, S. L. Lindenmayer J-P et al. Effect of a Haloperidol Challenge on Regional Brain Metabolism in Neuroleptic-Responsive and Nonresponsive Schizophrenic Patients. Am J Psychiatry (1998). , 155, 337-343.

[84] Buchsbaum, M. S, Potkin, S. G, Marshall, J. F, Lottenberg, S, Teng, C. Y, Heh, C. W, Tafalla, R, Reynolds, C, Abel, L, & Plon, L. Bunney WE Jr: Effects of clozapine and thiothixene on glucose metabolic rate in schizophrenia. Neuropsychopharmacology (1992). , 6, 155-164.

[85] Buchsbaum, M. S, & Potkin, S. G. Siegel BV Jr, Lohr J, Katz M, Gott~schalk LA, Gulasekaram B, Marshall JF, Lottenberg S, Teng CY, Abel L, Plon L, Bunney WE Jr: Striatal metabolic rate and clinical response to neuroleptics in schizophrenia. Arch Gen Psychiatry (1992). , 49, 966-974.

[86] Evans LEJBeumont PJV, Luttrell B. Prolactin response as a guide to neuroleptic treatment of schizophrenia. Prog Reprod Biol (1980). , 6, 260-263.

[87] Van Putten, T, Marder, S. R, & Mintz, J. Serum prolactin as a correlate of clinical response to haloperidol. J Clin Psychopharmacol (1991). , 11(6), 357-361.

[88] Green, A. I, Alam, M. Y, & Boshes, R. A. Watern aux C, Pappalardo KM, Fitzgibbon ME et al. Haloperidol response and plasma catecholamines and their metabolites. Schizophr Res (1993). , 10(1), 33-37.

[89] Sharma, R. P, Javaid, J. I, Janicak, P. G, Davis, J. M, & Faull, K. Homovanillic acid in the cerebrospinal fluid: patterns of response after four weeks of neuroleptic treatment. Biol Psychiatry (1993). , 34(3), 128-134.

[90] Akiama, K, Tsuchid, A K, Kanzaki, A, Ujike, H, Hamamura, T, Kondo, K, et al. Plasma homovanillic acid levels and therapeutic outcome in schizophrenics: comparisons of neuroleptic-naive first-episode patients and patients with disease exacerbation due to neuroleptic discontinuance. Biol Psychiatry (1995). , 38(1), 639-648.

[91] Davila, R, Gonzalez, M. A, Zumarra, M, Andia, I, Guimon, J, Silva, R. R, et al. Plasma prolactin and plasma homovanillic acid: predictors of clinical response in schizophrenia. Biol Psychiatry (1995). , 38, 267-269.

[92] Chang, W. H, Hwu, H. G, Chen, T. Y, Lin, S. K, Lung, F. W, Chen, H, et al. Plasma homovanillic acid and treatment response in a large group of schizophrenic patients. Schizophr Res (1993). , 10(3), 259-265.

[93] Van Kammen, D. P, et al. d-Amphetamine-induced heterogeneous changes in psychotic behavior in schizophrenia. Am J Psychiatry (1982). , 139, 991-997.

[94] Meltzer, H. Y, et al. Growth hormone and prolactin response to apomorphine in schizophrenia and the major affective disorders. Arch Gen Psychiatry (1984). , 41, 512-519.

[95] Light, G. A, & Braff, D. L. Mismatch negativity deficits are associated with poor functioning in schizophrenia patients. Arch Gen Psychiatry. (2005). , 62, 127-136.

[96] Dawson, M. E, & Schell, A. M. What does electrodermal activity tell us about prognosis in the schizophrenia spectrum? Schizophr Res. (2002). Mar 1;54(1-2):87-93.

[97] Perkins, D. O, Gu, H, Boteva, K, & Lieberman, J. A. Relationship between duration of untreated psychosis and outcome in first-episode schizophrenia: a critical review and meta-analysis. Am J Psychiatry. (2005). Oct;, 162(10), 1785-804.

[98] Sheitman, B. B, & Lieberman, J. A. The natural history and pathophysiology of treatment resistant schizophrenia. J Psychiatr Res. (1998). May-Aug;32(3-4):143-50.

[99] Lieberman, J. A. Neuroprotection: a new strategy in the treatment of schizophrenia. Neurobiological basis of neurodegeneration and neuroprotection. CNS Spectr. (2007). Oct;12(10 Suppl 18):4-6.

[100] Lieberman, J. A, Alvir, M. A, Koreen, A, Geisler, S, & Chacos, M. Sheitman B at al. Psychobiologic correlates of treatment response in schizophrenia. Neuropsychopharmacology (1996). S-21S.

[101] Lieberman, J. A, Koreen, A. R, Chakos, M, et al. Factors influencing treatment response an doutcome of first-episode schizohrenia: implications for understanding the pathophysiology of schizophrenia. J Clin Psychiatry (1996). suppl 9): 5-9.

[102] Robinson, D. G, & Woerner, M. G. Alvir JMJ, Geisler S, Koreen A, Sheitman B et al. P redictors of treatment response from a first episode of schizophrenia or schizoaffective disorder. Am J Psychiatry (1999). , 156, 544-549.

[103] Andreasen, N. C. Carpenter WT Jr, Kane JM, Lasser RA, Marder SR, Weinberger DR. Remission in schizophrenia: proposed criteria and rationale for consensus. Am J Psychiatry. (2005). Mar;, 162(3), 441-9.

[104] Van Os, J, Burns, T, Cavallaro, R, Leucht, S, Peuskens, J, Helldin, L, Bernardo, M, Arango, C, Fleischhacker, W, Lachaux, B, & Kane, J. M. Standardized remission criteria in schizophrenia. Acta Psychiatr Scand. (2006). Feb;, 113(2), 91-5.

[105] Keefe RSEFrescka E, Apter SH, Davidson M, Macaluso JM, Hirschowitz J, et al. Clinical characteristics of Kraepelinian schizophrenia: Replication and extension of previous findings. American Journal of Psychiatry (1996). , 153, 806-811.

[106] Roy, M. A, Merette, C, & Maziade, M. Subtyping schizophrenia according to outcome or severity: A search for homogeneous subgroups. Schizophrenia Bulletin (2001). , 27, 115-138.

[107] Melle, I, Larsen, T. K, Haahr, U, Friis, S, Johannessen, J. O, Opjordsmoen, S, et al. Reducing the duration of untreated first episode psychosis. Effect on clinical presentation. Arch Gen Psychiatry. (2004). , 61, 143-150.

[108] Mcgorry, P. D, Yung, A. R, Phillips, L. J, Yuen, H. P, Francey, S, Cosgrave, E. M, et al. Randomized controlled trial of interventions designed to reduce the risk of progression to first episode psychosis in a clinical sample with suthreshold symptoms. Arch Gen Psychiatry. (2002). , 59, 921-928.

[109] Cannon, T. D, & Huttunen, M. O. DahlstrÖm M, Larmo I, Räsänen P,Juriloo A. Antipsychotic drug treatment in the prodromal phase of schizophrenia. Am J Psychiatry (2002). , 159, 1230-1232.

[110] Sablier, J, Stip, E, & Franck, N. Cognitive remediation and cognitive assistive technologies in schizophrenia. Encephale. (2009). Apr;, 35(2), 160-7.

[111] Cho, R. Y, Ford, J. M, Krystal, J. H, Laruelle, M, Cuthbert, B, & Carter, C. S. Functional neuroimaging and electrophysiology biomarkers for clinical trials for cognition in schizophrenia. Schizophr Bull (2005). , 31(4), 865-869.

[112] Lenroot, R, Bustillo, J. R, Lauriello, J, & Keith, S. J. Integrated treatment of schizophrenia. Psychiatr Serv. (2003). Nov;, 54(11), 1499-507.

[113] Goff, D. C. Coyle JT: The emerging role of glutamate in the pathophysiology and treatment of schizophrenia. American Journal of Psychiatry (2001). , 158, 1367-1377.

[114] Milev, P, Ho, B-C, & Andreasen, N. Predictive values of neurocognition and negative symptomes on functional outcome in schizophrenia: A longitudinal first-episode study with 7 year follow-up. Am J Psychiatry (2005). , 162, 495-506.

Anxiolytics Use in the Families with (Non)dependent Member: Relation to Dependence Indicators, Self and Family Perceptions Including Social Neuroscience Perspective

Maja Rus-Makovec, Karin Sernec and Velko S. Rus

Additional information is available at the end of the chapter

1. Introduction

Social neuroscience seeks to explain social behavior in terms of information processing mechanisms that motivate and guide social behavior and in terms of neurobiological mechanisms (genetic, hormonal, biochemical, physiological) that underline social behavior [1]. Social neuroscience could be defined quite broadly as exploration of interdependence between processes, traditionally belonging to social psychology and particular neurological factors [2]. Because of the complexity of human social interaction (exchange, communication), social neuroscience needs to combine and integrate multi–level analysis across different domains [1, 2]. It's worth repeating Cacioppo & Berntson [3] connecting multi – level approach: "The doctrine of multilevel analysis specifies that microanalyses of a psychological phenomenon can be particularly effective when pursued in addition to or in conjunction with molar analyses." Relation "brain – culture" could be defined also as a typical thematic part of social anthropo – psychology, expression, etymologically and recognizably showing to fields of thematically origin. Particular aspects of social neuroscience are connected also with some new areas of contemporary social psychology, with the questions of (bio) - psycho - social evolution, the questions of mate preferences included [4]; it's also connected with social psychosomatics, particularly with social cognition and with a view of the person's information – processing capability [5]. Three routes of social cognition are distinguished: capacity to mentalize, to mimic and understand others' motor actions and our capacity to empathize [6]. The social environment is multifaceted and compromises a dynamic set of environmental and behavioral interactions that influence the connections among individuals such as parent and child, husband and wives, groups etc. These connections from the social network can have an impact on brain development and function and can be both a risk and a protective factor against drug abuse [7]. Social neuroscience perspective seems to be one of the most suitable disciplines for understanding the field of psychotropic substance use and abuse. That is why we tried to introduce the social neuroscientific perspective in the field of anxiolytic (ab)use by parents in families with and without dependent family member in our research.

1.1. Brains and social psychology: Social neuroscience, social psychology and interdisciplinary perspectives

According to Illeris [8], inseparability of emotional and cognitive functions regarding the brain basis of their location seems to be one of the prevailing contemporary beliefs of contemporary neuroscience. Social psychological contributions to the neurosciences served to the intensive development of the psychoneuroimunological field and immune responses are strongly influenced by the central nervous system (CNS) [9].

Social behavior could be connected with the brain functions and even structure also indirectly. Factually, we can hypothesize some connection, deriving from some evident and experimentally proved information. One of them is, for example, association between learning - cognitive style and hemisphericity. Torrance associated learning styles (left - more analytical, right - more synthetic and integrative hemispheric), characteristic also for social learning with dominant specialized functions of brain hemispheres [10]. Sphere only prevails, while the brain functions as a whole. More generally, we can conclude, that social neurosciences phenomena results in different outputs of activity, work, performance (effectiveness, efficacy), group structure and processes, climate, culture, communication and evaluation as interactive function of CNS activity. Information processing and decision making seem to be an important part of (social) neuroscience. According to Klavora [11], factors influencing information processing are the quality of sensory input information, the quality and effectiveness of sensory receptors, the speed of processing the stimulus information. Psychophysiological background and socio – psycho – neuro – logical relevancy of such a multilevel approach has been systematically developed by Cacioppo and collaborators [3, 8, 12]. The area of psychophysiology is connected with different efforts of neurophysiologists, experimental psychologists, psychiatrists and different technical professions [12]. Understanding behavioral flexibility, especially in the form of cultural variation, demands the understanding of the whole psychological "architecture", which guides social interaction [13].

1.2. Factual beginnings of social neuroscience? Eysenck, Moscovici, Personnaz

Pieces of mosaic of social neuroscience had existed already before. H. J. Eysenck's model, explanation of extra – introversion is such a possible example [14]. Habitually heightened level of central activation is supposed to be connected with introvert, and lowered level with extravert. That's why the extravert people, according to Eysenck, search new exogenous information and attempt to maintain ample social network of social relations and communications. Hypothetical construct of the balance between excitation and inhibition is reticular formation (RF). Psychotropic depressants (alcohol, benzodiazepines) and stimulants (caffeine, amphetamine) have direct influence on different parts of RF. According to Eysenck, depressants have extravert and stimulants have introvert effect, both being also typical patterns of social behavior.

Other piece of mosaic of the important de facto neuro scientific research, had been the research connecting active and consistent minorities and their influence on majority judgments and (sensory) perception, using the phenomenon of negative after effect [15] as the final dependent variable [16, 17]. Results of these experiments showed, although the dependent variable was the visual illusion, but illusion, based on central intervention, that also centrally determined phenomena could be influenced by minority (active and consistent) influence and that conversion could be sometimes additionally explained with complementary neuro – physiological consequences.

1.3. Listing of some social psychological thematic, differently connected with factual parts of social neuroscience

If we neglect so brutal and evident causes like head damage, which is also an exclusive element of behaviorist learning definition, elements of factual »social neuroscience« could be found also in many other cases, lets mention only research and applied phenomena of ideomotoric/visualization; than many aspects of NLP (neuro–linguistic programming); socio– and psycho–pathology of dependence behavior; sleeping and dreams, including different interpretations (metaphorical symbolism of dreams in classical Freudian psychoanalysis, archetype conception in Jung's concept of collective subconsciousness); associacionist antecedents of contemporary social cognition [18-20]; a great deal of EEG classical research and applied practice; cognitive theories of emotion, respective any theory of emotion, including the function of limbic system; brain and body reactions; alpha learning conditions; biofeedback; conditioning (Pavlov, Sokolov, Teplov) and (neo)behaviorist approaches, also on the domain of social behavior; placebo–effects, particularly researches in the last years, proving activation of relevant brain areas as consequence of persuasive/suggestive placebo effect; bio–psycho–social aspects of aggression and aggressiveness; different psychoanalytic conceptions connected with unconscious brain processes (Freud, Jung, Adler, Lacan, Erikson, Klein); screening of organic brain damage related to alcohol abuse as important for treatment planning [21]. Mentioned damage is highly connected also with degree and duration of alcohol dependence. That's why we decided to take into account the very slight approximation of this probability in the sense of AUDIT (Alcohol Use Disorder Identifying Test) [22] estimation of intensity of alcohol dependence abuse. This estimation was treated as co–variate in the design, where the hypothesis about the differences in self perceptions regarding the anxiolytics usage status was taken into account.

From this point of view, the whole classical behaviorism could be interpreted as introduction into the social neuroscience, while social behavior is interpreted as more or less direct function of centrally positioned associations Stimulus – Response, which are the basic point of any behavioral pattern.

1.4. Brain, behavior and social interaction in mood and dependence disorders

Ernst Fehr and collaborators [23] report about neurologic basis of social interactions, even on economic field (neuroeconomy). Such an approach could be helpful in explaining some irrational moments in otherwise rational cost – benefit dilemma resolution. According to Fehr, it even seems, that hormone oxytocin influences the experience of trust. Depression and anxiety is also a standard covariate of psychotropic medication treatments. That's why it's understandable, that psychopharmaceutical medications could have, in any group, an impact on different areas, levels and aspects of social interactions (communication, social exchange). Regarding alcohol dependence an understanding of action of alcohol on central gamma – amino butyric acid (GABA) receptors may significantly contribute to the incentive side of explanation of this disorder [3].

Although alterations in brain function can influence the symptoms which seem to be functional personality change, the inverse process is also possible. Depression, as an example of non–organic personality change, can result in symptoms, which are similar to alterations in brain functions - pseudo dementia, for example - which can disappear, when patients are treated with antidepressant medication. The relation between the psychopharmaceutical medications (non)use and different social representations of self and social environments, being an essential part of any social interaction (communication, social exchange and influence), is not at all one – way process. Anyway, in actual research, such a complexity of relations was not elaborated, while also the existent empirical methodology in behavioral sciences does not yet dispose with models, permitting analysis of two way processes, resulting in different effects of mutual partially simultaneous, partially sequential influences. However, it is well known, that epigenetic effects during development lead to a cascade of neurobiological changes, including enhanced emotionality [24].

Psychopharmaceutical medications affect brain neurotransmission processes for therapeutic purposes; however, psychotropic substances can be abused and alter behavior into non-functional/non-adaptive one. Altered brain neurobiology is the basis of dependence syndrome, with profound alteration on cognition, emotion and behavior of dependent person, which influence one's social interaction profoundly [25]. Mood and anxiety disorders are the most frequent cooccurent mental disorders accompanying dependence syndrome and most frequent symptoms in important others of dependent patients [26]. Mood and anxiety disorders and dependence syndrome are most frequently treated by antidepressants and anxiolytics as psychopharmaceutical medications [27].

Progression on to drug dependence after the exposure appears to be genetically influenced; however, dependence is both a biological disorder and a cultural category [28]. The addictive process is introduced as an interaction of impairments in three functional systems: motivation-reward, affect regulation, and behavioral inhibition. From a cultural perspective, drug dependence is seen as being related to peer pressure and conformity as well as to economic and cultural factors [29].

The net effects of inhibiting the diffuse GABA are anxiety reduction, behavioral disinhibition, sedation and euphoria, what is all connected also with interpersonal communication, family perception, perceived depression and self – concept. That's why we can expect, that chosen psychopharmaceutical medications can at least partially influence (facilitate or inhibit) particular social behavioral patterns, particularly connecting (declared) depression, interpersonal relations in primary social environment and social implications of some other dependence behavior. These implications, manifested in different complex social situations could be quite subtle, sometimes hidden in "social mimicry", mostly connected with alcohol and other psychoactive substances abuse. One of the very opportune measures of such implications, according to our opinion, could be (sub) scores of SASSI (Substance Abuse Subtle Screening Inventory) instrument, which is declared to be the instrument which "breaks through denial" [30].

It seems that relations between concrete forms and contents of social interaction (complex patterns of cooperation, competition, conformism, cohesiveness, role learning, group decision, leadership, conflicts, negotiations, mediations) and CNS (re) actions are yet to be researched. That's why the choice of family social climate has two advantages: we treat it as a kind of experiential common denominator of different social interaction effects, while climate is an integrating experience, deriving from diversified processes of social interaction. Inducing climate as dependent variable, we focus on one of most relevant and integrating level of social experience. Simultaneously, (perceived) climate is one of the most essential parts of micro culture. Analyzing climate, we simultaneously analyze an important part of family culture. On the other side, evaluation of climate is inseparably connected with different self concepts (esteem, confidence, consciousness, efficacy belief) and self – evaluation. In actual text "functional" is supposed to be such a category of self – evaluation, when personal bipolar attributes express the continuum of everyday adaptive/functional behavior. We suppose that psychopharmaceutical medications (anxiolytics) contribute to the change of retrograde functional self – evaluations, while medicaments are supposed to be a reason of improvement of mood level.

That's why in actual article, we'd like to analyze possible relations between psychopharmaceutical medications (anxiolytics) usage (in the last year) status and some other relevant perceptions: evaluation of own family, self – esteem, self – perceived depression and substance abuse indicators. We can express the general level of our research problem with the question: Which are the relations between A. last year psychopharmaceutical medications use status and B. particular perceptions, connecting family, self and substance abuse dependence? The question about (anxiolytics) usage (in the last year) has been formulated as follows: "Did you use prescribed psychopharmaceutical medications such as anxiolytics because of your emotional problems in last year?"

We formulated three expectations:

H.1: we hypothesized, that self–esteem, evaluation of own family and level of depression as predictors significantly differentiate, regardless co–variate inclusion, between users and non–users of anxiolytic pills in the last year, so in the case of mothers, as in the case of fathers.

H.2: we expect, that the change of self–evaluation in last few years significantly differ between users and non–users, so in the case of fathers, as in the case of mothers.

H.3: we also hypothesized, that the groups of users and non–users significantly differ in correspondent SASSI subscores, so in the case of mother, as in the case of fathers.

In families, having a dependent member, dependence is also the main area of different perceptions, social representations and social interactions. That's why, in our research, the estimated dependence of each family member was included, where possible, as covariate. In our case, the alcohol dependence aspect was identified and taken into account as co–variate in sense of AUDIT estimated seriousness of alcohol dependence.

2. Method

2.1. Participants

There were three types of families, each type attempting to "mirror" approximate proportion of such a type in Slovene society: a. families with no referred dependent member, neither parents, nor adolescent (about 56% of the whole sample); b. families with drug dependent children (about 16% of the whole sample) and c. families with alcohol dependent father (about 28% of the whole sample). If there were more than one adolescent child in the same family, only the eldest one was included. The average age of adolescents was M = 17.22 years, with SD = 1.27 years, with 45 percents of female and 55 percents of male respondents. From n = 183 valid cases (families) and excluding all missing, N = 159 "valid" mothers (mean age M = 42.85, SD = 4.68) and n = 147 fathers (with mean age M = 45.47, SD = 4.68) appeared in calculations.

It's worth underlining, that neither by mothers, nor by fathers, significant differences were found in age (users – no: n = 157, M = 42.70, SD = 4.66; users – yes: n = 22, M = 44.00, SD = 4.64; t(177) = - 1.21, p = 0.23 for mothers and users – no: n = 141, M = 45.56, SD = 5.06, users – yes: n = 16, M = 44.94, SD = 4.65; t(155) = 0.47, p = 0.64 for fathers) and education (t(179) = 1.54, p = 0.12 for mothers and t(155) = 0.87, p = 0.38 for fathers) and that no significant covariate effect of age had appeared neither by mothers (Pillai F = 0.57, p = 0.63), nor by fathers (Pillai F = 0.97, p = 0.41). On the other side, significant covariate effect of education was found for mothers (Pillai F = 6.32, p = 0.00, $\eta^2 = 0.10$), but not changing the significancy level of the independent variable (Pillai F = 2.62, p = 0.05, $\eta^2 = 0.046$); contrary to mothers, no such an effect was found for fathers (Pillai F = 1.35, p = 0.26, $\eta^2 = 0.03$).

2.2. Instruments

Relatively comprehensive questionnaire with 567 variables was applied, measuring different status and personal, subjective and objective characteristics (mothers and fathers 225 variables each, adolescents 117 variables). The whole questionnaire was applied so in individual, as in small group conditions. It seems that the conditions of data collecting influenced the number of missing, more of them being in small group conditions. The main thematic area of the questionnaire, which contains different information about demographic, socio – economic and socio – cultural status, anamnesis information about health status in different periods of life cycle, life style information, about suicidal ideation, exposure to different kinds of violence, different dependence behaviors (alcohol, nicotine, drugs …), info about intra – familiar processes, climate and, partially, culture, retrograde and actual self – evaluation, level of self-esteem and depression, evaluation of family climate, experiences with psychopharmacological treatment etc.. Validity was identified not only with coefficient of internal consistency (Table 1), which assures only the construct validity: from previous researches [31] validity of majority of summative scales was verified also with chosen outer criterion, consecrating almost equally needed time to construction as to validation of the instrument.

In actual report the following scales and questions from the total questionnaire were included into research: Zung's self – rating depression scale - 20 items [32], Rosenberg's self – esteem scale - 10 items [33]; original semantic differential for estimation of the climate in the proper family (15 bipolar continuums, selected according the demands of summative scale construction). Semantic differential - evaluation of the social climate in own family contained the following bipolar attributes on 7 – point bipolar continuums: good/bad, relaxed/ not-relaxed, aggressive/non-aggressive, pleasant/unpleasant, tolerant/intolerant, unorganized/organized, non-conflicting/conflicting, not-developing/developing, enjoying/not- enjoying, with insight/without-insight, with future/without future, charged/uncharged, not understanding/ understanding, without support/with support, with love/without love.

Actual and retrograde (»How do you evaluate yourself in time point about five years ago?«) functional self – evaluation bipolar attributes of self – evaluation scale: nervous/ calm, optimistic/pessimistic, with problems/without problems, lonely/with friends, independent/ dependent, with insight/without insight, mainly reposed/mainly tired, satisfied with/dissatisfied with, with bad habits/with good habits, successful in learning/unsuccessful in learning, non-creative/creative, self-conscious/self-unconscious, no-communicative/ communicative.

According the authors belief about data validity, the missing values were not substituted with missing values.

Also the missing values appeared which influence different number of valid cases in certain final reports and so diminish a little bit even the generalization on the basis of initial sample.

For the occasion of this research, the Substance Abuse Subtle Screening Inventory SASSI [9] was for the first time applied in Slovenia. Instrument has two forms, for adolescents and for the parents. SASSI identify two probability categories of dependence: high and low substance dependence probability. SASSI was adapted to Slovene version according to all demands of forward – backward translation.

AUDIT (Alcohol Use Disorder Identifying Test) [21] approach to identify the (alcohol) dependence degree of fathers was also applied. According to value = 8, two categories were obtained, one of the expressing low probability for alcohol connected problems, another expressing high probability for alcohol use which is hazardous or harmful to the health. So as

SASSI, also the AUDIT validity could be tested regarding the classification by the side of experts (therapists). The rates of agreement between the experts and decision rules are described also as data validation [9]. In our research, both kinds of estimation almost perfectly coincided with classificational distinction from the side of experts –therapists (SASSI: χ^2 (2, n = 161) = 1.27, p = ns for nondependent mothers, but with 50 % of cells with expected counts less than 5; χ^2 (2, n = 167) = 91, p = 0.00 for (non)dependent children, with 16.7% of cells with expected counts < 5, and χ^2 (2, n = 139) = 84.90, p = 0.00, with 0% of expected counts < 5, for (non)dependent fathers).

Evaluations from the side of father	**No of items**	Alpha Group 1	Alpha Group 2	Alpha Group 3
Actual self evaluation	14	0.84	0.67	0.79
Retrograde self evaluation	14	0.80	0.84	0.85
Perceived family climate	15	0.89	0.92	0.83
Self – esteem	10	0.87	0.93	0.82
Perceived own depression	20	0.90	0.95	0.90
Evaluations from the side of mother				
Actual self evaluation	14	0.82	0.82	0.71
Retrograde self evaluation	14	0.79	0.75	0.86
Perceived family climate	15	0.93	0.91	0.87
Self – esteem	10	0.83	0.82	0.80
Perceived own depression	20	0.88	0.87	0.76

Note: group 1 = family without dependent member (n = 104); 2 = family with dependent adolescent child (n = 29); 3 = family with alcohol dependent father (n = 52)

Table 1. Internal Consistency – Cronbach's Alpha Coefficients – For Summative Scales, Responded from the Side of Fathers and Mothers for Each of Three Groups/Family Types

The following sub scores are obtained with SASSI 3: FVA = face valid alcohol; FVOD = face valid other drugs; SYM = symptoms; OAT = obvious attributes; SAT = subtle attributes; DEF = defensiveness; SAM = supplemental addiction measure; FAM = family vs. controls; COR = correctional. Maja Rus Makovec had obtained also a permission for back – translation/adaptation and research use of SASSI from the author.

Kolmogorov – Smirnov test showed, that almost all summative scores (actual and retrograde self perception; evaluation of own family climate; self – esteem) did not differ significantly from normal distribution (p>.05), while for SASSI subscores the alternative hypotheses were accepted. Internal consistency of almost all (except one version of self – evaluation) summative scores was satisfactory (all Cronbach alphas mostly > 0.85).

Research was approved from the side of Ethical commission of Health Ministry of Slovenia.

3. Results

Arithmetic Means and Standard Deviations of mothers' dependent variables are shown in Table 2.

	anxiolytics	M	SD	n
family climate	no	75.46	19.93	152
	yes	63.52	22.07	21
self-esteem	no	40.06	6.59	152
	yes	35.95	7.39	21
depression	no	37.56	8.21	152
	yes	43.05	10.63	21

Note: family climate = evaluation of climate in own family – mothers (higher score means more positive evaluation); self-esteem = Rosenberg's self – evaluation score – mothers (higher score means higher self – esteem); Zung's depression score – mothers; covariate = SASSI estimation of dependence seriousness by mothers.

Table 2. Arithmetic Means and Standard Deviations for Dependent Variables Regarding Usage vs. Non-Usage of Anxiolytics in the Last Year - Mothers

One factor MANOVA, exploring differences in self – esteem, perceived depression and family climate by parents as a function of their anxiolytic usage status (usage: yes vs. no) was applied for successive inclusion of one (mothers), two (mothers and fathers) and three (mothers, fathers, children) covariates (AUDIT for parents and therapists' estimation (TE) of dependence intensity for adolescents). Multivariate effect was found as significant (Pillai's, Wilks, Hotelling, all $p = 0.14$ and all Levene tests of equality of error variances with $df1 = 1$ and $df = 171$ were highly un–significant, $p >>.05$ ($p = ns$)); Box M test was significant ($F = 3.79$, $p = 0.001$), what means, that demand of equality of covariances (multivariate analogy with homogeneity of variances in univariate approaches) was not satisfied. Because F test is the robust one, we anyway continued with data analyses. Mothers' AUDIT estimation covariate effect was found as non – significant ($F = 0.57$, $p = 0.63$ ($p = ns$)).

Univariate access showed significant differences ($p < 0.05$) for each of three dependent variables, expressing significantly more positive evaluation of own family climate ($F (1,172) = 5.01$, $p = 0.026$), higher self – esteem ($F (1,172)$, $p = 0.01$) and lower degree of perceived depression ($F (1,172 = 7.35$, $p = 0.007$) for mothers non – users of anxiolytic pills, than for correspondent users.

Discriminate analysis was computed also in order to estimate the relative contribution of studied variables to the discrimination of mothers, users and non – users of psychotropic pills. Taking into account no other covariates, the first and the only one extracted discriminate functions was highly significant (Wilks Lambda = 0. 94, $\chi^2 (3) = 10.98$, $p = 0.01$. The null hypothesis about the homogeneity of covariance's was not accepted (Box's M = 27.21, $F = 4.28$, $p = 0.00$).

Structure matrix showed relatively rare structure of relative predictive importance of independents/predictors. All coefficients of correlations between constructed (summative scores) manifest variables and discriminate functions were relatively very high and almost equal (climate (0.81), self – esteem (0.81), perceived depression (0.82)).

According to the values of group centroids for significant ($p < 0.05$) discriminate function, it could be suggested, that the discriminate function differentiates "strongly" between female (non) users of anxiolytics.

MANOVA was found as significant also when additional AUDIT and TE covariates (for fathers and children) were successively included into analysis (Pillai, Wilks, Hotelling, Roy, all $p = 0.00$). Anyway, risk level of the effect of independent variable ((non)anxiolytic usage status) changed: having mothers' ($F = 0.50$, $p = 0.68$, $\eta^2 = 0.009$) and fathers' ($F = 2.91$, $p =.036$, $\eta^2 = 0.05$) AUDIT as covariates, it was $F = 3.43$, $p = 0.02$, $\eta^2 = 0.06$, and adding children's TE ($F = 6.33$, $p = 0.00$, $\eta^2 = 0.106$), it was $F = 2.25$, $p = 0.08$, $\eta^2 = 0.04$.

One factor MANOVA, exploring differences in self – esteem, perceived depression and family climate by parents as a function of their anxiolytic usage status (usage: yes vs. no) was applied for successive inclusion of one (mothers), two (mothers and fathers) and three (mothers, fathers, children) covariates (AUDIT for parents and therapists' estimation (TE) of dependence intensity for adolescents). Multivariate effect was found as non - significant (Roy's, Pillai's, Wilks, $p >.05$). Box's M test of equality of covariance matrices was highly non - significant ($F = 0.93$, $p = 0.47$ ($p = ns$)), what confirmed the equality of co – variances. Fathers' AUDIT estimation covariate effect was found as non – significant ($F = 0.05$, $p = 0.98$ ($p = ns$)).

Univariate access, of course, only confirmed non - significant differences ($p >> 0.05$) for each of three dependent variables, for perceived climate ($F(1, 151) = 0.76$, $p = 0.38$), level of self – esteem ($F(1, 151) = 0.39$, $p = 0.53$ ($p = ns$)) and level of depression ($F (1,151 = 0.68$, $p = 0.41$) for fathers non – users of psychotropic pills, than for correspondent users (Table 3).

	anxiolytics	M	SD	n
family climate	no	74.69	19.07	136
	yes	75.81	19.36	16
self-esteem	no	39.18	6.87	136
	yes	39.50	7.80	16
depression	no	36.47	7.08	136
	yes	38.62	7.91	16

Note: family climate = evaluation of climate in own family – mothers (higher score means more positive evaluation); self-esteem = Rosenberg's self – evaluation score – mothers (higher score means higher self – esteem); Zung's depression score – mothers; covariate = SASSI estimation of dependence seriousness by fathers.

Table 3. Arithmetic Means and Standard Deviations for Dependent Variables Regarding Usage vs. Non- usage of Anxiolytics in the Last Year - Fathers

Discriminate analysis was also computed in order to estimate the relative contribution of studied variables to the discrimination of fathers, users and non – users of anxiolytic pills. The first and the only one extracted discriminate functions was non – significant with (Wilks Lambda = 0.97, Chi sq. (3) = 3.78, p = 0.29). The null hypothesis about the homogeneity of covariance's was otherwise accepted (Box's M = 6.02, F approx = 0.93, p =.47), but the further analysis was omitted.

MANOVA was found as non - significant also when additional AUDIT and TE covariates (for fathers and children) were successively included into analysis (Pillai, Wilks, Hotelling, Roy, all p > 0.00 (p = ns)). Risk level of the effect of independent variable (anxiolytic usage status) did not change in sense of significancy (p > 0.05). Having mothers' (F = 0.17, p =.91) and fathers' (F = 15.79, p = 0.00, $\eta^2 = 0.24$) AUDIT as covariates, it was F = 1.33, p =.27, $\eta^2 = 0.03$, and adding children's TE (F = 4.07, p =.01, $\eta^2 = 0.08$), it was F = 1.81, p =.15, $\eta^2 = 0.04$).

No significant differences were found between mothers users vs. non – users of in fathers' perceived difference between actual and retrograde self – evaluation, but significant difference (p = 0.05) was found in perceived difference between actual and retrograde self – evaluation for mothers. Similar, but non – significant trend was found also for difference between relative fathers' differences regarding mothers' anxiolytics usage, and yet interestingly: in both cases the difference is negative, what means that retrograde summative functional self – evaluation was more positive than the actual one after about one year long period of its usage (Table 4).

	anxiolytics mothers	**M**	**SD**	**n**	**t- test**	**P**
E1-E2 mothers	no	0.20	11.41	157		
	yes	- 5.19	14.75	21	1.96	0.05
E1-E2 fathers	no	- 0.69	9.30	128		
	yes	- 4.78	11.42	14	1.53	0.13

Note: Levene F for mothers = 3.04, p = 0.08, for fathers F = 0.19, p = 0.66

E1 = actual self – evaluation (higher score means more positive self – evaluation); E2 = retrograde ("five years ago") self – evaluation

Table 4. Arithmetic Means and Standard Deviations for Differences Between "Actual" and "Retrograde" Self – evaluation for Mothers and for Fathers Regarding the Anxiolytics(Non) Usage by Mothers

No significant differences were found between fathers users vs. non – users of anxiolytics fathers' perceived difference between actual and retrograde self – evaluation and also not in perceived difference between actual and retrograde self – evaluation for mothers (Table 5).

	anxiolytics fathers	M	SD	n	t- test	P
E1-E2 mothers	no	0.36	10.80	126		
	yes	0.07	8.95	15	0.10	0.92
E1-E2 fathers	no	- 0.81	8.82	135		
	yes	- 0.19	17.89	16	- 0.14	0.89

Note: Levene F for mothers = 0.14, p = 0.71 (p = ns), for fathers Levene F = 11.74, p = 0.01.

E1 = actual self – evaluation (higher score means more positive self – evaluation); E2 = retrograde ("five years ago") self – evaluation

Table 5. Arithmetic Means and Standard Deviations for Differences Between "Actual" and "Retrograde" Self – evaluation for Mothers and for Fathers Regarding the Anxiolytics(Non) Usage by Fathers

Significant differences ($p<0.05$) by fathers were found for other drugs' use FVODf, for category »symptoms« SYMf, and for obvious attributes OATf. Differences were not found for other subscores of SASSI (Table 6).

SASSI	anxiolytics usage	n	Mean Rank	Z	p
FVAf	no	141	77.94		
	yes	16	88.34	- 0.87	0.38
FVODf	no	141	77.20		
	yes	16	94.88	- 2.66	0.01
SYMf	no	141	76.30		
	yes	16	102.78	- 2.29	0.02
OATf	no	141	76.47		
	yes	16	101.28	- 2.09	0.04
SATf	no	141	77.71		
	yes	16	90.41	- 1.09	0.28
DEFf	no	141	80.93		
	yes	16	62.00	- 1.59	0.11
SAMf	no	141	77.29		
	yes	16	94.09	- 1.41	0.16
FAMf	no	141	79.14		
	yes	16	77.75	- 0.12	0.91

SASSI	anxiolytics usage	n	Mean Rank	Z	p
CORf	no	141	77.70		
	yes	16	90.44	- 1.07	0.28
RAPf	no	141	80.06		
	yes	16	69.69	- 0.93	0.35

Note: FVA = face valid alcohol; FVOD = face valid other drugs; SYM = symptoms; OAT = obvious attributes; SAT = subtle attributes; DEF = defensiveness; SAM = supplemental addiction measure; FAM = family vs. controls; COR = correctional; f = fathers.

Table 6. Results of Mann Whitney Nonparametric Test for SASSI Subscores for Fathers

Significant differences (p<0.05) by mothers were found for category »symptoms« SYMm, obvious attributes OATm, correctional CORm and supplemental addiction measure SAMm. Differences were not found for other subscores of SASSI (Table 7).

SASSI	anxiolytics usage	n	Mean Rank	Z	p
	no				
FVAm	yes	159	90.01		
	no	22	98.16	- 0.70	0.48
FVODm	yes	159	90.31		
	no	22	95.95	- 0.96	0.34
SYMm	yes	159	88.58		
	no	22	108.45	- 1.96	0.05
OATm	yes	159	87.43		
	no	22	116.82	- 2.49	0.01
SATm	yes	159	90.40		
	no	22	95.36	- 0.43	0.67
DEFm	yes	159	92.80		
	no	22	78.02	- 1.25	0.21
SAMm	yes	159	87.52		
	no	22	116.16	- 2.43	0.01
FAMm	yes	159	92.17		
	no	22	82.55	- 0.82	0.41
CORm	yes	159	88.20		
	no	22	111.25	- 1.96	0.05

SASSI	anxiolytics usage	n	Mean Rank	Z	p
RAPm	yes	159	89.86		
		22	99.25	- 0.89	0.37

Note: FVA = face valid alcohol; FVOD = face valid other drugs; SYM = symptoms; OAT = obvious attributes; SAT = subtle attributes; DEF = defensiveness; SAM = supplemental addiction measure; FAM = family vs. controls; COR = correctional; m = mothers.

Table 7. Results of Mann Whitney Nonparametric Test for SASSI Sub scores for Mothers

4. Discussion

An example of the principle of multiple determinism of the social neuroscience can be found in the extensive literature on drug abuse. Endogenous brain opioid receptor systems represent the neurophysiologic basis for cognitive, psychological and affective actions. The proximate and powerful determinants of drug abuse include the social factors of family dynamics, economics and different other social environments [3]. It's what we had tried to begin to analyze in our article.

Interactions between social processes and the underlying neural substrates facilitate the understanding of the holistic consequences of the drug administration. Molar features of phenomenon (like self and own family perceptions) have also their micro – molecular correlations (like presumed anxiolytic pills influence/function), as complements of the multilevel approach.

In our research, for self and family climate perceptions, we rejected all alternative hypotheses in the case of fathers, while by mothers they were mostly accepted. The only exception was, when children's TE (therapists' estimation of drug abuse) was included as co – variate, when multivariate effect was significant on $p = 0.08$ risk level and univariate approach showed significant differences ($p < 0.05$) between mothers anxiolytics (non)users only for level of self esteem. Results suggest, that children's TE could be maybe treated as new independent variable and that anxiolytics (non)use effects on self and family perceptions by mothers' in families with dependent member depend more on children than on husbands health (dependence) status. Taking into account relatively small number ($n = 21$) of anxiolytics users mothers and non – significant, but relatively low risk level, $p = 0.08$, we can infer, that children dependence status could be interpreted more as relatively most important factual reason of anxiolytics' usage by mothers, what both effect mothers' self and family perceptions.

In the framework of this research design, this general trend could not be persuasively formulated more in detail. Anyway, it seems that patterns of social behavior, expressed by SASSI (sub) scores specifically enough express the connections with anxiolytics (none) usage. In the case of SASSI (sub) scores, hypotheses were partially accepted, partially rejected, but mostly in accordance with our expectations.

We can say, that all results together show important differences between male and female participants. Female participants show the evident trend of significant differences in their family climate and in self (esteem/depression) perceptions, while the male participants in our research do not. It seems that mothers with emotional problems communicate about them with medical doctors (which prescribe them anxiolytics), and fathers do not.

By mothers, for example, we did not find significant differences between the (non)users in face valid other drugs scores (FVOD); higher score on either scale means that clients acknowledge usage, consequences of usage and loss of control. Higher scores mean that the client is willing to admit to having a problem with alcohol/drugs. The face valid items are relatively easy for clients to manipulate. Results show, that female participants do not perceive anxiolytics as "other drugs", but fathers do. It can be said that fathers show more critical view towards anxiolytics use. However, in a Norwegian population-based cohort study of anxiety, depression and sleep, benzodiazepine (anxiolytics) were associated with a higher risk of severe anxiety, depression and sleep outcomes; benzodiazepine use was not found to be associated with a higher risk of problematic alcohol use [34]. Results of our small (clinical) study are similar in way: in fathers there has been a group with alcohol problem, but it did not associate with anxiolytic use, but mood problems (in mothers) did.

Perspectives from multiple perspectives are required to fully understand individual vulnerability to addictions [6]. Our small piece of work points to vulnerability of mothers with drug abusing children to anxiolytic (ab) use. On the other hand, in primates social rank (dominant to subordinate) has been found inversely related to locomotor activity and cocaine self administration. In other words, monkey with high levels of locomotor activity tend to be subordinate in rank and self-administer cocaine avidly. PET imaging showed also, that there was an inverse relationship between Dopamine D_2 receptor availability and cocaine self administration [35]. – It would be interesting to research the connection between mothers' social status in family with/without dependence problem, brain neurotransmitters availability and their proness to anxiolytic abuse.

We perceive the following advantages of our research: it seems that the research problem have been up to date quite rarely investigated; the research contributed to some aspects of so called decision rule validation of SASSI (sub scores), while just the anxiolytics (non) usage could be one of those approach approximation for chosen sub scores, defined as chemically determined; difference between the actual and retrograde self – evaluation (of functionality in the everyday life) seems to be quite a suitable measure of relative subjective success/failure; including the AUDIT and TE covariates of dependence seriousness, we tried to assure the necessary minimum of (a posteriori) statistical control and partial interpretability in the sense of consequences; users and non – users of anxiolytics did not significantly differ in age and education, what, together with AUDIT covariates, eventually contributes to attempt of more clear identification of anxiolytics effects; families with dependent member represented quite an adequate environment for anxiolytics usage effect study.

Weaknesses of our research could be the following: research design is quasi – experimental, a kind of "ex post facto", without (direct) systematic and sensible manipulation of independent variable, without relevant control of (eventual) extraneous variables. That's why relations between chosen dependents and independent could not be interpreted in the pure sense of causal relation. Effect sizes (eta square) are mostly (very) low; neurobiological effects are taken into account only indirectly, without sophisticated technological measurements. Also the distributions of AUDIT covariate estimations significantly differed from the normal one, what is normal taking account the character and purpose of the instrument. Internal consistency of instruments, as the additional demands for statistic calculations (homogeneity of covariance) were not ulimatively respected. The structure of demographic, socio – economic and socio – cultural status of target participants do not permit spreader societal or cultural generalizations.

Anyway, results could be discussed also from the aspects of personal and micro – group (family) culture. According to Trice and Beyer [36], social climate is one of the essential parts (elements) of micro and macro group culture. From this point of view, also the individualistic – collectivistic orientation could be treated not only relatively, as underlined from some authors in last decade [37], but also on different micro and macro levels. Attachment to the values of the secondary family could mean also a typical micro–collectivistic orientation [38], without any anticipation of positive or negative connotations. In our research, evaluation of family climate is a central psychological variable, which correlate with some other indicators of group/family culture, like characteristic ways of communication, habits and rituals, perceived distribution of power/ influence, relevant social representations etc. From this aspect, we can conclude, that family culture is partially connected with brain – anxiolytics usage by females in Slovenia as representative part of Central European culture.

5. Conclusion

Social neuroscience finally ends one of the important phases of the developing of social psychology, which intensely obtained quantitative and qualitative accelerations in »eighties«, with applied social psychology, partially derived from societal and cross-cultural trends of development, what resulted in new relations to new interdisciplinary areas, and from social cognition, which revitalized the importance of social interaction, language/linguistic, social knowledge, taxonomy of meaning and categorization processes with prototypical perceptions. Neuroscience researches could be guided by different definitions of the field. One of the main objectives, goals, and purposes is only to understand better the relation between the brain, its related systems and social interaction. According to them, the instruments of social neuroscience are limited only by the imagination of the researcher: so creative uses of traditional approaches, as developments of new techniques are welcome [2]. That's why we see our research as a micro attempt of the contribution to this field.

Author details

Maja Rus-Makovec[1*], Karin Sernec[2] and Velko S. Rus[3]

1 University Psychiatric Hospital Ljubljana & School of Medicine, University Ljubljana, Slovenia

2 University Psychiatric Hospital Ljubljana, Slovenia

3 Department of Psychology, Faculty of Arts, University Ljubljana, Slovenia

References

[1] Ochsner KN, Lieberman MD. The emergence of social cognitive neuroscience. American psychologist 2001; 56: 717-34.

[2] Decety J, Keenan JP. Social neuroscience: A new journal. Social Neuroscience 2006; 1: 1-4.

[3] Cacioppo JT, Berntson GG. Social psychological contributions to the decade of the brain: doctrine of multilevel analysis. In. Kruglanski A, Higgins T (eds.). Social psychology. New York: Psychology Press; 2003. p 9 – 22.

[4] Buss DM. Mate preferences in 37 cultures. In: Kruglanski A, Higgins T (eds.). Social psychology. New York: Psychology Press; 2003. p 3 – 8.

[5] Taylor SE, Brown JD. Illusion and well being: a social psychological perspective on mental health. Psychological Bulletin 1988; 103(2): 193-210.

[6] Singer T. The past, present and future of social neuroscience: A European perspective. NeuroImage 2012; 61: 437 - 9.

[7] Schnur P, Shurtleff D. Social neuroscience: Application to addiction. Drug and Alcohol Dependence 2008; 94: 285-90.

[8] Illeris K. How we learn. (2nd edition). New York: Routledge; 2007.

[9] Caccioppo JT, Berntson GG, Lorig TS, Norris CJ, Rickett E, Nusbaum H. Just because you're imaging the brain doesn't mean you can stop using your head: a primer and set of first principles. Journal of Personality and Social Psychology 2003; 85: 650–661.

[10] Torrance EP. Hemisphericity and creative functioning. Journal of Research of Development and Education 1983; 15: 29 – 37.

[11] Klavora P. Foundations of kinesiology – studying human movement and health. Toronto: Sport books publishers; 2008.

[12] Cacioppo JT, Petty RE, Tassinary LG. Social Psychophysiology: A New Look. Sociophysiology: A new look. In L. Berkowitz (Ed.). Advances in experimental social psychology (Vol. 22). Kent, UK: Harcourt; 1989. p 39-91.

[13] Gangestad SW, Simpson JA. The evolution of human mating: trade – offs and strategic pluralism. Behavioral and Brain Sciences 2000; 23: 573-587.

[14] Eysenck HJ. The biological basis of personality. Springfield: Charles & Thomas; 1967.

[15] Hayes N. Foundation of psychology. London, New York: Routledge; 1994.

[16] Moscovici S, Personnaz B. Studies in social influence V: minority influence and conversion behavior in a perceptual task. Journal of experimental social psychology 1981; 16: 270 – 282.

[17] Personnaz B. Study in social influence using the spectrometer method: dynamic of the phenomena of conversion and correctness in perceptual responses. European Journal of Social Psychology 1981; II: 431–438.

[18] Anderson JR, Bower GH. Human associative memory. Washington: Winston and Sons; 1973.

[19] Collins AM, Loftus EF. A spreading activation theory of semantic processing. Psychological Review 1975; 82: 407–428.

[20] Hayes–Roth B. Evolution of cognitive structures and processes. Psychological Review 1977; 84: 270–278.

[21] Wagner EF, Sobell M, Sobell LS. Substance related disorders: alcohol. In: Hersen M., Turner SM, Beidel DC (eds.). Adult Psychopathology and diagnosis (5th ed.). Hoboken, NJ: Wiley; 2007. p 166 – 200

[22] Allen JP, Litten RZ, Fertig JB, Babor T. A review of research on the Alcohol Use Disorders Identification Test (AUDIT). Alcoholism: Clinical and Experimental Research 1997; 21(4): 613-619.

[23] Kossfeld M, Heinrichs M, Zak P, Fishbacher U, Fehr E. Oxytocin increases trust in humans. Nature 2005; 435: 673–676.

[24] Curley JP, Jensen CL, Mashood R, Champagne FA. Social influences on neurobiology and behavior: Epigenetic effects during development. Psychoneuroendocrinology 2011; 36: 352-71.

[25] Koob GF, Le Moal M. Neurobiology of Addiction. London: Elsevier; 2006.

[26] Brady KT, Sinha R. Co-occurring mental and substance use disorders: the neurobiological effect of chronic stress. Am J Psychiatry 2005; 162: 1483-1493.

[27] Stahl SM. Stahl's Essential Psychopharmacology. Cambridge: Cambridge University Press; 2008.

[28] Goodman A. Neurobiology of addiction. An integrative review. Biochemical Pharmacology 2008; 75: 266-322.

[29] Boyarsky BK, Dilts S, Frances RJ et al. Responsibility and Choice in Addiction. Psychiatric Services 2002; 53 (6): 707-13.

[30] Miller FG, Miller M, Knot R, Renn W. Breaking through denial – The SASSI-3 a new addiction measure. The SASSI-3 Institute. News & Reports, vol. 1. Bloomington: The SASSI institute; 1994.

[31] Rus VS. Sociopsihologija kot sodobna paradigma socialne psihologije (Sociopsychology as contemporary paradigm of social psychology). Ljubljana: Univerza v Ljubljani, Filozofska fakulteta; 1999.

[32] Zung WA. Self – rating depression scale. Arch Gen Psychiatry 1965; 12: 63–70.

[33] Rosenberg M. Society and the adolescent self – image. Princeton: Princeton University Press; 1989.

[34] Nordfjaern T. A population-based cohort study of anxiety, depression, sleep and alcohol outcomes among benzodiazepine and z-hypnotic users. Addictive Behaviors 2012; 37: 1151-7.

[35] Nader MA, Czoty PW. PET imaging of dopamine D_2 receptors in monkey models of cocaine abuse: genetic predisposition environmental modulation. Am J Psychiat 2005; 162: 1473-82.

[36] Trice HM, Beyer JM. The Cultures of Work Organizations. New Jersey: Englewood Cliffs; 1993.

[37] Oyserman D, Coon H, Kemmelmeier M. Rethinking individualism and collectivism: Evaluation of theoretical assumptions and meta-analyses. Psychological Bulletin 2002; 128(1): 3-72. doi: 10.1037/0033-2909.128.1.3

[38] Rus VS. Socialna in societalna psihologija (z obrisi sociopsihologije) (Social and societal psychology (with frames of sociopsychology)). Ljubljana: Univerza v Ljubljani, Filozofska fakulteta; 1997.

Chapter 5

Management of Delirium

Narong Maneeton and Benchalak Maneeton

Additional information is available at the end of the chapter

1. Introduction

Delirium is categorized in the cognitive disorders, characterized by acute onset, global impairment in cognitive, emotional, mental, and behavioral functioning, fluctuating level of consciousness, attention impairment, decreased or increased psychomotor activity and the disturbance of sleep-wake cycle. Emotional and behavioral abnormalities are common presented with some neurological manifestations, e.g., tremor, asterixis, nystagmus, incoordination, urinary incontinence.

Delirium is a behavioral disturbance and serious complication commonly found in consultation-liaison psychiatry. Its prevalence and incidence rates are varied, possibly depend on severity of illness, patient population, the method of assessment and the diagnostic criteria. Prevalence of delirium ranges from 10% to 30% and its incidence is between 3% and 29% for patients admitted in general hospitals (Siddiqi et al., 2006, Maneeton et al., 2007a, Praditsuwan et al., 2012). High prevalence and incidence are noted in elderly and severely ill patients. For instance, the prevalence of delirium in elderly and ICU patients are up to 40% and 80%, respectively (Bledowski and Trutia, 2012, Praditsuwan et al., 2012).

An occurrence of delirium is associated with miserable clinical outcomes. It often increases morbidity, mortality, length of hospitalization, institutionalization, and poor functional outcome (Siddiqi et al., 2006, Cole et al., 2009, Fong et al., 2012). The mortality rate is higher in patients with hypoactive subtype of delirium (Yang et al., 2009).

Delirium is often under recognized by health professionals. There are many faces for the clinical presentation of delirium. It can be caused by a variety of etiology. To prevent and minimize the consequences of delirium, physician should prompt intervenes for this condition (Attard et al., 2008).

This chapter aims to summarize current strategies for managing and preventing delirium caused by a variety of etiology, except substance withdrawal delirium. In addition, etiologies, clinical manifestations and risk factors are also addressed.

2. Definition

According to the *Diagnostic and Statistical Manual of Mental Disorders, fourth edition, text revision* (DSM-IV-TR), delirium due to a general medical condition is defined by four criteria: a. disturbance of consciousness (i.e., reduced clarity of awareness of the environment) with reduced ability to focus, sustain, or shift attention; b. a change in cognition (such as memory deficit, disorientation, language disturbance) or the development of a perceptual disturbance that is not better accounted for by a preexisting, established, or evolving dementia; c. the disturbance develops over a short period of time (usually hours to days) and tends to fluctuate during the course of the day; d. there is evidence from the history, physical examination, or laboratory findings that the disturbance is caused by the direct physiological consequences of a general medical condition(American Psychiatric Association, 2005).

For the ICD-10, delirium not induced by alcohol and other psychoactive substances is defined as an etiologically nonspecific organic cerebral syndrome characterized by concurrent disturbances of consciousness and attention, perception, thinking, memory, psychomotor behavior, emotion, and the sleep-wake schedule. The duration is variable, and the degree of severity ranges from mild to very severe (World Health Organization, 1993).

3. Clinical manifestation

The hallmark of delirium is rapid and fluctuated disturbance of consciousness, orientation and global cognitive functioning.

3.1. Prodromal phase

Prodromal symptoms may be observed for hours to a few days in some patients. These symptoms include restlessness, anxiety, irritability, hypervigilance, drowsiness, transient hallucination, nightmare and etc. Because these symptoms are not specific for delirium, they may be overlooked by health care providers.

3.2. Fluctuating course

Most patients have rapidly changes of emotion and cognition. The diurnal fluctuation is common. Because the patient's condition is usually worse at night time, this clinical feature may be called "sundowner's syndrome". During thi speriod of time, delusion, hallucination, depression, irritability and anxiety are frequently prominent.

3.3. Disorientation

Most patients are disoriented to time, place and/or person.

3.4. Sleep-wake cycle abnormality

Sleep-wake disturbance is usually noted in delirium. The patients may be sleepy during the day and stay awake at night. The sleep pattern is characterized by brief and fragmented periods of sleeping time.

3.5. Psychomotor disturbance

Arousal disturbance is common and usually related to the abnormality of reticular activating system. Currently, psychomotor behavior of delirium is categorized into four subtypes, including normal, hypoactive, hyperactive, and mixed (Yang et al., 2009). Hyperactive delirium is characterized by agitation, restlessness and hypervigilance. Lethargy, somnolence, apathy, depression, catatonia and quiet confusion are common for hypoactive delirium. For the mixed subtype, it manifests both psychomotor hypoactivity and hyperactivity.

3.6. Perceptual disturbance

Because most delirious patients cannot discriminate and integrate the sensory stimuli around them, illusions and hallucinations are common in this population. The patients are easily frustrated or distracted when they encounter new information.

3.7. Dysfunction of higher cortical function

Although the DSM IV-TR does not include language difficulties, most patients have speech abnormality, such as rambling, irrelevancy and incoherent. Impairment of memory, especially the short-termone, can be found in most patients. The impaired short-term memory may be explained by the loss of concentration, perceptual disturbance, and/or malfunction of the hippocampus. Since delirium is a global cerebral dysfunction, higher cortical dysfunction such as dysphasia, dyspraxia, dysgraphia, is also common. In addition, the patients may have other neurological signs, e.g., tremor, asterixis, incoordination and urinary incontinence.

4. Predisposing and risk factors

Individuals are differently susceptible to delirium. Despite the exposing to the same causative factor, individuals are not equally prone to develop delirium. Predisposing and risk factors appear to play a role in the susceptibility to delirium. There have been numerous studies on predisposing and risk factors of delirium. For instance, Inouye and Charpentier (1996) demonstrated the five independent precipitating factors for delirium, including use of physical restraints, malnutrition, more than three medications taken, use of bladder catheter and any iatrogenic event. Recently, risk factors for delirium have been established in four domains, including patient characteristics, chronic pathology, acute illness, and environmental factors (Van Rompaey et al., 2009). Another study in elderly patients receiving hip surgery found that early symptoms of memory impairments, incoherence, disorientation and underlying somatic illness were predictors of delirium (de Jonghe et al., 2007).

In general, the common predisposing and risk factors for delirium that have been recognized are age of 60 years or over, brain damage (e.g., stroke, brain injury), chronic organic brain syndrome (e.g., dementia of Alzheimer type), postoperative patients, history of delirium, diabetes, malignancy, sensory impairment (e.g., blindness, deafness) and HIV infection.

5. Etiology

Common causes of delirium include central nervous system (CNS) diseases, systemic diseases, intoxication or withdrawal from substance and toxic agent. Most delirious patients often encounter with multiple causes.

5.1. Medications

The use of medication is one of the most common causes of delirium. Medications that have been identified are antibiotics, antidepressants, antihistamines, anticholinergic agents, antiparkinson agents, antipsychotic medications, antineoplastics, anticonvulsants, antituberculosis agents, cardiac drugs, diuretics, non-steroidal anti-inflammatory drugs, L-dopa, lithium, opiates, sedative-hypnotics, steroids, sympathomimetic agents. It has been found that the administration of three medications or more is a risk factor for delirium. Because elderly patients tend to take multiple medications, they are a population at particular risk for delirium (Inouye, 2004, Clegg and Young, 2011, Catic, 2011).

5.2. Neurological causes

Delirium is a state of global cerebral dysfunction. Therefore, any pathology in the CNS may cause this syndrome. Common neurological contributors for delirium consist of head injury, stroke, hypertensive encephalopathy, intracranial neoplasm and epilepsy (Ramirez-Bermudez et al., 2006, Martin, 2012).

5.3. Infection

Infection, in particular sepsis, can be a cause of delirium (Rahkonen et al., 2000, Srinonprasert et al., 2011, Zampieri et al., 2011). Other infectious diseases commonly found, including CNS infection (Ramirez-Bermudez et al., 2006); meningitis, encephalitis, brain abscess, neurosyphilis, HIV encephalopathy and other systemic infection (Warshaw and Tanzer, 1993, Eriksson et al., 2011, van Gool et al., 2010).

5.4. Metabolic disorders

Metabolic disturbances are frequently associated with delirium (Khurana et al., 2011, Grover et al., 2012). Common metabolic abnormalities consist of hepatic encephalopathy, hypo- or hyperglycemia, hypoxia, hypo- or hypernatremia, hypo- orhypercalcemia, hypo- orhyper-magnesemia, acidosis, uremia and metabolic acidosis (Aldemir et al., 2001, Khurana et al., 2011).

5.5. Vitamin deficiency

Vitamin deficiency, such as thiamine, B12, nicotinic acid, folic acid, is a common factor contributing to the development of delirium (Kane et al., 1993, O'Keeffe et al., 1994, Harrington et al., 2011).

5.6. Endocrine abnormalities

Several lines of evidence suggest that endocrine disturbances may be a cause of delirium (Olsson, 1999, Grover et al., 2012). Common abnormalities include hypo- or hyperthyroidism, hypo- or hyperparathyroidism, Cushing's syndrome, Addison's disease, pheochromocytoma and hypopituitary diseases (Olsson, 1999, Maldonado, 2008a).

5.7. Withdrawal syndrome

The withdrawal of some drugs or substances could precipitate the phenomena of delirium. Those possible causative agents are alcohol, benzodiazepines, barbiturates, other sedatives and hypnotics (Saitz, 1998, Trevisan et al., 1998, Maldonado, 2008a, Yu et al., 2012).

5.8. Substance abuse

Numerous substances, for instance methamphetamine, cocaine, hallucinogens, inhalants, opioids and bath salts may be a cause of delirium (Nakatani and Hara, 1998, Maldonado, 2008a, Fadel and Serra, 2009, Kasick et al., 2012 Burapakajornpong et al., 2012).

5.9. Toxin exposure

Toxin exposure is also a significant contributor in the development of delirium. Example toxic agents are heavy metals and toxins (Maldonado, 2008a).

6. Pathophysiology

Since there have been only a few studies on the mechanism of delirium, its pathophysiology are still poorly understood. However, some recent findings suggest several mechanisms possibly related to the development of delirium, including abnormality in neurotransmitters, inflammatory response, the blood-brain barrier permeability, cerebral oxidative metabolism and the hypothalamic-pituitary adrenal axis (Flacker and Lipsitz, 1999, van der Mast,

1998, Gunther et al., 2008, Marcantonio et al., 2006). However, the heterogeneity of the delirium syndrome and the populations are the major challenges. The mechanism may differ in the various clinical settings and individual risk factors (Chaput and Bryson, 2012).

6.1. Neurotransmitter abnormalities

According to the neurotransmitter hypothesis, delirium is a result of complex interacting neurotransmitter systems that modulate the control of cognition, behavior, and emotion and pathologic processes. The decreased oxidative metabolism of the brain causes cerebral dysfunction due to abnormalities of many neurotransmitter systems. Various symptoms and clinical manifestations of delirium may be associated with numerous neurotransmitter activities (van der Mast, 1998). More specifically, the pathogenesis of delirium may include the decreased cholinergic activity; both decreased and increased serotonergic and gamma-aminobutyric acid activities and excessive release of dopamine, norepinephrine and/or glutamate (Flacker and Lipsitz, 1999).

6.2. Reduction of cerebral oxidative metabolism

Impaired oxidative metabolism is related to the development of delirium (Seaman et al., 2006). Its dysfunction is often associated with a decrease of oxygen supply to the brain, which leads to the widespread of cerebral dysfunction. Therefore, patients with oxygen exchange dysfunction, such as cardiac diseases, intraoperative hypotension, perioperative factors, intrinsic lung diseases and anemia may be important causes of delirium (Maldonado, 2008b, Ali et al., 2011).

6.3. Inflammatory response

Delirium is high prevalence in patients with systemic inflammatory diseases, including infection, malignancy, and the postoperative state (Marcantonio et al., 2006). Recent findings suggest the association between cytokines and the development of delirium. Cytokine dysregulation can cause neuronal injury by means of (1) abnormal neurotransmission, (2) apoptosis and (3) activation of microglia and astrocytes producing free radicals, complement factors, glutamate, and nitric oxide (Wilson et al., 2002, Simone and Tan, 2011).The cytokines considered as proinflammatory factors (e.g., interleukin-1, interleukin-6 and interleukin-8, tumor necrosis factor-alpha, interferon gamma and C-reactive protein) and anti-inflammatory factors (e.g., interleukin receptor antagonist and insulin-like growth factor -1) have been hypothesized as factors related to the pathogenesis of delirium (Gunther et al., 2008, van den Boogaard et al., 2011).

6.4. Increased activity of the hypothalamic-pituitary adrenal axis

The disturbance of hypothalamic-pituitary-adrenal (HPA) axis is another hypothesis relevant to the pathogenesis of delirium. It has been known that excessive cortisol or glucocorticoid affect memory and mood in delirium (Maldonado, 2008b). The association between delirium and disturbance of dexamethasone suppression (DST) has been noted (Robertsson et al., 2001). In addition, the elevation of cerebrospinal fluid (CSF) and plasma cortisol levels observed in hip fracture patients with delirium also support the hypothesis that high brain cortisol levels are related to delirium development (Pearson et al., 2011).

7. Management

Once delirium is diagnosed, prompt and appropriated interventions should be implemented. Other than the DSM IV-TR criteria for delirium, several measures are helpful to confirm the diagnosis and determine the progress of illness course. Since common causes of delirium are medical/surgical conditions and medications, priority should be given to specific treatment for the removal of these causes. Frequently, delirium is associated with multi-factorial etiology, all possible causes, therefore, should be investigated and corrected. Because behavioral and other psychiatric disturbances are also common, psychopharmacological and psychosocial interventions are also needed in most patients. Those include the control of behavioral disturbances, preventing complications (e.g., accident, falling) and supporting functional needs (Burns et al., 2004).

7.1. Assessment

Physicians should review all possible contributed factors for the development of delirium, including histories of medical/psychiatric illness, prescribed or over-the-counter medications and substance uses. Physical examination should address in all systems, especially the one possibly causing or contributing to the development of delirium. Mental status examination should focus on cognitive function, such as orientation, memory, concentration, attention, language ability, mood/affect and psychotic symptoms.

The use of screening tests or tools prior to the occurrence of delirium or in patients suspected of having delirium is very helpful for the early detection of delirium. In addition, some measures can be used to determine the progress of delirium. Bedside cognitive screening tests, such as the three-item registration, the three-item delayed recall test, the clock drawing test, the problem-solving task and the ability of abstraction, can determine the cognitive impairment (de Wet et al., 2007). Example measures of delirium are the Mini-Mental State Examination (MMSE), the original and revised versions of Delirium Rating Scale (DRS and DRS-98), the Memorial Delirium Assessment Scale (MDAS) and the Confusion Assessment Method (CAM) recommended (Breitbart et al., 1997, Trzepacz et al., 2001, Salawu et al., 2009, Wongpakaran et al., 2011, Inouye et al., 1990).

To identify the causes of delirium, laboratory studies are essential. Generally, basic investigation for delirium includes a routine blood test, including complete blood count, electrolytes, glucose levels, liver function test, thyroid function test, renal function test, blood alcohol, blood ammonia, calcium/magnesium/phosphate levels, pulse oximetry, urinalysis, urine drug screen, electrocardiogram (ECG), CSF study, radiological studies (e.g., chest x-ray and computed tomography (CT) the head) (Salawu et al., 2009, Lorenzl et al., 2012). However, further studies to verify infection, hypoxia and etc are also important for some patients. In equivocal case, electroencephalography (EEG) can be helpful. While the EEG pattern of alcohol or sedative withdrawal delirium usually presents with the prominence of beta activity, diffuse bilateral slowing records are typical for delirium due to a general medical condition. This later pattern of the EEG is also helpful for being used as a confirm test for the delirious state (Jacobson and Jerrier, 2000, Salawu et al., 2009, Sidhu et al., 2009).

7.2. Specific and supportive treatment

The specific treatment for delirium is the removal of all possible causes. Therefore, the precipitating factors must be promptly addressed and corrected (Burns et al., 2004). However, the etiology may not be identifiable when the patient is diagnosed, sometimes cannot be identified until the patient is recovery, and, for rare cases, cannot be identified at all. Consequently, the initially supportive and symptomatic treatments are, therefore, essential in all patients with delirium.

7.3. Psychopharmacological treatment

7.3.1. Antipsychotics

7.3.1.1. Typical antipsychotics

To our knowledge, only two RCTs of typical antipsychotics, including haloperidol and chlorpromazine, have been carried out.

7.3.1.1.1. Haloperidol

Haloperidol, a dopamine antagonist, has been used in various neuropsychiatric conditions. It is considered as a first-line medication for the symptom control of delirium (American Psychiatric Association, 1999). The advantages of this medication are that it can be administered through several routes. In addition, it has fewer active metabolites, less anticholinergic effect and fewer sedative or hypotensive effects compared with other antipsychotics (Attard et al., 2008).

Breitbart et al. (1996) conducted an RCT to compare the efficacy and safety among haloperidol, chlorpromazine and lorazepam in adult AIDS patients with delirium. Thirty patients met the DSM-III-R criteria for delirium and scored 13 or more on the DRS. The measures used included the DRS, the Mini-Mental State and the extrapyramidal symptoms (EPS). The sample size was relatively small (n's for haloperidol = 11,chlorpromazine = 13 and lorazepam = 6). Based on the DRS scores, haloperidol (2.8±2.4 mg)and chlorpromazine (50±23.1 mg) were significantly superior to lorazepam for controlling the symptoms of delirium in the first 24 hours, usually before the underlying medical causes of delirium could be identified. The improvement of delirious symptoms was continued until the study end. The doses of haloperidol from day 2 to the study end were decreased for an average of 1.4±1.2 mg/day. While cognitive improvement, as measured by the Mini-Mental State, was observed as soon as day 2 of haloperidol or chlorpromazine treatment, no cognitive improvement was found in the lorazepam group. At the study end, cognitive function of the haloperidol group was significantly improved. No patient developed extrapyramidal symptoms.

Several RCTs have been conducted in comparing the efficacy and tolerability between haloperidol and atypical antipsychotic medications. An RCT compared the efficacy and safety of haloperidol and olanzapine for the treatment of delirium in the medical and surgical intensive care unit. A total of 80 delirious patients were randomized to receive either haloperidol or olanzapine, administered orally. Measured by Delirium Index, the findings indicated that haloperidol (a mean dose of 6.5 mg/day, range: 1–28 mg), was as effective as olanzapine (a mean dose of 4.54 mg/day, range: 2.5–13.5 mg) in the treatment of delirium. However, the EPS measured by Ross-Chouinard and Angus-Simpson scales was significantly more severe in the haloperidol group (Skrobik et al., 2004).

There was a double-blind trial comparing haloperidol and risperidone for the treatment of delirium. A total of 28 patients with delirium were enrolled and randomly assigned to receive either a flexible-dose regimen of haloperidol or risperidone for 7 days. The measure in efficacy is the reduction of the MDAS scores. Significant reduction of delirious symptoms was observed in both haloperidol and risperidone groups. The average resolution times, measured by the MDAS score of 13 or lower, were 4.22±2.48 days in the haloperidol group and 4.17±2.14 days in the risperidone group. At the study end, the mean daily doses of the haloperidol and the risperidone groups were 1.71±0.84 and 1.02±0.41mg, respectively. No patient reported clinically significant side effects, except one patient in the haloperidol group experienced mild akathisia (Han and Kim, 2004).

Grover et al. (2011) conducted an RCT to compare the efficacy and safety of haloperidol, olanzapine and risperidone in medical and surgical in patients with delirium. A total of 64 patients (20 in the haloperidol group, 21 in the risperidone group and 23 in the olanzapine group) participated in the study. The patients were randomly assigned to receive the flexible dose regimens, including 0.25 to 10 mg of haloperidol, 0.25 to 4 mg of risperidone and 1.25 to 20 mg of olanzapine. The efficacy measures were the DRS-R 98 and MMSE. The mean doses of haloperidol, olanzapine and risperidone were 0.88±0.98 mg (range: 0.25–5 mg), 3.05±1.44 mg (range: 1.25–10 mg) and 0.95±0.28 mg (range: 0.5-2 mg), respectively. According to DRS-R98 and MMSE scores, haloperidol was significantly superior for the reduction of delirious symptoms on day 6. However, the efficacy of all three regimens was not significantly different from other days. Four patients in a haloperidol group had some side effects.

Maneeton and colleagues conducted an RCT comparing the efficacy and tolerability between quetiapine and haloperidol in delirious inpatients. All participants, aged 18-75 years, were delirious patients who were consulted to a psychiatric department. The diagnoses of all patients with DSM-IV delirium were confirmed by using the CAM. The primary efficacy outcome was the DRS-R-98. The other efficacy measures were the Clinical Global Impression (CGI) and hours of night sleep. The EPS was assessed by using the Modified (9-item) Simpson-Angus Scale (MSAS). All measures were applied daily. Thirty-eight patients were randomly to receive either a flexible dose regimen of quetiapine and haloperidol. Mean (SD) doses of the quetiapine and haloperidol groups were 34.0±12.8 and 0.9±0.5 mg/day, respectively. Based on the DRS-R-98 and CGI scores, both haloperidol and quetiapine significantly reduced the symptoms of delirium from baseline to day 7. The mean hours of night-time sleep in haloperidol and quetiapine group were 6.9±3.5 and 7.8±1.8 hours (not significantly different). In the respect of EPS, the MSAS scores were not significantly different between groups (Maneeton et al., 2011).

Intravenous (IV) haloperidol should be used only if the oral administration is unlikely accessible, or a rapid resolution is needed. Although some previous findings suggest the use of IV haloperidol in these patients, most studies have low methodological quality. Two prospective studies with small sample sizes demonstrated the efficacy of intravenous haloperidol in disturbed behavioral control. The patients experienced a low risk of EPS (Menza et al., 1987, Moulaert, 1989). Another prospective, controlled study of EPS in delirious patients found that the combination of IV haloperidol and IV benzodiazepine reduced a risk of EPS compared with IV haloperidol mono therapy (Menza et al., 1988).

Although IV haloperidol appears to be effective for delirium, it should be used with great caution. Its incidence of QT prolongation (QTP) and torsades de pointes (TdP) has been increasing reported.

Meyer-Massetti et al. (2010) summarized 54 and 42 cases with intravenous haloperidol-related TdP and QTP, respectively. A cumulative dose in TdP cases ranged from 5 to 645 mg, while a that in patients with QTP alone was 2 to 1540 mg. this serious adverse event frequently occurred in the patients with concomitant risk factors. These findings suggest that a total cumulative dose of IV haloperidol less than 2 mg appears to be safely administered. At this cumulative dose range (<2 mg), ECG monitoring may not be needed for delirious patients who have no concomitant risk factors.

The administration of IV haloperidol may not be possible in severe delirious and aggressive patients. Therefore, intramuscular injection (IM) may be an alternative route for this condition. In addition, several settings cannot routinely monitor ECG in these cases. Based on some pharmacokinetic studies, IM haloperidol also had more rapid onset of action than that of oral administration (Schaffer et al., 1982, Froemming et al., 1989, Wang et al., 2012).

So far, there has been promising evidence that haloperidol is effective and safe for the management of delirium. However, a few patients may experience EPS. In the respect of efficacy, haloperidol is comparable to atypical antipsychotic medications (e.g., risperidone, olanzapine and quetiapine) but superior to lorazepam. Parenteral route for haloperidol is widely used for the management of acute delirium. Although the IV haloperidol may rapidly control disruptive behavior of delirious patients, it also increases the incidence of TdP and QTP. ECG monitoring may be needed for patients with concomitant risk factors or received a total cumulative dose of 2 mg or more for IV haloperidol. Alternatively, the administration of IM haloperidol is effective and safe for the treatment of severe delirium. Although it has been widely used, there has been no RCT comparing haloperidol and placebo in delirious patients. Further randomized, placebo-controlled trials are useful to confirm its efficacy and tolerability.

7.3.1.1.2. Chlorpromazine

Chlorpromazine is the first antipsychotic drug widely used in various psychotic disorders. The only one RCT demonstrated that it is effective for controlling delirious symptoms. Breitbart et al. (1996) suggested that the low doses of chlorpromazine (50±23.1 mg) may rapidly reduce the delirious symptoms in AIDS patients in the first 24 hours and continuously improved the symptoms until the study end. This efficacy was comparable to haloperidol but significantly superior to lorazepam. After the first 24 hours of treatment, the average dose of chlorpromazine from day 2 to the study end was decreased for 36±18.4 mg/day. Although the cognitive improvement could be observed in the first two days of chlorpromazine treatment, it is slightly declined from day 2 until the treatment end. This phenomenon may be caused by the high anticholinergic property of chlorpromazine. No patient developed clinically significant extrapyramidal symptoms.

These findings show that chlorpromazine is effective and tolerable for treating delirium. However, due to its anticholinergic effects, cognitive function and other anticholinergic side effects should be monitored.

7.3.1.2. Atypical antipsychotics

Although typical antipsychotic medications are the mainstay for managing behavioral disturbance in delirium, its side effects, in particular EPS and anticholinergic effects are an issue of concern. The use of atypical antipsychotic medications with less propensity to induce EPS or cause anticholinergic effects is, therefore, an alternative. Several studies have demonstrated the efficacy and tolerability of atypical antipsychotic agents for controlling delirious symptoms.

7.3.1.2.1. Risperidone

Risperidone is probable the first atypical antipsychotic agent used for controlling delirious symptoms. An RCT comparing risperidone with haloperidol demonstrated that risperidone is as effective as haloperidol in reducing delirious symptoms. No patient receiving risperidone developed significant side effects (Han and Kim, 2004).

In a 7-day, RCT comparing the efficacy of risperidone and olanzapine in the treatment of delirium. The outcomes included the DRS-R-98, reported adverse events and EPS. Patients with dementia, serious hepatic problems, or bone marrow suppression, as well as those already taking antipsychotics for behavioral problems, were excluded. Thirty-two patients, aged 36-82 (median = 72) years, were included and randomly assigned to receive either risperidone (n = 17) or olanzapine (n = 15). Twenty-three patients had malignant cancer, and the rest had femur fracture, head trauma, or pneumonia. The mean initial doses of risperidone and olanzapine were 0.6±0.2 and 1.8±0.6 mg/day, respectively. However, the mean doses of risperidone and olanzapine at the last observation were 0.9±0.6 and 2.4±1.7 mg/day, orderly. With respected to the decreased DRS-R-98 scores, risperidone as well as olanzapine were significantly superior in reducing delirious symptoms over the 7 days of study. However, the response rates were not significantly different between groups (risperidone group:

64.7%, olanzapine group: 73.3%). The response to risperidone was poorer in the older age group. The median times to the recovery of delirium in the risperidone and olanzapine groups were 5 and 3 days, respectively. Risperidone, like olanzapine, was well tolerated. Although a few patients developed extrapyramidal symptoms, they were tolerable (Kim et al., 2010).

Another RCT conducted by Grover et al.(2011) compared the efficacy and safety of olanzapine, risperidone and haloperidol in medical and surgical inpatients with delirium. The findings indicated that risperidone, like olanzapine, was as effective as haloperidol.

Several findings support that low doses of risperidone are effective and tolerable for delirious patients. Its efficacy is comparable to other typical and atypical antipsychotic medications. To our knowledge, there has not been a randomized, placebo-controlled trial of risperidone in delirious patients.

7.3.1.2.2. Quetiapine

Quetiapine is an atypical antipsychotic agent approved for the treatment of schizophrenia, bipolar disorder and major depressive disorder. However, its evidence in controlling delirious symptoms has been increased. There have had several RCTs conducted to determine the efficacy and safety of quetiapine in the management of delirium.

There was a randomized, double-blind, placebo-controlled trial of quetiapine in critically ill patients with delirium. A total of 36 delirious adult patients admitted in intensive care units were enrolled. All patients had a score of 4 or more on the Care Delirium Screening Checklist, were tolerable to enteral nutrition and had no neurologic condition. The patients were randomly assigned to receive either quetiapine 50 mg every 12 hours (n = 18) or placebo (n = 18). The doses of quetiapine were increased every 24 hours for up to 200 mg/day. The results showed that quetiapine was superior to placebo in the respects of time to resolution of delirium, [1.0 (0.5-3.0) vs. 4.5 days (2.0-7.0), p =0.001], duration of delirium [36 (12-87) vs. 120 hours (60-195, p =0.006], and duration of agitation [6 hours (0-38) vs. 36 hours (11-66), p =0.02)]. However, the length of hospitalization was similar in both groups (16 days vs. 16 days). The incidence of QTc prolongation and EPS were not significant different between groups. However, somnolence was more common in the quetiapine groups (22% vs. 11%, p =.66). In addition, the rate of discharge to home or rehabilitation was greater in the quetiapine group (89% vs. 56%, p =0.06) (Devlin et al., 2010).

Tahir et al. (2010) conducted an RCT to investigate the efficacy and acceptability of quetiapine for the control of delirious symptoms. Forty-two patients (21 in each group) were randomly received either quetiapine or placebo. The DRS-R-98 was used as the primary outcome. The results demonstrated that improvement for quetiapine, as measured by DRS-R-98 severity score, was faster than that of placebo. Based on DRS-R-98 severity score, the quetiapine group recovered faster than the placebo group (P=0.026). In addition, the non-cognitive items of the DRS-R-98, including restlessness, agitation, thought disorder and perceptual impairment in the quetiapine group were significantly improved faster than that of placebo group (p=0.048).

Lee et al. (2005) conducted an open, randomized, prospective trial to investigate the effectiveness and tolerability of quetiapine and amisulpride in delirious patients. Forty patients with delirium were randomly assigned to receive a flexible dose of amisulpride or quetiapine. Outcome measures included the DRS-R-98 and CGI-Severity (CGI-S), the total sleep time and the quality of sleep. The mean doses of quetiapine and amisulpride were 113 mg/day and 156.4 mg/day, respectively. The DRS-R-98 scores of both groups decreased over time. Time to recovery for the quetiapine group was 7.4±4.1 days. The quality of sleep and the total sleep time were not significantly different between groups. Both quetiapine and amisulpride were well tolerated.

After the reveal of promising benefits of quetiapine for delirium in an open-label study (Maneeton et al., 2007b), Maneeton and colleagues conducted an RCT to compare the efficacy and tolerability of quetiapine and haloperidol in the management of delirium. Based on the DRS-R-98 and CGI scores, quetiapine was as effective as haloperidol in the treatment of delirium. The mean of night time sleep was 7.8±1.8 hours for the quetiapine group. Quetiapine and haloperidol were well tolerated. In addition, the incidence rates of extrapyramidal side effects were very low in both groups (Maneeton et al., 2011).

The above mentioned findings suggest that low doses of quetiapine are effective and safe in the treatment of delirium. Its efficacy is, at least, comparable to typical and other atypical antipsychotic agents. Compared with other antipsychotic agents, only quetiapine has been shown its superiority to placebo in the management of delirium. It also causes only few adverse events, including EPS and QTc prolongation, which may be comparable to placebo.

7.3.1.2.3. Olanzapine

Olanzapine is, also, an atypical antipsychotic medication approved in the treatment of schizophrenia and bipolar disorder. There have been a few RCTs of this agent in patients with delirium.The RCT carried out by Skrobik et al. (2004) compared the safety and efficacy of olanzapine and haloperidol in delirious patients admitted in a critical care unit. The results indicated that olanzapine was as effective as haloperidol in controlling delirious symptoms. Olanzapine was a safe alternative agent, especially for delirious patients contraindicated to haloperidol.

The study of Kim and colleagues demonstrated that olanzapine was effective for delirium. This agent also had low incidence of adverse events, especially EPS. Its efficacy is equal to the effects of risperidone (Kim et al., 2010).

Elsayem et al. (2010) conducted a prospective, open-label study to investigate the safety, tolerability and efficacy of subcutaneous (SC) olanzapine for hyperactive or mixed delirium in the cancer patients. The subjects had the MMSE scores of 24 or higher and agitation with Richmond Agitation Sedation Scale (RASS) score of 1 or more. In addition, they were those who had not responded to 10 mg or more of parenteral haloperidol over 24 hours. All subjects received olanzapine 5mg SC every eight hours for three days and continued haloperidol for controlling agitation. Twenty-four patients, aged 49 to 79, were evaluated. The findings indicated that the patients tolerated well with the SC olanzapine. In the respect of agitation, only 37.5% of the subjects were rated as responders.

There was an RCT comparing the efficacy of olanzapine, risperidone and haloperidol in delirious patients. The findings suggested that olanzapine was comparable to risperidone and haloperidol (Grover et al., 2011).

Olanzapine appears to be an effective and tolerable antipsychotic medication in the control of delirious behavior. It can be administered in several routes, such as oral, intramuscular and subcutaneous administration. Further well-defined studies should be conducted to confirm these findings.

7.3.1.2.4. Aripriprazole

Aripiprazole is a dopamine partial agonist approved in the treatment of schizophrenia and bipolar disorder. Similar to other antipsychotic medications, it is widely used for controlling the behavioral disturbances and psychotic symptoms in patients with dementia and delirium. As an agent with little sedative and anticholinergic effects, it may have a few adverse effects on attention, concentration and sleep-wake cycle. In addition, it may be beneficial for hypoactive delirium (Straker et al., 2006). However, only a few studies of this agent have been carried out in delirious patients.

The study of Boettger et al. (2011) compared the efficacy and tolerability between aripiprazole and haloperidol for the reduction of delirious symptoms. The subjects were 21 delirious patients treated with aripiprazole and 21 case-matched, delirious patients treated with haloperidol. The measures consisted of the MDAS, the Karnofsky Performance Scale (KPS) and the abbreviated Udvalg Kliniske Undersogelser Side Effect Rating Scale (UKU). With respect to the MDAS, both groups improved significantly from baseline to day 7. The resolution rates of delirium were 76.2% for both groups. Both hypoactive and hyperactive deliriums significant improved. For those with hypoactive delirium, the rates of delirium resolution in the aripiprazole and haloperidol groups were 100 and 77.8%, respectively. For those with hyperactive delirium, such rates were 58.3% and 75%, respectively. However, the haloperidol group had more side effects.

Boettger and Breitbart (2011) conducted an open-label study to determine the efficacy and safety of aripiprazole for controlling delirious symptoms in hospitalized cancer patients. Twenty-one patients were treated with aripiprazole. Based on the changed MDAS scores, the aripiprazole group improved significantly. The mean dose of aripiprazole was 18.3 (range 5-30) mg/day at the end of study. The rates of delirium resolution were 100% for hypoactive delirium and 58.3% for hyperactive delirium. The patients with pre-morbid cognitive deficits and the hyperactive subtype of delirium did not respond well to aripiprazole treatment. The clinically significant adverse events were not found.

The case series of Straker et al. (2006) also demonstrated the efficacy of aripiprazole in the treatment of delirium. Fourteen patients, aged 18 to 85 and met DSM-IV-TR criteria for a diagnosis of delirium, were included. The results found that 12 patients had ≥ 50 % reduction in DSR-R-98, and 13 patients showed improvement on the CGI scores. The mean dose of aripiprazole was 8.9±3.5 mg/day. The adverse events were rare.The finding suggested that aripiprazole appeared to be effective and safe in the treatment of hypoactive delirium.

The above-mentioned findings demonstrate that aripiprazole is safe and effective for delirium. As a non sedating antipsychotic agent, it may be suitable for hypoactive delirium. However, its evidence in delirious patients is still limited.

7.3.1.2.5. Amisulpride

Amisulpride is an atypical antipsychotic agent used for the treatment of psychoses and manic episode. Its low doses may be effective for the treatment of depression. However, some studies have been carried out to examine its efficacy for controlling delirious symptoms.

There was an RCT comparing the efficacy, tolerability and sleep quality of amisulpride and quetiapine in controlling delirious symptoms. The findings showed that, similar to quetiapine, amisulpride was safe and effective for delirious patients. The mean time to stabilization in the amisulpride group was 6.3±4.4 days (Lee et al., 2005). The finding suggested that amisulpride, like quetiapine, appear to be effective and tolerable for the management of delirium. However, further studies are still needed to confirm its efficacy and safety.

Drug	Treatment route	Resolution or response time (days)	Level of evidence*	Comments
Haloperidol	Oral, IM, IV	4	Ib	IV administration increases risk of the QT prolongation and torsades de pointes
Chlorpromazine	Oral	-	Ib	worsen the cognitive impairment
Risperidone	Oral	4-5	Ib	as effective as haloperidol
Olanzapine	Oral, SC	3	Ib	limited efficacy in agitated delirium for SC administration
Quetiapine	Oral	1-7	Ib	effective with low risk of EPS
Amisulpride	Oral	6	Ic	
Aripriprazole	Oral	-	IIIb	effective in hypoactive delirium

* Gray and Taylor (2010), IM: intramuscular injection; IV: intravenous injection; SC; subcutaneous injection

Table 1. Summary of evidence on antipsychotic agents for managing delirium

7.3.2. Benzodiazepine

Lorazepam is primary used as hypnotics and anxiolytics. It has rapid onset and shorter duration of action, a low risk of accumulation and no major active metabolites. Its bioavailability is predictable when it is administered either orally or intramuscularly (Attard et al., 2008). Due to these preferable pharmacokinetic profiles, it is alternatively administered for controlling disruptive behavior in several clinical settings.

There was a prospective study suggested that intravenously administration of benzodiazepine added haloperidol can reduce the risk of EPS (Menza et al., 1988). An RCT of lorazepam monotherapy (3.0±3.6 mg for first 24 hours and 4.6±4.7 mg/day after day 2) did not show its efficacy in controlling delirious symptoms in AIDS patients. In addition, it continuously decreased cognitive function, as measured by the MMSE. Due to these preliminary results, this study was prematurely stopped (Breitbart et al., 1996).

Based on the results of a systematic review, there has been no adequate RCT to support the use of benzodiazepines in the management of non-alcohol withdrawal related delirium in patients admitted in the hospital (Lonergan et al., 2009). Although benzodiazepines are the first-line treatment for alcoholic withdrawal delirium, their evidence in the treatment of non-alcoholic delirium is very limited.

7.3.3. Cholinesterase inhibitors

Presumably, cholinergic deficiency (Mussi et al., 1999, Trzepacz, 2000) is postulated as neurochemical correlates of delirium. In addition, anticholinergic medications are correlated to drug-induced delirium (Han et al., 2001), and cholinergic medications can reduce symptoms of delirium in dementia (Wengel et al., 1998). It has been hypothesized that cholinesterase inhibitors may be beneficial for treating cholinergic deficiency in delirium.

Overshott et al. (2010) conducted a double-blind, placebo-controlled randomized trial of rivastigmine in the management of delirious patients hospitalized in medical settings. Patients (age≥ 65 years) were diagnosed as delirium by using the CAM. After entry, the patients in each group were assessed by using the CAM daily. Patients with delirium were randomly assigned to receive either rivastigmine 1.5 mg once a day and increased to 1.5 mg twice a day after seven days or an identical placebo (two tablets after seven days). A total of 15 patients were included in the study. Eight patients received rivastigmine, and seven patients received placebo. With regarded to the CAM scores, all patients in the rivastigmine group and 3 patients in the placebo group had a resolution of delirium when they exited the trial. However, there was no significant difference between groups on the duration of delirium (rivastigmine group 6.3 days versus placebo group 9.9 days).

There was an RCT comparing the efficacy and tolerability of donepezil and placebo. A total of 80 patients were randomly assigned to orally administered donepezil 5 mg once a day or a placebo capsule once a day, commenced 14 days before the surgery and continued taking for 14 days following the surgery. The delirium was identified with the Delirium Symptom Interview, the CAM, daily medical record, nurse-observation reviews, and the DSM-IV diagnostic criteria for delirium. With respect to DSM-IV criteria, patients diagnosed as delirium were suggested to receive a double dose of donepezil or placebo treatments. No measure outcome was used to assess in severity of delirium. The mean duration of postoperative delirium for the donepezil and placebo groups were 1.0 and 1.3 days, respectively (Liptzin et al., 2005, Overshott et al., 2008).

Marcantonio et al. (2011) conducted an RCT comparing the efficacy and safety of donepezil and placebo in reduction of the prevalence and severity of delirium in older adults undergoing hip fracture repair. Seventeen patients aged 70 or more were randomized to receive a daily donepezil 5 mg or placebo, initiated on the day before surgery or unless possible, administered within 24 hours after surgery. The treatment was continued for 30 days, unless side effects occurred. The presence and severity of delirium were measured by using the CAM and MDAS. Patients in the donepezil group had significantly more adverse events. With regard to delirium presence over time or the CAM scores over time, there were no significant differences between the donepezil and placebo groups in terms of delirium incidence or severity.

A pilot study of Oldenbeuving et al. (2008) investigated the efficacy and tolerability of rivastigmine in the treatment of delirium after stroke. Seventeen patients with delirium (DRS≥12) were treated with oral rivastigmine within the dose range of 3-12 mg a day. Based on the DRS scores, 16 of 17 patients had a decrease in severity of delirium after rivastigmine treatment. The mean duration of the delirium for 16 patients was 6.7 (2-17) days. No significant adverse event was observed.

Based on the findings, there has been no strong evidence supporting the use of cholinesterase inhibitors in the treatment of delirium. Conversely, these agents may cause a greater risk of adverse events in this population. Further studies should be carried out.

Delirious symptoms are likely to be improved by themselves after the recovery of underlining diseases. Judgment on the severity of these behavioral symptoms is easily biased by raters. In addition, placebo effects are noted in all area of therapeutic approach (Kradin, 2011). The percentage of placebo effect on psychiatric illness, such as anxiety and depression is often high (Raz et al., 2011). According to the nature of this medical condition, a randomized, placebo-controlled trial of a medication for controlling delirious symptoms is desperately needed to assess the efficacy and safety of a particular agent.

Among the medications mentioned above, only quetiapine has been examined in a placebo-controlled study. The superiority of quetiapine to placebo may suggest that the agents may be considered as first-line treatment for controlling the disruptive behavior of delirium. Low dose of other typical and atypical antipsychotics may be also effective. The evidence so far also suggests that haloperidol may be associated with EPS, and chlorpromazine has a risk for anticholinergic side effects. Other atypical antipsychotics that appear to be effective and tolerable in the management of delirium are risperidone, olanzapine, amisulpride and aripiprazole. Only aripiprazole may be effective for hypoactive delirium. Although benzodiazepine, especially lorazepam, is widely used in delirium, there is no evidence supporting its efficacy for the treatment of non-withdrawal delirium. Therefore, the use of benzodiazepine should be limited to alcohol or benzodiazepine withdrawal delirium only. Similarly, there has not been evidenced to demonstrate the efficacy of cholinesterase inhibitors, including donepezil and rivastigmine, in the treatment of delirium.

7.4. Environmental intervention

The reticular formation and its connections, the main sites of arousal and attention, are involved in delirium. Dysfunction of this system may affect the perception and interpretation of environmental stimuli in delirious patients. The reduction or over activity of the environmental factors may exacerbate the symptoms of delirium. Several studies, especially multi-component programs, have supported that an environmental intervention is also effective in the management of delirium.

Cole et al. (1994) conducted an RCT to determine a systematic intervention in elderly inpatients with DSM-IV delirium. Eighty-eight patients, aged 75 years or more, were enrolled in the study. The patients were randomized to either the treatment group (n=42) or the control group (n=46). Each treatment patient received a consultation by a geriatric internist or psychiatrist and followed up by a liaison nurse. Regular medical care was provided in the control group. The environmental intervention, used in this study, was the nursing intervention protocol, including the interventions for (1) environment: appropriate sensory input, only one stimulus or task background stimulation at a time, and medication not interrupting sleep, (2) orientation: environmental cues, such as clock, calendar and etc., verbal reminders of time, place and person, and needs of eye glasses or hearing aids, (3) familiarity: familiar possession from home, family members to stay with the patients, and the same staff to care for them (4) communication: clear, slow paced, simple and repetitive instructions and explanations, use of face-to-face contact, a warmth attitude and kind firmness, identification by name and information, acknowledgement of their emotions and encouragement of verbal expression, (5) activities: avoidance in physical restraint, free movement, provision of safety, encouragement of self-care and other personal activities. Two weeks after hospitalization, as measured by the Short Portable Mental Status Questionnaire (SPMSQ), the improvement was observed in the intervention group, while deterioration was observed in the control group. However, the difference was not reported by the end of 8-week period. There were statistically significant differences between the groups in terms of the use of restraints, length of hospital stay, discharges to a setting providing more care than needed before admission or mortality rate.

Milisen et al. (2001) developed and investigated the effectiveness of a nurse-led interdisciplinary intervention program for delirium. A total 120 participants (60 for intervention cohort, 60 for a usual care/non-intervention cohort) were included. The intervention protocol consisted of education for the nursing staff; systematic cognitive screening; consultative services by a delirium resource nurse, a geriatric nurse specialist, or a psychogeriatrician; use of a scheduled pain protocol. The findings showed that the intervention cohort group had shorter duration of delirium (p=0.3), less severity of delirium (p=0.049) and less memory impairment (p=0.046) than those of the control group. The length of hospital stay tended to be decreased in the intervention cohort compared with the control (p=0.09). The study suggested that this intervention was beneficial for older hip-fracture patients with delirium.

Cole et al. (2002) conducted an RCT to investigate the effectiveness of systematic detection and multidisciplinary care of delirium in reducing time to improvement of cognitive status in older patients admitted to general medical settings. Two hundred twenty-seven patients with high prevalent or incident delirium participated in the study. Significant differences between groups were not observed within the eight weeks after enrolment in terms of time to and rate of improvement of the Delirium Index, the Barthel Index, length of stay, rate of discharge into the community, living arrangements after discharge or survival. Based on the findings, systematic detection and multidisciplinary care of delirium did nots how a benefit over usual care for elderly patients in medical settings.

A prospective intervention study conducted by Lundstrom et al. (2005) determine an education program and a reorganization of nursing and medical care for improving the symptoms of delirium in elderly patients. A total of 400 patients, aged 70 or older, were consecutively admitted to either an intervention or a control ward. The intervention program composed of staff education emphasizing on the assessment, prevention, and treatment of delirium, as well as caregiver-patient interaction. The Organic Brain Syndrome Scale and the MMSE were used as outcome measures. Fewer patients in the intervention ward had delirious symptoms on day 7 compared with the control group (30.2% vs 59.7%, p=0.001). The mean length of hospitalization was significantly shorter in the intervention patients as compared with the control ones (9.4±8.2 vs 13.4±12.3 days, P< 0.001), especially for the delirious patients (10.8±8.3 vs 20.5±17.2 days, P< 0.001).

Inouye et al. (2006) conducted a cross-sectional survey of the Hospital Elder Life Program (HELP) dissemination in 17 study sites. The trained interdisciplinary teams assessed and intervened on six delirium risk factors, including orientation, therapeutic activities, early mobilization, vision/hearing optimization, oral volume repletion and sleep enhancement. The finding that the HELP improved hospital outcomes in delirium was promising in this population.

There was a prospective analysis to determine the pattern and frequency of implementation of environmental intervention in managing delirious patients admitted in an acute hospital service. Forty-six patients meeting the ICD-10 criteria for delirium were studied. The patients were categorized into hyperactive, hypoactive or mixed subtypes of delirium. The environmental strategies were the eight basic nursing strategies for delirium, including (1) frequent observation; (2) efforts by staff to re-orientate the patient to the surroundings; (3) effort made to avoid excessive staff changes; (4) nurse in single room; (5) uncluttered nursing environment; (6) use of an individual night light; (7) specific effort to minimize noise levels and (8) relatives or friends specifically requested to visit regularly in an effort to enhance re-orientation. The study found that these environmental strategies were more beneficial in the management of behavioral difficulties, such as overall severity of delirium, agitation, mood lability and sleep-wake cycle disturbance, than the core features of delirium, such as severity of disorientation, disturbed perception/thinking (Meagher et al., 1996).

The above-mentioned studies suggest the benefits ofthe environmental interventions for delirium, and, therefore, should be recommended in all patients with delirium. Those interventions aim to correct or reduce the sensory impairment, and to improve the patient's perception, by using eyeglasses and hearing aids. Optimal sensory stimulation is helpful to decrease the behavioral disturbance of delirium. While sensory deprivation may exacerbatethe behavioral disturbance, over stimulation, such as loud noise, should be also avoided.

Providing environmental cues, such as calendar, clock, family pictures, windows, should be encouraged to facilitate orientation. In addition, supportive interventions, including re-orientation, reassurance and explanation about delirium, could reduce fear and anxiety.

8. Prevention

Once a patient with high risks of delirium is hospitalized, all risks should be addressed, followed by the employment of effective preventive strategies (Salawu et al., 2009). Some studies have shown the benefits of some preventive interventions for delirium. In general, those strategies usually include the multidisciplinary and psychopharmacological interventions.

8.1. Non-pharmacological interventions

Multi-factors, including patient vulnerabilities, predisposing factors at admission and precipitating factors during hospitalization can interactively cause syndrome of delirium.

Inouye (2000) conducted a controlled clinical trial in 852 subjects to prevent delirium in elderly inpatients. Significant predisposing factors for delirium included vision impairment, severe illness, cognitive impairment and dehydration. Precipitating factors were physical restraint use, malnutrition, adding more than three drugs, bladder catheter use, and any iatrogenic event. The findings showed that the incidence of delirium was significantly reduced in the intervention group compared with usual care (9.9% vs. 15.0%, 95% CI: 0.39-0.92). The total number of days and episodes of delirium were also significantly smaller in the intervention group. These findings suggested that delirium prevention is useful and could reduce the morbidity and mortality associated with delirium in elderly patients.

Colombo et al. (2012) conducted a two-stage prospective observational study to determine the epidemiology, risk factors and predictors of delirium. The subjects were all patients admitted to the ICU settings over a year. The first phase was the observational stage, while the second one was the interventional phase. Delirium assessment was performed by using of the CAM twice daily after the sedation interruption. For the second phase, the patients were received both a re-orientation and environmental manipulations (e.g., acoustic and visual stimulation). The patients in phase 1 and 2 were 170 and 144, respectively. The incidence rate of delirium was significantly lower in the interventional group (phase-I vs. phase-II: 22% vs. 35.5%, p = 0.020). Based on the Cox's Proportional Hazard model, the use of re-orientation strategy was the strongest protective factor of delirium: (HR 0.504, 95% C.I. 0.313-0.890, p=0.034), while age (HR 1.034, 95% CI: 1.013-1.056, p=0.001) and sedation with midazolam plus opiate (HR 2.145, 95% CI: 2.247-4.032, p=0.018) were negative predictors.

Milisen et al. (2001) conducted a systemic review to investigate the characteristics and efficacy of various multicomponent programs for managing older patients with delirium admitted in hospitals. Three RCTs, three controlled trials and one before-after study were included in the review. The multicomponent strategies for preventing delirium appear to be the most efficacious in reducing the incidence, both in surgical and medical patients. In addition, some additional effects of preventive intervention were observed in the duration and severity of delirium, as well as functional status. The review suggested that multicomponent strategies are effective for preventing delirium.

Yang et al. (2008) conducted a prospective cohort study to investigate the mediating role of activity participation between educational attainment and risk of delirium. The contributions of participation in specific activities for the development of delirium were also determined. Seven hundred seventy-nine newly admitted patients without dementia, aged 70 or older, were studied. The findings showed that activity participation before hospitalization mediated the relationship between education and risk for delirium in elderly persons without dementia. It also suggested that participation in regular exercise was a significantly protective factor of delirium.

Another study examined the efficacy of multicomponent intervention for preventing delirium. Inpatients with an intermediate or high risk for delirium were randomly assigned to receive either a non-pharmacological intervention delivered by family members (144 patients) or standard management (143 patients). The outcome measure was the occurrence of delirium during hospitalization. The incidence rates of delirium in the intervention group and the control group were 5.6% and 13.3% (relative risk:0.41; 95% CI: 0.19–0.92; P = 0.027), respectively. The findings suggested that the non-pharmacological prevention of delirium given by family members, as compared with standard management, could reduce the patients' risk of delirium (Martinez et al., 2012).

These findings suggest that non-pharmacological interventions can reduce the incidence of delirium. Effective interventions, including multicomponent approach frequently focuses on predisposing factors in an individual patient. However, environmental prevention, such as re-orientation and environmental stimulation, are also effective for preventing delirium. A strong protective factor against delirium is the routinely participation in exercise. The use of multicomponent interventions by family members can also reduce the risk of delirium.

8.2. Psychopharmacological interventions

There have been several studies examining the effectiveness of antipsychotic medications for preventing delirium. Kalisvaart et al. (2005) conducted an RCT comparing haloperidol and placebo for preventing postoperative delirium in elderly hip-surgery patients, who were at risk for delirium. A number of 430 hip-surgery patients, aged 70 and older, at risk for postoperative delirium were randomly assigned to receive haloperidol 1.5 mg/d or placebo, started before surgery and continued for up to 3 days after surgery. The incidence rates of postoperative delirium in both groups were not significantly different (haloperidol vs placebo, 15.1% vs. 16.5%). The means of delirium duration in haloperidol and placebo treatment groups were 5.4 vs 11.8 days, orderly (mean difference 4.0, 95% CI=2.0-5.8, P<.001), and the means of hospital stay were 17.1±11.1 and 22.6±16.7 days, respectively (mean difference 5.5 days, 95% CI=1.4-2.3; P<.001). The adverse events were not significantly different between groups. These results suggested that low doses of haloperidol might not be able to prevent postoperative delirium. However, it is safe and can decrease the severity, duration, and the length of hospitalization for these patients.

Wang et al. (2012) conducted an RCT to determine the efficacy and safety of intravenous haloperidol for preventing delirium in critically ill elderly patients who had undergone non-cardiac surgery. A total of 457 patients, aged 65 years older, who were admitted to the intensive care unit after non cardiac surgery, were included and randomized to receive either haloperidol (0.5 mg intravenous bolus injection followed by continuous infusion at a rate of 0.1 mg/h for 12 hours; n = 229) or placebo (n = 228). The incidence rates of delirium were significantly lower in the haloperidol group(15.3% vs 23.2%, p = 0.031) during the first seven day after surgery. No drug related adverse event was noted. A short-term, low-dose intravenous haloperidol prophylaxis appeared to reduce the incidence rate of postoperative delirium.

Prakanrattana and Prapaitrakool (2007) conducted an RCT to determine the effects of risperidone in preventing postoperative delirium after cardiac surgery with cardiopulmonary bypass. A total of 126 adult patients underwent elective surgery were randomized to receive risperidone 1 mg or placebo after regained consciousness. With regard to the using of CAM, the incidence of postoperative delirium in the risperidone group was significantly lower than that in the placebo group (11.1% vs. 31.7% respectively, P=0.009, relative risk: 0.35, 95% CI: 0.16-0.77).

Larsen et al. (2010) conducted an RCT comparing the efficacy of olanzapine and placebo in preventing postoperative delirium in elderly patients after joint-replacement surgery. A total of 400 elderly patients, aged 65 years or more, who had undergone elective knee- or hip-replacement surgery, were randomly assigned to receive either 5 mg of orally-disintegrating olanzapine or placebo before and after surgery. The findings showed that the olanzapine group had a significantly lower incidence of delirium.

There have been a few studies of cholinesterase inhibitors for preventing delirium. Liptzin et al. (2005) conducted an RCT comparing donepezil and placebo for the prophylaxis of postoperative delirium in elderly patients, who had undergone elective total joint-replacement surgery. Eighty patients without dementia were randomly assigned to receive either donepezil or placebo for 14 days before surgery and 14 days afterward. The findings did not show any benefit of donepezil in preventiong delirium in this population.

Gamberini et al. (2009) conducted an RCT to compare rivastigmine and placebo for preventing delirium in elderly patients during the first six days after elective cardiac surgery. A total of 120 patients, aged 65 or older, underwent the surgery with cardiopulmonary bypass were randomized to receive either placebo or rivastigmine. The incidence rates of delirium were not significantly between groups (30% vs 32%, p = 0.8). The findings did not support a short-term oral administered rivastigmine for delirium prophylaxis in this population.

Drug	Route administration	Dose	Level of evidence*	Comment
Haloperidol	IV	0.1 mg/hr	1b	0.5 mg intravenous bolus injection followed by continuous infusion at a rate of 0.1 mg/h for 12 hrs
Risperidone	Oral	1 mg/day	1b	
Olanzapine	Oral	5 mg/day	1b	
Melatonin	Oral	0.5 mg/day	1b	Administer at night

* Gray and Taylor (2010)

Table 2. Summary of evidences relevant to the pharmacological prophylaxis of delirium

There was a randomized, double-blinded, placebo-controlled trial of low dose exogenous melatonin in preventing delirium. A total of 145 patients, aged 65 years or older, hospitalized in a medical unit were randomly assigned to receive either 0.5 mg of melatonin or placebo every night for 14 days or until discharge. Based on the CAM, the incidence rate of delirium in the melatonin group was significant lower than that in the placebo group (12% vs 31%, p=0.014). The findings suggested that exogenous low dose melatonin may be of benefit in preventing delirium in this population (Al-Aama et al., 2012).

The above-mentioned findings demonstrate the benefits low-dose risperidone and olanzapine in preventing delirium. While they can reduce the incidence rate of delirium, their adverse events, in particular EPS, appear to be comparable to placebo. Similarly, exogenous low-dose melatonin administered at night time may be able to prevent delirium. Although haloperidol can reduce severity, duration and length of hospital stay in postoperative delirium, it might not be able to prevent the occurrence of this condition. However, cholinesterase inhibitors, including donepezil and rivastigmine may have no efficacy in this regard. Therefore, at low doses, high-potency antipsychotic agents, atypical antipsychotic medications or exogenous melatonin may be beneficial for the prevention of delirium in patients at high risk or subsydrome of delirium.

9. Further studies

Several lines of evidence indicate that pharmacological and environmental interventions are effective in the management and prophylaxis of delirium. However, those studies still have some limitations, including methodological weakness, small sample sizes, lack of placebo control in several studies and the specific patients. Further randomized, placebo-controlled trials and systemic reviews with well-defined methodology, large sample sizes, consistent outcomes and various clinical settings may be helpful in clarifying the benefits of these interventions.

10. Conclusion

Delirium is a condition in medical emergency, common in medical or surgical settings and highly incident in intensive care units. Several causative factors for the development of delirium have been identified. Specific treatment for curing or removing the causes is an effective approach. Initially, the precipitating factors are often overlooked or unidentified. Therefore, supportive and symptomatic managements are beneficial. For hyperactive type of delirium, all antipsychotic medications may help relief the behavioral disturbance, including psychotic symptoms. Although haloperidol is considered as the first-line treatment, it may increase the risk of adverse events, especially EPS. Alternatively, atypical antipsychotic agents, which have low propensity to induce EPS, may be useful in this condition. Intravenous haloperidol may be associated with QT prolongation and torsades de pointes. To avoid these serious adverse events, only low doses of IV haloperidol (a total cumulative dose < 2 mg) should be administered in delirious patients without concomitant risk factors. Based on its pharmacokinetic profile, IM haloperidol can be an alternative for the behavioral control of acute or severe delirium. For hypoactive delirium, only aripriprazole, a non sedative antipsychotic agent, is evidently beneficial. In addition to psychopharmacological interventions, environmental manipulation is also necessary in the management of delirium and should be used in all delirious patients. Preventing delirium is challenging. A number of studies demonstrate the efficacy of some interventions in preventing delirium. The multicomponent strategy, systemically focusing on predisposing factors in individual patients is one of the highly effective approaches. Pharmacological prophylaxis is another strategy in preventing delirium. The evidence so far suggests that risperidone, olanzapine and melatonin may be effective in preventing delirium.

Acknowledgement

We thank Professor Manit Srisurapranont, Department of Psychiatry, Faculty of Medicine, Chiang Mai University, Thailand for reviewing and editing this chapter.

Author details

Narong Maneeton and Benchalak Maneeton

Department of Psychiatry, Faculty of Medicine, Chiang Mai University, Thailand

References

[1] Al-Aama, T., Brymer, C., Gutmanis, I., Woolmore-Goodwin, S. M., Esbaugh, J. & Dasgupta, M. (2012). Melatonin decreases delirium in elderly patients: a randomized,

placebo-controlled trial. *International journal of geriatric psychiatry,* Vol. 26, No. 7, pp. 687-694, ISSN1099-1166

[2] Aldemir, M., Ozen, S., Kara, I. H., Sir, A. & Bac, B. (2001). Predisposing factors for delirium in the surgical intensive care unit. *Critical care,* Vol. 5, No. 5, pp. 265-270, ISSN1364-8535

[3] Ali, S., Patel, M., Jabeen, S., Bailey, R. K., Patel, T., Shahid, M., Riley, W. J. & Arain, A. (2011). Insight into delirium. *Innovations in clinical neuroscience,* Vol. 8, No. 10, pp. 25-34, ISSN 2158-8341

[4] American Psychiatric Association. (1999). American Psychiatric Association Practice guideline for the treatment of patients with delirium. *The American journal of psychiatry,* Vol. 156, No. supplement 5, pp. 1-20, ISSN 0002-953X

[5] American Psychiatric Association. (2005) *Diagnostic and statistical manual of mental disorders,* American Psychiatric Association, ISBN 0-89042-061-0, Washington, USA

[6] Attard, A., Ranjith, G. & Taylor, D. (2008). Delirium and its treatment. *CNS drugs,* Vol. 22, No. 8, pp. 631-644, ISSN 1172-7047

[7] Bledowski, J. & Trutia, A. (2012) A review of pharmacologic management and prevention strategies for delirium in the intensive care unit. *Psychosomatics,* Vol. 53, No. 3, pp. 203-211,ISSN 1545-7206

[8] Boettger, S. & Breitbart, W. (2011). An open trial of aripiprazole for the treatment of delirium in hospitalized cancer patients. *Palliative & supportive care,* Vol. 9, No. 4, pp. 351-357, ISSN 1478-9523

[9] Boettger, S., Friedlander, M., Breitbart, W. & Passik, S. (2011). Aripiprazole and haloperidol in the treatment of delirium. *The Australian and New Zealand journal of psychiatry,* Vol. 45, No. 6, pp. 477-482, ISSN 1440-1614

[10] Breitbart, W., Marotta, R., Platt, M. M., Weisman, H., Derevenco, M., Grau, C., Corbera, K., Raymond, S., Lund, S. & Jacobson, P. (1996). A double-blind trial of haloperidol,chlorpromazine, and lorazepam in the treatment of delirium in hospitalized AIDS patients. *The American journal of psychiatry,* Vol. 153, No. 2, pp. 231-237,ISSN 0002-953X

[11] Breitbart, W., Rosenfeld, B., Roth, A., Smith, M. J., Cohen, K. & Passik, S. (1997). The Memorial Delirium Assessment Scale. *Journal of pain and symptom management,* Vol. 13, No. 3, pp. 128-137, ISSN 0885-3924

[12] Burapakajornpong N., Maneeton, B. & Srisurapanont M. (2012) Pattern and risk factors of alcohol withdrawal delirium. *Journal of the Medical Association of Thailand,* Vol. 94, No. 8, pp. 991-997, ISSN 0125-2208

[13] Burns, A., Gallagley, A. & Byrne, J. (2004). Delirium. *Journal of neurology, neurosurgery, and psychiatry,* Vol. 75, No. 3, pp. 362-367, ISSN 0022-3050

[14] Catic, A. G. (2011). Identification and management of in-hospital drug-induced delirium in older patients. *Drugs & aging,* Vol. 28, No. 9, pp. 737-748, ISSN 1170-229X

[15] Chaput, A. J. & Bryson, G. L. (2012). Postoperative delirium: risk factors and management: continuing professional development. *Canadian journal of anaesthesia,* Vol. 59, No. 3, pp. 304-320, ISSN 1496-8975

[16] Clegg, A. & Young, J. B. (2011). Which medications to avoid in people at risk of delirium: a systematic review. *Age and ageing,* Vol. 40, No. 1, pp. 23-29, ISSN 1468-2834

[17] Cole, M. G., Ciampi, A., Belzile, E. & Zhong, L. (2009). Persistent delirium in older hospital patients: a systematic review of frequency and prognosis. *Age and ageing,* Vol. 38, No. 1, pp. 19-26, ISSN 1468-2834

[18] Cole, M. G., Mccusker, J., Bellavance, F., Primeau, F. J., Bailey, R. F., Bonnycastle, M. J. & Laplante, J. (2002). Systematic detection and multidisciplinary care of delirium in older medical inpatients: a randomized trial. *Canadian Medical Association journal,* Vol. 167, No. 7, pp. 753-759, ISSN 0820-3946

[19] Cole, M. G., Primeau, F. J., Bailey, R. F., Bonnycastle, M. J., Masciarelli, F., Engelsmann, F., Pepin, M. J. & Ducic, D. (1994). Systematic intervention for elderly inpatients with delirium: a randomized trial. *Canadian Medical Association journal,* Vol. 151, No. 7, pp. 965-970, ISSN 0820-3946

[20] Colombo, R., Corona, A., Praga, F., Minari, C., Giannotti, C., Castelli, A. & Raimondi, F. (2012). A reorientation strategy for reducing delirium in the critically ill. Results of an interventional study. *Minerva anestesiologica,*(July 6), ISSN 1827-1596,[Epub ahead of print]

[21] De Jonghe, J. F., Kalisvaart, K. J., Dijkstra, M., Van Dis, H., Vreeswijk, R., Kat, M. G., Eikelenboom, P., Van Der Ploeg, T. & Van Gool, W. A. (2007). Early symptoms in the prodromal phase of delirium: a prospective cohort study in elderly patients undergoing hip surgery. *The American journal of geriatric psychiatry,* Vol. 15, No. 2, pp. 112-121, ISSN 1064-7481

[22] De Wet, H., Levitt, N. & Tipping, B. (2007). Executive cognitive impairment detected by simple bedside testing is associated with poor glycaemic control in type 2 diabetes. *South African medical journal,* Vol. 97, No. 11, pp. 1074-1076, ISSN 0256-9574

[23] Devlin, J. W., Roberts, R. J., Fong, J. J., Skrobik, Y., Riker, R. R., Hill, N. S., Robbins, T. & Garpestad, E. (2010). Efficacy and safety of quetiapine in critically ill patients with delirium: a prospective, multicenter, randomized, double-blind, placebo-controlled pilot study. *Critical care medicine,* Vol. 38, No. 2, pp. 419-427, ISSN 1530-0293

[24] Elsayem, A., Bush, S. H., Munsell, M. F., Curry, E., 3rd, Calderon, B. B., Paraskevopoulos, T., Fadul, N. & Bruera, E. (2010). Subcutaneous olanzapine for hyperactive or mixed delirium in patients with advanced cancer: a preliminary study. *Journal of pain and symptom management,* Vol. 40, No. 5, pp. 774-782, ISSN 1873-6513

[25] Eriksson, I., Gustafson, Y., Fagerstrom, L. & Olofsson, B. (2011). Urinary tract infection in very old women is associated with delirium. *International psychogeriatrics,* Vol. 23, No. 3, pp. 496-502, ISSN 1741-203X

[26] Fadel, D. & Serra, H. A. (2009). Cocaine-induced agitated delirium, a different consequence of cocaine addiction. *Vertex,* Vol. 20, No. 84, pp. 85-92, ISSN 0327-6139

[27] Flacker, J. M. & Lipsitz, L. A. (1999). Neural mechanisms of delirium: current hypotheses and evolving concepts. *The journals of gerontology. Series A, Biological sciences and medical sciences,* Vol. 54, No. 6, pp. B239-246, ISNN 1079-5006

[28] Fong, T. G., Jones, R. N., Marcantonio, E. R., Tommet, D., Gross, A. L., Habtemariam, D., Schmitt, E., Yap, L. & Inouye, S. K. (2012). Adverse outcomes after hospitalization and delirium in persons with Alzheimer disease. *Annals of internal medicine,* Vol. 156, No. 12, pp. 848-856, ISSN 1539-3704

[29] Froemming, J. S., Lam, Y. W., Jann, M. W. & Davis, C. M. (1989). Pharmacokinetics of haloperidol. *Clinical pharmacokinetics,* Vol. 17,No. 6, pp. 396-423, ISSN 0312-5963

[30] Gamberini, M., Bolliger, D., LuratiBuse, G. A., Burkhart, C. S., Grapow, M., Gagneux, A., Filipovic, M., Seeberger, M. D., Pargger, H., Siegemund, M., Carrel, T., Seiler, W. O., Berres, M., Strebel, S. P., Monsch, A. U. & Steiner, L. A. (2009). Rivastigmine for the prevention of postoperative delirium in elderly patients undergoing elective cardiac surgery-a randomized controlled trial. *Crit Care Med,* Vol. 37, No. 5, pp. 1762-1768, ISSN 1530-0293

[31] Gray, G. E. & Taylor, C. B. (2010). Searching for answers, In: *How to practice evidence-based psychiatry: basic principles and case studies,* C. B. Taylor, (Ed.), 21-34, American Psychiatric Publisher, Inc., ISBN 978-1-58562-365-5, Arlington, USA

[32] Grover, S., Kate, N., Agarwal, M., Mattoo, S. K., Avasthi, A., Malhotra, S., Kulhara, P., Chakrabarti, S. & Basu, D. (2012). Delirium in elderly people: a study of a psychiatric liaison service in north India. *International psychogeriatrics,* Vol. 24, No. 1, pp. 117-127, ISSN 1741-203X

[33] Grover, S., Kumar, V. & Chakrabarti, S. (2011). Comparative efficacy study of haloperidol, olanzapine and risperidone in delirium. *Journal of psychosomatic research,* Vol. 71, No. 4, pp. 277-281, ISSN 1879-1360

[34] Gunther, M. L., Morandi, A. & Ely, E. W. (2008). Pathophysiology of delirium in the intensive care unit. *Critical care clinics,* Vol. 24, No. 1, pp. 45-65, viii, ISSN 0749-0704

[35] Han, C. S. & Kim, Y. K. (2004). A double-blind trial of risperidone and haloperidol for the treatment of delirium. *Psychosomatics,* Vol. 45, No. 4, pp. 297-301, ISSN 0033-3182

[36] Han, L., Mccusker, J., Cole, M., Abrahamowicz, M., Primeau, F. & Elie, M. (2001). Use of medications with anticholinergic effect predicts clinical severity of delirium symptoms in older medical inpatients. *Archives of internal medicine,* Vol. 161, No. 8, pp. 1099-1105, ISSN 0003-9926

[37] Harrington, A. L., Dixon, T. M. & Ho, C. H. (2011). Vitamin B(12) deficiency as a cause of delirium in a patient with spinal cord injury. *Archives of physical medicine and rehabilitation*, Vol. 92, No. 11, pp. 1917-1920,ISSN 1532-821X

[38] Inouye, S. K. (2000). Prevention of delirium in hospitalized older patients: risk factors and targeted intervention strategies. *Annals of medicine*, Vol. 32, No. 4, pp. 257-263, ISSN 0785-3890

[39] Inouye, S. K. (2004). A practical program for preventing delirium in hospitalized elderly patients. *Cleveland Clinic journal of medicine*, Vol. 71, No. 11, pp. 890-896, ISSN 0891-1150

[40] Inouye, S. K., Baker, D. I., Fugal, P. & Bradley, E. H. (2006). Dissemination of the hospital elder life program: implementation, adaptation, and successes. *Journal of the American Geriatrics Society*, Vol. 54, No. 10, pp. 1492-1499, ISSN 0002-8614

[41] Inouye, S. K. & Charpentier, P. A. (1996). Precipitating factors for delirium in hospitalized elderly persons. Predictive model and interrelationship with baseline vulnerability. *JAMA*, Vol. 275, No. 11, pp. 852-857, ISSN 0098-7484

[42] Inouye, S. K., Van Dyck, C. H., Alessi, C. A., Balkin, S., Siegal, A. P. & Horwitz, R. I. (1990). Clarifying confusion: the confusion assessment method. A new method for detection of delirium. *Annals of internal medicine*, Vol. 113, No. 12, pp. 941-948, ISSN 0003-4819

[43] Jacobson, S. & Jerrier, H. (2000). EEG in delirium. *Seminars in clinical neuropsychiatry*, Vol. 5, No. 2, pp. 86-92, ISSN 1084-3612

[44] Kalisvaart, K. J., De Jonghe, J. F., Bogaards, M. J., Vreeswijk, R., Egberts, T. C., Burger, B. J., Eikelenboom, P. & Van Gool, W. A. (2005). Haloperidol prophylaxis for elderly hip-surgery patients at risk for delirium: a randomized placebo-controlled study. *Journal ofthe American Geriatrics Society*, Vol. 53, No. 10, pp. 1658-1666, ISSN 0002-8614

[45] Kane, F. J., JR., Remmel, R. & Moody, S. (1993). Recognizing and treating delirium in patients admitted to general hospitals. *Southern medical journal*, Vol. 86, No. 9, pp. 985-988, ISSN 0038-4348

[46] Kasick, D. P., Mcknight, C. A. & Klisovic, E. (2012). "Bath salt" ingestion leading to severe intoxication delirium: two cases and a brief review of the emergence of mephedrone use. *The American journal of drug and alcohol abuse*, Vol. 38, No. 2, pp. 176-180, ISSN 1097-9891

[47] Khurana, V., Gambhir, I. S. & Kishore, D. (2011). Evaluation of delirium in elderly: a hospital-based study. *Geriatrics & gerontology international*, Vol. 11, No. 4, pp. 467-473, ISSN 1447-05941447-0594

[48] Kim, S. W., Yoo, J. A., Lee, S. Y., Kim, S. Y., Bae, K. Y., Yang, S. J., Kim, J. M., Shin, I. S. & Yoon, J. S. (2010). Risperidone versus olanzapine for the treatment of delirium. *Human psychopharmacology*, Vol. 25, No. 4, pp. 298-302, ISSN 1099-1077

[49] Kradin, R. L. (2011). Placebo response: a consideration of its role in therapeutics. *Current psychiatry reports,* Vol. 13, No. 1, pp. 37-42, ISSN 1535-1645

[50] Larsen, K. A., Kelly, S. E., Stern, T. A., Bode, R. H., JR., Price, L. L., Hunter, D. J., Gulczynski, D., Bierbaum, B. E., Sweeney, G. A., Hoikala, K. A., Cotter, J. J. & Potter, A. W. (2010). Administration of olanzapine to prevent postoperative delirium in elderly joint-replacement patients: a randomized, controlled trial. *Psychosomatics,* Vol. 51, No. 5, pp. 409-418, ISSN 1545-7206

[51] Lee, K. U., Won, W. Y., Lee, H. K., Kweon, Y. S., Lee, C. T., Pae, C. U. & Bahk, W. M. (2005). Amisulpride versus quetiapine for the treatment of delirium: a randomized, open prospective study. *International clinical psychopharmacology,* Vol. 20, No. 6, pp. 311-314, ISSN 0268-1315

[52] Liptzin, B., Laki, A., Garb, J. L., Fingeroth, R. & Krushell, R. (2005). Donepezil in the prevention and treatment of post-surgical delirium. *The American journal of geriatric psychiatry,* Vol. 13, No. 12, pp. 1100-1106, ISSN 1064-7481

[53] Lonergan, E., Luxenberg, J. & AreosaSastre, A. (2009). Benzodiazepines for delirium. *Cochrane database of systematic reviews (Online),* No. 4, pp. CD006379, ISSN 1469-493X

[54] Lorenzl, S., Fusgen, I. & Noachtar, S. (2012). Acute confusional States in the elderly-diagnosis and treatment. *DeutschesArzteblatt international,* Vol. 109, No. 21, pp. 391-400, ISSN 1866-0452 1866-0452

[55] Lundstrom, M., Edlund, A., Karlsson, S., Brannstrom, B., Bucht, G. & Gustafson, Y. (2005). A multifactorial intervention program reduces the duration of delirium, length of hospitalization, and mortality in delirious patients. Journal of the American Geriatrics Society, Vol. 53, No. 4, pp. 622-628, ISSN 0002-8614

[56] Maldonado, J. R. (2008a). Delirium in the acute care setting: characteristics, diagnosis and treatment. *Critical care clinics,* Vol. 24, No. 4, pp. 657-722, vii, ISSN 0749-0704

[57] Maldonadoaldonado, J. R. (2008b). Pathoetiological model of delirium: a comprehensive understanding of the neurobiology of delirium and an evidence-based approach to prevention and treatment. *Critical care clinics,* Vol. 24, No. 4, pp. 789-856, ix, ISSN 0749-0704

[58] Maneeton, B., Khemawichanurat, W. & Maneeton, N. (2007a). Consultation-liaison psychiatry in MaharajNakorn Chiang Mai Hospital. *ASEAN Journal of Psychiatry,* Vol. 8, No. 2, pp. 124-130, ISSN 2231-7805

[59] Maneeton, B., Maneeton, N. & Srisurapanont, M. (2007b). An open-label study of quetiapine for delirium. *Journal of the Medical Association of Thailand,* Vol. 90, No. 10, pp. 2158-2163, ISSN 0125-2208

[60] Maneeton, B., Maneeton, N. & Srisurapanont, M. (2011). A double-blind, randomised, controlled trial of quetiapine versus haloperidol for the treatment of delirium: a preliminary report. *European Neuropsychopharmacology,* Vol. 21, pp. s557

[61] Marcantonio, E. R., Palihnich, K., Appleton, P. & Davis, R. B. (2011). Pilot randomized trial of donepezil hydrochloride for delirium after hip fracture. *Journal of the American Geriatrics Society,* Vol. 59 Suppl 2, pp. S282-8, ISSN 1532-5415

[62] Marcantonio, E. R., Rudolph, J. L., Culley, D., Crosby, G., Alsop, D. & Inouye, S. K. (2006). Serum biomarkers for delirium. *The journals of gerontology. Series A, Biological sciences and medical sciences,* Vol. 61, No. 12, pp. 1281-1286, ISSN 1079-5006

[63] Martin, J. J. (2012). Confusion, agitation and delirium. *Frontiers of neurology and neuroscience,* Vol. 30, pp. 46-49, ISSN 1662-2804

[64] Martinez, F. T., Tobar, C., Beddings, C. I., Vallejo, G. & Fuentes, P. (2012). Preventing delirium in an acute hospital using a non-pharmacological intervention. *Age and ageing,* Vol. 41, No. 5, pp. 629-634, ISSN 1468-2834

[65] Meagher, D. J., O'Hanlon, D., O'Mahony, E. & Casey, P. R. (1996). The use of environmental strategies and psychotropic medication in the management of delirium. *The British journal of psychiatry,* Vol. 168, No. 4, pp. 512-515, ISSN 0007-1250

[66] Menza, M. A., Murray, G. B., Holmes, V. F. & Rafuls, W. A. (1987). Decreased extrapyramidal symptoms with intravenous haloperidol. *The Journal of clinical psychiatry,* Vol. 48, No. 7, pp. 278-280, ISSN 0160-6689

[67] Menza, M. A., Murray, G. B., Holmes, V. F. & Rafuls, W. A. (1988). Controlled study of extrapyramidal reactions in the management of delirious, medically ill patients: intravenous haloperidol versus intravenous haloperidol plus benzodiazepines. *Heart Lung,* Vol. 17, No. 3, pp. 238-241, ISSN 0147-9563

[68] Meyer-Massetti, C., Cheng, C. M., Sharpe, B. A., Meier, C. R. & Guglielmo, B. J. (2010). The FDA extended warning for intravenous haloperidol and torsades de pointes: how should institutions respond? *Journal of hospital medicine,* Vol. 5, No. 4, pp. E8-16, ISSN 1553-5606

[69] Milisen, K., Foreman, M. D., Abraham, I. L., De Geest, S., Godderis, J., Vandermeulen, E., Fischler, B., Delooz, H. H., Spiessens, B. & Broos, P. L. (2001). A nurse-led interdisciplinary intervention program for delirium in elderly hip-fracture patients. *Journal of the American Geriatrics Society,* Vol. 49, No. 5, pp. 523-532, ISSN 0002-8614

[70] Moulaert, P. (1989). Treatment of acute nonspecific delirium with i. v. haloperidol in surgical intensive care patients. *ActaanaesthesiologicaBelgica,* Vol. 40, No. 3, pp. 183-186, ISSN 0001-5164

[71] Mussi, C., Ferrari, R., Ascari, S. & Salvioli, G. (1999). Importance of serum anticholinergic activity in the assessment of elderly patients with delirium. *Journal of geriatric psychiatry and neurology,* Vol. 12, No. 2, pp. 82-86, ISSN 0891-9887

[72] Nakatani, Y. & Hara, T. (1998). Disturbance of consciousness due to methamphetamine abuse. A study of 2 patients. *Psychopathology,* Vol. 31, No. 3, pp. 131-137, ISSN 0254-4962

[73] O'Keeffe, S. T., Tormey, W. P., Glasgow, R. & Lavan, J. N. (1994). Thiamine deficiency in hospitalized elderly patients. *Gerontology,* Vol. 40, No. 1, pp. 18-24, ISSN 0304-324X

[74] Oldenbeuving, A. W., De Kort, P. L., Jansen, B. P., Kappelle, L. J. & Roks, G. (2008). A pilot study of rivastigmine in the treatment of delirium after stroke: a safe alternative. *BMC neurology,* Vol. 8, pp. 34, ISSN 1471-2377

[75] Olsson, T. (1999). Activity in the hypothalamic-pituitary-adrenal axis and delirium. *Dementia and geriatric cognitive disorders,* Vol. 10, No. 5, pp. 345-349, ISSN 1420-8008

[76] Overshott, R., Karim, S. & Burns, A. (2008). Cholinesterase inhibitors for delirium. Cochrane database of systematic reviews (Online),No. 1, pp. CD005317, ISSN 1469-493X

[77] Overshott, R., Vernon, M., Morris, J. & Burns, A. (2010). Rivastigmine in the treatment of delirium in older people: a pilot study. *International psychogeriatrics,* Vol. 22, No. 5, pp. 812-818, ISSN 1741-203X

[78] Pearson, A., De Vries, A., Middleton, S. D., Gillies, F., White, T. O., Armstrong, I. R., Andrew, R., Seckl, J. R. & Maclullich, A. M. (2011). Cerebrospinal fluid cortisol levels are higher in patients with delirium versus controls. *BMC research notes,* Vol. 3, pp. 33, ISSN 1756-0500

[79] Praditsuwan, R., Limmathuroskul, D., Assanasen, J., Pakdeewongse, S., Eiamjinnasuwat, W., Sirisuwat, A. & Srinonprasert, V. (2012). Prevalence and incidence of delirium in Thai older patients: a study at general medical wards in Siriraj Hospital. *Journal of the Medical Association of Thailand,* Vol. 95 Suppl 2, pp. S245-250, ISSN 0125-2208

[80] Prakanrattana, U. & Prapaitrakool, S. (2007). Efficacy of risperidone for prevention of postoperative delirium in cardiac surgery. *Anaesthesia and intensive care,* Vol. 35, No. 5, pp. 714-719, ISSN 0310-057X

[81] Rahkonen, T., Makela, H., Paanila, S., Halonen, P., Sivenius, J. & Sulkava, R. (2000). Delirium in elderly people without severe predisposing disorders: etiology and 1-year prognosis after discharge. *International psychogeriatrics,* Vol. 12, No. 4, pp. 473-481, ISSN 1041-6102

[82] Ramirez-Bermudez, J., Lopez-Gomez, M., Sosa Ana, L., Aceves, S., Nader-Kawachi, J. & Nicolini, H. (2006). Frequency of delirium in a neurological emergency room. *The Journal of neuropsychiatry and clinical neurosciences,* Vol. 18, No. 1, pp. 108-112, ISSN 0895-0172

[83] Raz, A., Campbell, N., Guindi, D., Holcroft, C., Dery, C. & Cukier, O. (2011). Placebos in clinical practice: comparing attitudes, beliefs, and patterns of use between academic psychiatrists and nonpsychiatrists. *Canadian journal of psychiatry,* Vol. 56, No. 4, pp. 198-208, ISSN 1497-0015

[84] Robertsson, B., Blennow, K., Brane, G., Edman, A., Karlsson, I., Wallin, A. & Gottfries, C. G. (2001). Hyperactivity in the hypothalamic-pituitary-adrenal axis in de-

mented patients with delirium. *International clinical psychopharmacology,* Vol. 16, No. 1, pp. 39-47, ISSN 0268-1315

[85] Saitz, R. (1998). Introduction to alcohol withdrawal. *Alcohol health and research world,* Vol. 22, No. 1, pp. 5-12, ISSN 0090-838X

[86] Salawu, F. K., Danburam, A. & Ogualili, P. (2009). Delirium: issues in diagnosis and management. *Annals of African medicine,* Vol. 8, No. 3, pp. 139-146, ISSN 0975-5764

[87] Schaffer, C. B., Shahid, A., Javaid, J. I., Dysken, M. W. & Davis, J. M. (1982). Bioavailability of intramuscular versus oral haloperidol in schizophrenic patients. *Journal of clinical psychopharmacology,* Vol. 2, No. 4, pp. 274-277, ISSN 0271-0749

[88] Seaman, J. S., Schillerstrom, J., Carroll, D. & Brown, T. M. (2006). Impaired oxidative metabolism precipitates delirium: a study of 101 ICU patients. *Psychosomatics,* Vol. 47, No. 1, pp. 56-61, ISSN 0033-3182

[89] Siddiqi, N., House, A. O. & Holmes, J. D. (2006). Occurrence and outcome of delirium in medical in-patients: a systematic literature review. *Age and ageing,* Vol. 35, No. 4, pp. 350-364, ISSN 0002-0729

[90] Sidhu, K. S., Balon, R., Ajluni, V. & Boutros, N. N. (2009). Standard EEG and the difficult-to-assess mental status. *Annals of clinical psychiatry,* Vol. 21, No. 2, pp. 103-108, ISSN 1547-3325

[91] Simone, M. J. & Tan, Z. S. (2011). The role of inflammation in the pathogenesis of delirium and dementia in older adults: a review. *CNS neuroscience & therapeutics,* Vol. 17, No. 5, pp. 506-513, ISSN 1755-5949

[92] Skrobik, Y. K., Bergeron, N., Dumont, M. & Gottfried, S. B. (2004). Olanzapine vs haloperidol: treating delirium in a critical care setting. *Intensive care medicine,* Vol. 30, No. 3, pp. 444-449, ISSN 0342-4642

[93] Srinonprasert, V., Pakdeewongse, S., Assanasen, J., Eiamjinnasuwat, W., Sirisuwat, A., Limmathuroskul, D. & Praditsuwan, R. (2011). Risk factors for developing delirium in older patients admitted to general medical wards. *Journal of the Medical Association of Thailand,* Vol. 94 Suppl 1, pp. S99-104, ISSN 0125-2208

[94] Straker, D. A., Shapiro, P. A. & Muskin, P. R. (2006). Aripiprazole in the treatment of delirium. *Psychosomatics,* Vol. 47, No. 5, pp. 385-391, ISSN 0033-3182

[95] Tahir, T. A., Eeles, E., Karapareddy, V., Muthuvelu, P., Chapple, S., Phillips, B., Adyemo, T., Farewell, D. & Bisson, J. I. (2010). A randomized controlled trial of quetiapine versus placebo in the treatment of delirium. *Journal of psychosomatic research,* Vol. 69, No. 5, pp. 485-90, ISSN 1879-1360

[96] Trevisan, L. A., Boutros, N., Petrakis, I. L. & Krystal, J. H. (1998). Complications of alcohol withdrawal: pathophysiological insights. *Alcohol health and research world,* Vol. 22, No. 1, pp. 61-66, ISSN 0090-838X

[97] Trzepacz, P. T. (2000). Is there a final common neural pathway in delirium? Focus on acetylcholine and dopamine. *Seminars in clinical neuropsychiatry,* Vol. 5, No. 2, pp. 132-148, ISSN 1084-3612

[98] Trzepacz, P. T., Mittal, D., Torres, R., Kanary, K., Norton, J. & Jimerson, N. (2001). Validation of the Delirium Rating Scale-revised-98: comparison with the delirium rating scale and the cognitive test for delirium. *The Journal of neuropsychiatry and clinical neurosciences,* Vol. 13, No. 2, pp. 229-242, ISSN 0895-0172

[99] Van Den Boogaard, M., Kox, M., Quinn, K. L., Van Achterberg, T., Van Der Hoeven, J. G., Schoonhove, L. & Pickkers, P. (2011). Biomarkers associated with delirium in critically ill patients and their relation with long-term subjective cognitive dysfunction; indications for different pathways governing delirium in inflamed and noninflamed patients. *Critical care,* Vol. 15, No. 6, pp. R297, ISSN 1466-609X

[100] Van Der Mast, R. C. (1998). Pathophysiology of delirium. *Journal of geriatric psychiatry and neurology,* Vol. 11, No. 3, pp 138-45; discussion 157-158, ISSN 0891-9887

[101] Van Gool, W. A., Van De Beek, D. & Eikelenboom, P. (2010). Systemic infection and delirium: when cytokines and acetylcholine collide. *Lancet,* Vol. 375, No. 9716, pp. 773-775, ISSN 1474-547X

[102] Van Rompaey, B., Elseviers, M. M., Schuurmans, M. J., Shortridge-Baggett, L. M., Truijen, S. & Bossaert, L. (2009). Risk factors for delirium in intensive care patients: a prospective cohort study. *Critical care,* Vol. 13, No. 3, pp. R77, ISSN 1466-609X

[103] Wang , W., Li, H. L., Wang, D. X., Zhu, X., Li, S. L., Yao, G. Q., Chen, K. S., Gu, X. E. & Zhu, S. N. (2012). Haloperidol prophylaxis decreases delirium incidence in elderly patients after noncardiac surgery: a randomized controlled trial*. *Critical care medicine,* Vol. 40, No. 3, 731-739, ISSN 1530-0293

[104] Warshaw, G. & Tanzer, F. (1993). The effectiveness of lumbar puncture in the evaluation of delirium and fever in the hospitalized elderly. *Archives of family medicine,* Vol. 2, No. 3, pp. 293-297, ISSN 1063-3987

[105] Wengel, S. P., Roccaforte, W. H. & Burke, W. J. (1998). Donepezil improves symptoms of delirium in dementia: implications for future research. *Journal of geriatric psychiatry and neurology,* Vol. 11, No. 3, pp. 159-161, ISSN 0891-9887

[106] Wilson, C. J., Finch, C. E. & Cohen, H. J. (2002). Cytokines and cognition--the case for a head-to-toe inflammatory paradigm. *Journal of the American Geriatrics Society,* Vol. 50, No. 12, pp. 2041-2056, ISSN 0002-8614

[107] Wongpakaran, N., Wongpakaran, T., Bookamana, P., Pinyopornpanish, M., Maneeton, B., Lerttrakarnnon, P., Uttawichai, K. & Jiraniramai, S. (2011). Diagnosing delirium in elderly Thai patients: utilization of the CAM algorithm. *BMC family practice,* Vol. 12, pp. 65, ISSN 1471-2296

[108] World Health Organization. (1993). *The ICD-10 Classification of Mental and Behavioural Disorders: Diagnostic Criteria for Research,* World Health Organization, ISBN 92-4-154422-8, Geneva, Switzerland

[109] Yang, F. M., Inouye, S. K., Fearing, M. A., Kiely, D. K., Marcantonio, E. R. & Jones, R. N. (2008). Participation in activity and risk for incident delirium. *Journal of the American Geriatrics Society,* Vol. 56, No. 8, pp. 1479-1484, ISSN 1532-5415

[110] Yang, F. M., Marcantonio, E. R., Inouye, S. K., Kiely, D. K., Rudolph, J. L., Fearing, M. A. & Jones, R. N. (2009). Phenomenological subtypes of delirium in older persons: patterns, prevalence, and prognosis. *Psychosomatics,* Vol. 50, No. 3, pp. 248-254, ISSN 1545-7206

[111] Yu, Y. H., Chen, A. C., Hu, C. C., Hsieh, P. H., Ueng, S. W. & Lee, M. S. (2012). Acute Delirium and Poor Compliance in Total Hip Arthroplasty Patients With Substance Abuse Disorders. *The Journal of arthroplasty,* Vol. 27, No. 8, pp. 1526-1529, ISSN 1532-8406

[112] Zampieri, F. G., Park, M., Machado, F. S. & Azevedo, L. C. (2011). Sepsis-associated encephalopathy: not just delirium. *Clinics (Sao Paulo, Brazil),* Vol. 66, No. 10, pp. 1825-1831, ISSN 1980-5322

Chapter 6

Rethinking Dissociation in an Age of Virtual Worlds

Gregory Patrick Garvey

Additional information is available at the end of the chapter

1. Introduction

My previous research sought to address the general question of whether the use of virtual worlds and video games may induce experiences that fit the language used to describe dissociative disorders. The method of investigation was the development of a survey instrument based on the Structured Clinical Interview for Depersonalization – Derealization Spectrum (Mula et al., 2008). The new survey was in turn administered to a population of users of the virtual world *Second Life*. While results from this initial study provided some provisional insights the question that motivated this research remains worthy of further attention. In fact this question was originally arose from a consideration of a more general question: how do we distinguish what it real from what is virtual? From this initial question it is possible to tease out a number of questions deserving of further investigation.

A significant number of people spend a significant amount of time using virtual worlds for gaming and entertainment. According to the market research company KZERO WORLDWIDE (http://www.kzero.co.uk/) the cumulative total of registered accounts for virtual worlds, MMOs (massive multi-player online games) and social gaming stands at 1.92 billion. The Entertainment Software Association (http://www.theesa.com/facts/index.asp) reports that 72 percent of American households play computer or video games. According to the Pew Research Center 97 percent of teens in the United States play videogames of some sort. (Pew Research Center 2008).

Edward Castronova argues that virtual worlds and games attract our attention because they offer more positive experiences than the real world. This places the real and the virtual in competition for people's time and attention. Castronova invokes simple economic theory to claim, that "the real world is going to lose." (Castronova 2008). With Castronova's exodus people are "moving their attention, not their bodies, and they are moving back and forth all the time."

If Castronova is right and the data on the growing numbers of users of games and virtual worlds appear to support his speculations, then we need to understand how is it that people "are moving back and forth all the time" but manage not to confuse the real and the virtual. We need to understand why and how "reality testing is intact" as people migrate back and forth from the real to the virtual.

The use of virtual worlds is no longer an activity at the margins of society. It is now a part of the cultural fabric. Yet we have a poor understanding of the impact of this activity on the psychological well being of players. More to the point we do not understand how human beings sort out the differences between virtual experiences and real life experiences. How is it that most people easily recognize and separate these two domains of experience?

In the near future this ability will be challenged. Rapid advances in wearable computing (compact computational and sensing devices molded to comfortably fit the human body) have introduced new viewing devices that promise to further blur the lines between the real and the virtual. Announced in April 2012 Goggle's Project Glass introduces augmented reality eyewear that offers anywhere, anytime connectivity (Hill 2012). The display visible with the eyewear merges together a view of the real world with the overlay of the capabilities of web browsers and smartphones.

The *Rift Project* developed by Oculus will introduce Virtual Reality goggles in early 2013 that feature an extremely high resolution display with head motion tracking for the home market for games. As video gaming experiences become increasingly realistic, engaging and immersive how will users/players distinguish real experiences from virtual experiences? What of their long-term memories of these experiences? Will those memories of virtual experiences intermingle with memories of "real" experiences? What of dreams? Anecdotal accounts suggest that players do have dreams about gaming experiences.

With augmented reality the distinction between the real and the virtual collapses and becomes a single unified experience. A person viewing the Grand Canyon through augmented reality glasses might a see text overlay identifying prominent features of that landscape. It seems quite unlikely that someone might confuse this text overlay as part of the observed reality as they can simply take off the glasses and view the natural world as it is. But what if that overlay includes a video conferencing feature similar to Skype? The individual sees a Park Ranger (who is not physically there) and hears the voice of the Ranger through their ear buds (headphones built into the glasses). The Park Ranger responds to questions, gestures to geological features in the environment (much like the weather man or woman against a green screen), engages in conversation and can even make eye contact.

For all intents and purposes this experience is real, feels real to the viewer and will be remembered just as vividly (perhaps even more so?) as the experience of talking to a person standing next to him or her on the South Rim. What is substantively different about this experience is that it is a broadband, information rich, real time interaction. This experience completely engages the participant in the visual, auditory domains and more importantly in the realm of human social affairs.

A determined materialist might argue that this is simply a pseudo question and concern. We know the physics and electrical engineering of how the bits and bytes are represented as electrical impulses and stored on a hard drive. The engineering is well established for how the data is read, parsed into instructions and the algorithms are executed, while user input is processed resulting in the real time display of 3D computer graphics along with the playback of stereo sound. We know a great about the systems of visual and auditory processing, from the anatomy of the eye and ear to the neural correlates in the brain. The reductionist can confidently say that we objectively know what is out there, is real. We thoroughly understand the science and engineering how the virtual worlds are generated. The light from a pattern of pixels that hits the retina is just as "real" as light coming from the "real" or natural world. We even understand a great deal about perception, both how the brain creates the world out there from sensory inputs to even how the brain processes illusions.

But that is not the point. This reductionist argument is like trying to explain the experience of reading a novel by describing the technology of papermaking, publishing and printing. The real question centers on that human capacity to imagine fictitious worlds when hearing or reading stories or watching a play or film or play a game.

What is happening when we experience the "suspension of disbelief"? What is this capacity to simultaneously know that the experience (reading fiction, watching a play or movie) is not real but still responding as if it were real? When dreaming one's motor control is suppressed. When we read a book, watch a play or film we remain seated. When we play a video game we interact within the constraints defined by the interface. Historically game interaction has been accomplished by use of a mouse and keyboard, or with the buttons on a game controller. More recently motion tracking and motion sensing technologies motion used with the Wii or Microsoft Kinect make it possible to interact using one's whole body.

There is also the temptation to dismiss this as a topic best suited for an introductory class in philosophy. After all the question of what is the reality of the virtual is an epistemological one. Yet this does not mean that such questions have to be abandoned and left to metaphysics. Testing a series of questions and gathering data using quantitative and qualitative methods can provide meaningful results. To return to the question suggested at the onset of this chapter, does the language used to describe the diagnostic criteria for dissociative disorders specifically from the *Diagnostic and Statistical Manual of Mental Disorders*: Fourth Edition, Text Revision (2000), apply to experience of using virtual worlds or playing games?

In the DSM–IV–TR dissociative disorders are described as the "disruption in the usually integrated functions of consciousness, memory, identity, or perception of the environment" and "partial or complete loss of the normal integration between memories of the past, awareness of identity and immediate sensations, and control of bodily movements." Why is it that frequent migrations between the real and virtual do not trigger a "disruption in the usually integrated functions..."? If a subject presents symptoms of dissociation in real life do these symptoms carry over or are aggravated by use of a virtual world like *Second Life* (http://secondlife.com/)?

The DSM-IV-TR acknowledges that dissociative states "occur frequently and are not inherently pathological" and are even "sought-after experiences as part of long standing religious and cultural rituals and practices." Many conditions present similar clusters of symptoms, yet the language used in the DSM for the diagnostic criteria for depersonalization and derealization is a fitting description for how avatars (the user's onscreen representation in a virtual world or game) look "unreal" and one's surroundings looks "unreal" in a virtual worlds like the *SIMS, The World of Warcraft* or *Second Life*. These virtual worlds are all computer generated 3D computer graphics simulations that in spite of considerable advances in real time rendering fall well short of photo-realism and still look fake and cartoonish.

The DSM-IV-TR uses the following criteria for derealization: "The perception or experience of the external world so that it seems strange or unreal; Feeling as though one's environment is lacking in spontaneity, emotional colouring and depth." In *Second Life* the objects, architecture and avatars representing other residents appear "strange and unreal" and are "lacking in spontaneity, emotional coloring (especially other avatars) and depth."

The diagnostic criteria for Item 300.6 Depersonalization Disorder specifies the following: "Persistent or recurrent feelings of being detached from one's mental processes or body; as if an observer; During depersonalization, reality testing is intact." In *Second Life* users see their avatars from a default point-of-view (POV) slightly above and behind their "in world" avatar. This is not unlike descriptions of out-of-body experiences. Users can also use a viewing technique called mouse-look which makes it possible for a user to view his or her own avatar as if it were someone else. Avatars controlled by other users can "seem unfamiliar or mechanical" or "robotic".

Updated in DSM-IV-TR, Dissociative Identity Disorder (DID) refers to the "presence of two or more distinct identities or personality states" that "recurrently take control" of a person's behavior. It is a common practice for *Second Life* users to have multiple "in-world" avatars (known as alts) that can be of a different gender. The user effectively takes on a different personality and behavior when employing a different avatar.

2. A Survey and results

It is an informal observation to say that the language of the diagnostic criteria of the DSM is an apt description of the experience using a virtual world like *Second Life*. To say that a computer generated simulation of a world looks "strange, unreal" or that the avatars in that virtual world "seem unfamiliar or mechanical" or "robotic" is a matter-of-fact statement. Similarly asserting that for most users and players "reality testing is intact" is likewise an uncontroversial truism.

To suggest that users and players who have multiple avatars may experience something akin to dissociative identity disorder is another matter. These terms and phrases have real import when used as part of the diagnostic criteria for dissociative disorders. If users self-report and respond in the affirmative to a self-administered questionnaire related to the diagnostic criteria then there may be something worth further scrutiny. In order to conduct a more systematic investigation the development of a survey instrument and its deployment was required.

The Structured Clinical Interview for Depersonalization – Derealization Spectrum (SCI-DER) (Mula et al., 2008) was chosen as a model for a new survey. Questions were selected on the basis of how well they applied to the experience of using *Second Life*. Those questions that referenced situations that could only be experienced in "real life" were not used. Some questions were used as is or were minimally rewritten to clearly reference the experience of using *Second Life*. This newly created survey instrument was administered to a select population of users of *Second Life*. A parsimonious interpretation of the initial results, suggest that a significant number of survey respondents agreed that the descriptions of dissociative experiences based on the diagnostic criteria of the DSM-IV-TR do apply to the experience of using virtual worlds.

The SCI-DER introduces the survey questions with this general question: "Have you ever experienced just for a few seconds or for days or months. ..." After that each of the specific questions follow such as the first: ... *that the outside world was strange and unreal?*

This preface from the SCI_DER is rewritten for the new survey as: "While in Second Life have you ever experienced just for a few seconds or for a longer period of time…" The first question is modified as follows to refer directly to the experience of being logged into *Second Life*.

…that the virtual world was strange and unreal?"

Questions were added that addressed gender, age and length of time spent as a registered user (resident) of Second Life. In the end the new survey instrument comprised a total of 23 questions. Respondents answered Yes or No to each. While the SCI-DER is considered a validated instrument with high reliability, this new survey does not make any such claims. Additionally this new survey was not intended to be used for the purposes of diagnosis. The survey was administered by the Social Research Foundation (http://www.socialresearchfoundation.org/) to a sample population of 110 "residents" of Second Life. Respondents completed the survey online anonymously. The following charts show sample results of this new survey using questions modified from the SCI-DER. As noted above the list of twenty-three questions is prefaced by this general question:

While in Second Life have you ever experienced just for a few seconds or for a longer period of time…

…that the virtual world was strange and unreal?

Question 1 uses the descriptive phrase directly from the diagnostic criteria of the DSM-IV-TR and corresponds to the first domain of questions in the SCI-DER. Items in this domain focus on derealization or "referring to an altered experience of the external world (Mula et al., 2008)." Question 2 is another example of this domain. Survey responses suggest that it is "normal" and expected to view other avatars and objects as "not real" when logged into *Second Life*. Indeed it is likely a desirable and sought after experience whereas to experience the "real" world as "strange and unreal" is disturbing and potentially disabling.

... having the feeling that other avatars, objects, and the 'in-world' environment around you were not real?

Question 12 references the *Somatopsychic depersonalization* domain which "describes a variety of changes in body experience such as lack of body ownership feelings, feelings of disembodiment, which can range from a nonspecific feeling of not being in the body to out-of-body experiences and autoscopic hallucinations (Mula et al., 2008)."

... that you were not in charge of your avatar's movements, so that you felt "automatic" and mechanical as if you were a robot?

Questions 17 and 18 reference the third domain of Auto Psychic depersonalization which includes "unfamiliarity of the self in terms of sensation of being an outside observer of one's mental process, not being 'in charge' of their own behavior or mental processes, the automaton-line experience and anomalous subjective recall." Yes responses are not surprising given that the default viewpoint in *Second Life* is from a vantage point slightly above and behind their "in-world" avatar. In fact residents often use *Mouse Look* (Second Life Wikia, n.d.) where it is possible to move the camera representing their avatar's point-of-view, independent of the location of their avatar. This makes it possible to observe their own avatar as if they were "detached from one's body;" as if "an observer."

... that you were a "detached observer"?

Question 18 references the déjà vu experience. Sims (simulations) in Second Life have a sameness to them because of the basic technology consists of complex shapes built out of primitive shapes with simple texture maps. Question 18 also references item 300.13 Dissociative Fugue in the DSM-IV-TR where the "predominant disturbance is sudden, unexpected travel away from home or one's customary place of work, with inability to recall one's past."

... that when in a new situation, you had been there before?

Question 23 references the DSM-IV-TR category 300.14 *Dissociative Identity Disorder*. Male and female responses differ by only 1.5 percentage points. These results suggest that nearly half of the population of residents use "alts" or alternative avatars that have "distinct personalities." It is not clear from these responses if these personalities take control but most Second Life users enact or "perform" their avatar in a way consistent with its appearance. Item 300.14 Dissociative Fugue is also implicated here as it involves "Confusion about personal identity, or the assumption of a new identity, (partial or complete)."

... that you use two or more distinct avatars having different personalities?

Some value lies in this survey's potential to define and recognize potential manifestations that (weakly) correlate to DSM-IV diagnostic criteria. This has led to further research questions (as noted above) that suggest the development of new instruments and methodologies.

3. Other considerations

Digital games conjure up virtual worlds by means of graphical displays. Play further establishes the divide between the real and the virtual by demarcating what play theorists call the magic circle. First described by Huizinga in his seminal work on play (1955) the magic circle is a place set apart for not only play but also much more:

"All play moves and has its being within a play-ground marked off beforehand either materially or ideally, deliberately or as a matter of course. Just as there is no formal difference between play and ritual, so the 'consecrated spot' cannot be formally distinguished from the play-ground. The arena, the card-table, the magic circle, the temple, the stage, the screen, the tennis court, the court of justice, etc., are all in form and function play-grounds, i.e. forbidden spots, isolated, hedged round, hallowed, within which special rules obtain. All are temporary worlds within the ordinary world, dedicated to the performance of an act apart."

Gregory Bateson (1972) links play to Goffman's frame analysis (1974): "play occurs within a delimited psychological frame, a spatial and temporal bounding of a set of interactive messages." Goffman himself aims at a certain granularity of experience by using the term "strip" by which he means "any arbitrary slice or cut from the stream of ongoing activity, including here sequences of happenings, real or fictive, as seen from the perspective of those subjectively involved in sustaining an interest in them (Goffman 1974)." In a similar fashion Zerubavel (1991) speaks of "mental fences," which "delimit geographical areas, historical events, people, ideas, and so on that appear to be contiguous, similar, functionally related, or otherwise associated." Zerubavel, (1991) reminds us that boundaries allow us to "visually as well as mentally to grasp any entity at all."

Salen and Zimmerman (2003) link Huizinga's (1955) notion of the 'magic circle' to Bateson's analysis of play as a frame that "delimits the peculiar space of play." When someone engages in play, he/she crosses a boundary (into the magic circle) that separates the artificial world of the game from "real life." The magic circle is a frame that sets a thick boundary between real life and the make believe of game play. This cognitive frame establishes the "reality" of the game. Anthropologist Tom Boellstroff (2008) suggests that the "magic circle"– may constitute a virtual world meaningful in its own right. Bateson points out that this is a paradoxical state of mind (Bateson 1972, p. 84). For the player the game is simultaneously real and not real. This boundary is likewise thin–the player can easily stop and step instantly back into "real life."

Work-family-life border/boundaries theories (Ashforth 2000; Clark 2000) likewise make use of the concepts of boundaries and borders to understand how daily life is "sliced" into discrete domains. These theories study the conflicts and interactions that arise between the domains of work, family life and what is termed third places defined as social activities outside the home or work place. This partitioning makes it possible for "one to concentrate more on whatever domain is currently salient and less on other domains."

These borders can be both flexible and permeable. Behavior can spill over from one domain into another when flexible boundaries allow a role to "be enacted in various settings as various times (Ashforth et al. 2000)." Flexible borders or boundaries can be characterized by the "degree to which the spatial and temporal boundaries are pliable." A role having flexible boundaries "can be enacted in various settings and at various times". Permeability can be measured as "the degree to which a role allows one to be physically located in the role's domain but psychologically and/or behaviorally involved in another role (Ashforth et al. 2000)."

The framework of border/boundary theory does not take into account domains beyond so-called third places. I have argued elsewhere (Garvey 2010) that the virtual should be considered as a fourth place. The analytical tool set of work-family-life border/boundary theories does not capture the full dynamic of the phenomena of immersion in the domains of virtual worlds and video games. These theories as currently formulated have little to say about how gamers are "quite facile at juggling roles" and how gamers can easily and quickly navigate back and forth between the domains of play (the virtual) and real life.

4. Toward a new survey

The foregoing discussion suggests that a number a new survey instruments could be devised that would examine the notion of the magic circle, paradoxical states of mind as manifested in game play, role-playing and boundaries. Goffman's notion of frames has enormous intuitive appeal but suffers from an awkwardness of how to design experimental questions that get at this idea, that are testable and indeed quantifiable. Boundaries and borders have likewise a certain conceptual appeal. But as discussed above the border/boundary framework suffers from certain limitations when we try to apply this framework beyond the work/family balance framework.

The Boundary Questionnaire (Hartmann, 1991; Hartmann, Harrison and Zborowski 2001) offers another approach to using the notion of boundaries as an investigative tool. The BQ is a 138-item instrument that covers 12 categories of boundaries. Hartmann et al. point out that there is a long tradition in the field of psychology of investigating "perceptual boundaries, boundaries related to thoughts and feelings, boundaries between states of awareness or consciousness, sleep-dream-wake boundaries, boundaries related to memory, body boundaries, interpersonal boundaries, boundaries related to sexual identity and other forms of identity, group boundaries, and boundaries in opinions and judgments." Hartmann et al. (1991; 2001), distinguish thick (solid) boundaries from thin or permeable boundaries. They have also developed a theory of dreams based on a "wake-dreaming continuum (Hartman 1989; Hartmann & Kunzendorf 2007)." This continuum begins on one end with "focused waking thought" having thick boundaries characterized by "solid, divisions, categorizations." On the other end of the continuum is "Dreaming" having "thin boundaries" characterized as "merging, condensation, loosening of categories." Hartmann et al. (2001) introduces the following table compiling types of boundaries:

Perceptual boundaries
Between sensory inputs
Sensory focus or "bandwidth"
Around perceptual entities
Boundaries related to thoughts and feelings
Between two thoughts or two feelings
Between thought and feeling
Around thoughts and feelings (free association)
Boundaries between states of awareness or states of consciousness
Sleep-dream-wake boundaries
Between sleep and waking
Between dreaming and waking
In and around the dream
Daydreaming
Boundaries related to play
Boundaries related to memory
Early memories
Recent memories and memory organization
Personal past
Future plans
Boundaries around oneself (body boundaries)
Barriers against stimuli
The skin as a boundary
Posture and musculature as boundaries
Personal space
Interpersonal boundaries
Boundaries between conscious and unconscious and between id, ego, and superego
Defense mechanisms as boundaries
Boundaries related to identity
Sexual identity
Age identity: Between adult and child
Constancy of identity
Group boundaries
Boundaries in organizing one's life
Boundaries in environmental preferences
Boundaries in opinion and judgments
Boundaries in decision making and action

Table 1. Types of Boundaries (Hartmann et al. 2001)

The Boundary Questionnaire (BQ) organizes those various kinds of boundaries into twelve categories (Hartmann et al. 2001):

Category 1: Sleep/Dream/Waking
Category 2: Unusual Experiences
Category 3: Thoughts/Feelings/Moods
Category 4: Childhood/Adolescence/Adult
Category 5: Interpersonal
Category 6: Sensitivity
Category 7: Neat/Exact/Precise
Category 8: Edges/Lines/Clothing
Category 9: Opinions re Children, etc.
Category 10: Organizations
Category 11: Peoples/Nations/Groups
Category 12: Beauty/Truth

Table 2. Categories of Boundaries (Hartmann et al. 2001)

Hartmann et al. (2001) argue that "thick vs. thin boundaries appears to be a robust personality measure, which can be considered an important dimension of personality." Boundaries related to "sexual identity" and "constancy of identity" are of direct relevance in a discussion of the use of avatars in virtual worlds and games. Thus the BQ might serve as a model for a new survey. In order to make such an instrument relevant to the target population the questions in the BQ could be slightly revised in a similar fashion to the approach described above with the SCI-DER.

The following table (Hartmann et al. 2001) lists the each of the twelve categories of boundary types. Under each category are two sample items from original the BQ followed by revisions of each items modified in such a way that it applies to the experience of using the virtual world *Second Life*. Subjects are given instructions to rate each of the statements on a scale from 0 to 4, where "0" indicates either the subject thinks the statement does not apply to him/her (not at all or not at all true of me). A "4" indicates that the subject thinks the statement definitely applies (true of me).

Category 1: Sleep/Dream/Waking

1. When I awake in the morning, I am not sure whether I am really awake for a few minutes.

37. I spend a lot of time daydreaming, fantasizing, or in reverie.

Agreement with these questions are indicative of thin boundaries. Question 1 and 37 could be modified as follows:

1. When I awake in the morning, I am not sure for a few minutes whether I am logged into Second Life or really awake.

37. I spend a lot of time daydreaming, fantasizing, or in reverie about Second Life.

Category 2: Unusual Experiences

61. At times I have felt as if I were coming apart.

100. I have had déjà vu experiences.

The modified questions are:

61. At times while using Second Life I have felt as if I were coming apart.

100. In Second Life I have had déjà vu experiences.

Category 3: Thoughts/Feelings/Moods

15. Sometimes I don't know whether I am thinking or feeling.

74. I can easily imagine myself to be an animal or what it might be like to be an animal.

In Second Life users can change the appearance of their avatar. A large group of users choose to be furries – avatars that have animal heads, tails and paws. The modified questions are:

15. Sometimes while using Second Life I don't know whether I am thinking or feeling.

74. In Second Life I can easily imagine myself to be a furry or what it might be like to be a furry.

Category 4: Childhood/Adolescence/Adult

4. I am very close to my childhood feelings.

40. I have definite plans for my future. I can lay out pretty well what I expect year by year for the next few years.

The modified questions are:

4. I am very close to my childhood feelings when using Second Life.

40. I have definite plans for my future logins in Second Life. I can lay out pretty well what I expect year by year for the next few years.

Category 5: Interpersonal

53. When I get involved with someone, we sometimes get too close.

103. I am a very open person.

The modified questions are:

53. When I get involved with someone in Second Life, we sometimes get too close.

103. In Second Life I am a very open person.

Category 6: Sensitivity

6. I am very sensitive to other people's feelings.
42. I am unusually sensitive to loud noises and bright lights.
The modified questions are:
6. While in Second Life I am very sensitive to other avatar's feelings.
42. While in Second Life I am unusually sensitive to loud noises and bright lights.
Category 7: Neat/Exact/Precise
19. I keep my desk and work table neat and well organized.
43. I am good at keeping accounts and keeping track of my money.
In *Second Life* each user account has an inventory where the user can store various items such as clothing or objects. The currency of Second Life is called Lindens and can be purchased using real money. Questions 19 and 43 can be modified as:
19. With my Second Life account I keep my inventory and folders neat and well organized.
43. I am good at keeping accounts and keeping track of my Lindens in Second Life.
Category 8: Edges/Lines/Clothing
32. I like heavy, solid clothing.
44. I like stories that have a definite beginning, middle, and end.
The modified questions are:
32. When in Second Life I like clothing to have a heavy, solid look.
44. I like stories that have a definite beginning, middle, and end.
Category 9: Opinions re Children, etc.
33. Children and adults have a lot in common. They should give themselves a chance to be together without any strict roles.
56. I think a good teacher must remain in part a child.

Table 3. Sample Items by Category

The following modification is problematic as Linden Labs (makers of *Second Life*) found it necessary to age segregate users by creating a separate but equal version of *Second Life* for teens. In fact underage role-playing is prohibited in Second Life for adults. The modified questions are:

33. Children and adults have a lot in common. In Second Life they should give themselves a chance to be together without any strict roles.

56. I think a good mentor must remain in part a child.

Category 10: Organizations

10. In an organization, everyone should have a definite place and a specific role.

58. A good relationship is one in which everything is clearly defined and spelled out.

The modified questions are:

10. In Second Life, everyone should have a definite place and a specific role.

58. In Second Life, a good relationship is one in which everything is clearly defined and spelled out.

Category 11: Peoples/Nations/Groups

11. People of different nations are basically very much alike.

105. There are no sharp dividing lines between normal people, people with problems, and people who are considered psychotic or crazy.

The modified questions are:

11. In Second Life people from different sims, groups and regions are basically very much alike.

105. In Second Life there are no sharp dividing lines between normal people, people with problems, and people who are considered psychotic or crazy.

Category 12: Beauty/Truth

36. Either you are telling the truth or you are lying; that's all there is to it.

76. When I am in a new situation, I try to find out precisely what is going on and what the rules are as soon as possible.

The modified questions are:

36. Either you are telling the truth or you are lying; that's all there is to it.

76. When I am in a new sim in Second Life, I try to find out precisely what is going on and what the rules are as soon as possible.

A subject's score is obtained by adding up all the scores (0-4) for all items. Some items are scored backwards i.e. an answer of "0" is scored as 4, "1" is scored as 3, "2" is scored as 2, "3" is scored as 1, and "4" is scored as 0. A reverse logic is built in to the questionnaire design so respondents need to think about each response instead of answering mechanically. A subject with a low score is interpreted as having "Thick boundaries" and those with higher scores are determined to have "Thin boundaries."

The prediction would be that subjects with thick boundaries would keep the domains of the real and the virtual clearly separate. It would also be expected that subjects whose scores are low would be able to quickly navigate back and forth and still maintain the boundaries. Subjects with thin boundaries would possibly experience spill over effects from one domain to another. Subjects with thick boundaries will be on the "focused waking thought" end of the "wake-dreaming continuum" which is characterized by "solid, divisions, categorizations." Those subjects with thin boundaries are on the "Dreaming" end of the continuum characterized as "merging, condensation, loosening of categories." Hartmann et al. (2001) notes: "... people with thick boundaries spend more time and find themselves more comfortable at the left-hand end of our continuum involved in focused waking. They can be considered, "thought people," whereas the people with thinner boundaries are more comfortable at the other end of the continuum and can be thought of as "dream people," although these terms are obviously an over-simplification." The authors acknowledge at one time or another individuals can exhibit both thin and thick boundaries. Most individuals experience the different aspects of the "wake-dreaming continuum" during the course of entire day.

Subjects with thin boundaries might be predicted to experience spill over effects such as daydreaming about the virtual world or perhaps confusing dreams about the virtual world with actual experiences as a user of that virtual world. However the BQ is not able to determine exactly what those spill over effects might be, rather it predicts the tendency for a subject to behave in a manner consistent with thin or thick boundaries. In fact it really is a measure of self-assessment of attitudes in regard to each of the identified categories. To determine how a subject actually behaves, what they perceive, whether or not there are spill over effects with daydreams or dream recall between the domains of the real and virtual likely requires another research methodology. In related dream research Hartmann employs a qualitative approach where subjects provide written descriptions of dreams. Such methodologies may get at other details that quantitative measures miss.

As part of a theory of dreams Hartmann introduces the concept of a Central Image (Hartmann & Kunzendorf 2006-7) or Contextualizing Image (Hartmann et al. 2001) that dominates in "big" and generally memorable dreams. The CI is often the feature that is readily remembered about a dream. Individual with "thin boundaries" tend to remember their dreams while individuals with "thick boundaries" tend to not remember their dreams. Do users of virtual worlds with thin boundaries have dreams where there is a high intensity Central Image based on their experiences in Second Life?

5. Conclusion

To make real progress in understanding the complex nature of the borders and boundaries that separate the real from the virtual necessitates a multifaceted approach. A new "boundary questionnaire" is one step toward further study. There remains a broader question. In an age where new technologies such as augmented reality blur the boundaries of the real and virtual how do we achieve a consensus about norms of mental health against which we make judgments about what is to be considered deviations from that norm? Since the period of the enlightenment science has been the answer. But today we live in era of climate change denial, political campaigns that ignore "fact checkers", the rise of religious extremism where competing versions of reality clash. If we add on to this the overlay of virtual worlds and augmented realities, along the real possibility of malware and cyber attacks that might distort what is heard and seen, where does it leave the rational understanding of the "real?" How do we determine if "reality testing is intact?" And whose reality is it?

Author details

Gregory Patrick Garvey

Quinnipiac University, Hamden, USA

References

[1] American Psychiatric Association (2000). Diagnostic and Statistical Manual of Mental Disorders: DSM_IV_TR, Fourth Edition, Text Revision. Washington, DC: American Psychiatric Association.

[2] Ashforth, B. E., Kreiner, G. E. and Fugate, M. (2000). All in a day's work: Boundaries and micro role transitions. *Academy of Management. The Academy of Management Review.* 25 (3), p. 472-491.

[3] Bateson, G. (1972). "A Theory of Play and Fantasy" in Steps to an Ecology of Mind, Chicago: University of Chicago Press.

[4] Boellstorff, T., (2008). Coming of Age in Second Life: An Anthropologist Explores the Virtually Human. Princeton and Oxford: Princeton University Press.

[5] Castronova, E. (2008). Exodus to the Virtual World. New York, NY: Palgrave Macmillan.

[6] Clark, S. C. (2000). June. Work/family border theory: A new theory of work/family balance. *Human Relations.* 53 (6), 747-771.

[7] Entertainment Software Association. Retrieved 8/15/2012 from http://www.theesa.com/facts/index.asp)

[8] Garvey, G. (2010, Summer). Dissociation: A Natural State of Mind? *Journal of Consciousness Studies: Controversies in Science & the Humanities. Social Approaches to Consciousness II Special Issue.* Ed. Charles Whitehead. 17(7–8), 139-155.

[9] Goffman, E. (1974). Frame Analysis: An Essay on the Organization of Experience. London: Harper and Row.

[10] Hartmann, E., Harrison, R., Zborowski, M. (2001). Boundaries in the Mind: Past Research and Future Directions. *North American Journal of Psychology.* 3: 347-368.

[11] Hartmann, E., Kunzendorf, R. (2006–2007). Boundaries and Dreams. *Imagination, Cognition, and Personality,* 26, 101-115.

[12] Hartmann, E. (1989). Boundaries of dreams, boundaries of dreamers: thin & thick boundaries as a new personality dimension. *Psychiatric Journal of the University of Ottawa,* 14, 557-560.

[13] Hartmann, E. (1991). Boundaries in the Mind. New York: Basic Books.

[14] Hill, D. J., *Google Unveils Augmented-Reality Glasses, Its Vision Of The Post-PC Era.* April 5, 2012. Retrieved 9/2/2012. http://singularityhub.com/2012/04/05/google-unveils-augmented-reality-glasses-its-vision-of-the-post-pc-era/

[15] Huizinga, J. (1955). Homo Ludens: A Study of the Play Element in Culture. Boston: Beacon Press.

[16] KZERO WORLDWIDE Retrieved 8/5/2012 from http://www.kzero.co.uk/

[17] Mula, M., Pini, S., Calugi, S., Preve, M., Masini, M., Giovannini, I., Conversano, C., Rucci, P., and Cassano, G. B. (2008), Validity and reliability of the Structured Clinical Interview for Depersonalization–Derealization Spectrum (SCI-DER), *Neuropsychiatric Disease and Treatment,* 4(5), 977–986.

[18] Pew Research Center. (2008). Teens, Video Games and Civics. Retrieved 8/30/2012 from http://pewresearch.org/pubs/953/teens-video-games-and-civics. September 16, 2008.

[19] Salen, K. & Zimmerman, E. (2003). Rules of Play: Game Design Fundamentals. Cambridge: MIT Press.

[20] *Second Life.* Retrieved 7/19/2012 from http://secondlife.com/

[21] Second Life Wikia. (n.d.). Glossary. Retrieved 8/25/2012 from http://secondlife.wikia.com/index.php?title=Category:Glossary&until=Popular+Places

[22] Zerubavel, E. (1991). The fine line: Making distinctions in everyday life. New York: Free Press.

Chapter 7

Racism and Mental Illness in the UK

Apu Chakraborty, Lance Patrick and Maria Lambri

Additional information is available at the end of the chapter

1. Introduction

There is substantial evidence of differential outcomes for different racial and ethnic groups in many health, social and economic arenas in the United Kingdom today, ranging from disease prevalence and outcome, hiring and promotion in the labour workforce, to loan approvals in mortgage lending, to rate of arrest and detention in the criminal justice system. These disparities – and others – describe social conditions that most Britons believe deserve some measure of attention. To understand such conditions and to fashion appropriate responses, it is important to assess whether and how racism and racial discrimination, along with other factors, may contribute to observed disparities in mental health outcomes among racial and ethnic groups.

2. Race

The focus on measuring racial discrimination in this study raises an initial question of "what is race?" Defining race is a task far more complex than can be accomplished here. In fact, there is little consensus on what race actually means. The term "race" was used to distinguish populations in different areas on the basis of differing physical characteristics that had developed over time, such as the colour of skin, facial features, and other features (Zuckerman 1990).

2.1. Biological definition of race

Recently, genetics researchers have found evidence of genetic clusters that correspond to geographically similar populations and yield the kind of variations in phenotype that have been used to construct concepts of race. Recent developments in the fields of genetics and evolutionary biology have prompted a renewed focus on identifying the biological basis of human behaviour as well as ascertaining the historical relationships among different populations (Graves,2004). More important, developments in the structuring of an International HapMap, which maps clusters of genes, have revealed variations in strings of DNA that correlate with geographic differences in phenotypes among humans around the world (Olson, 2002). New genetic data has enabled scientists to re-examine the relationship between human genetic variation and 'race'. A review of the results of genetic analyses has shown that human genetic variation is geographically structured, in accord with historical patterns of gene flow and genetic drift (Jorde and Wooding 2004).

However, because they have been only partially isolated, human populations are seldom demarcated by precise genetic boundaries. Substantial overlap can therefore be seen to occur between populations, invalidating the concept that populations (or races) are discrete types.

In the meantime, race may in some cases provide useful information in biomedical contexts, just as other categories, such as gender or age, do. But the potential usefulness of race must be balanced against the potential hazards. Ignorance of the shared nature of population variation could lead to diagnostic errors or to inappropriate treatment. The general public, including policy-makers, may be seduced by typological thinking, and so they should be made aware of the genetic data that help to prove it wrong.

Race remains an inflammatory issue, both socially and scientifically. Fortunately, modern human genetics may deliver the salutary message that human populations share most of their genetic variation and that there is no scientific support for the concept that human populations are discrete, non-overlapping entities. Although not all scientists are in agreement (Crow 2002; Mayr 2002), many critics deny that meaningful distinctions among contemporary human groups can be derived from a notion of race based upon biology (Cavalli-Sforza 2000; Omi 2001). To date, science has not identified a set of genes that correspond with social conceptions of race.

It may be argued therefore that race is not a naturally occurring phenomenon. The belief in race as a biological concept struggles to withstand scrutiny on at least two bases. First, genetic differences between population groups may not support the belief that there are genetic differences that justify racial groups (Nei & Roychoudhury 1983). There appear to be genetic differences among groups of people but these population groupings are not the same as racial groupings. The genetic distinctiveness of population groups appears to be a function of geography more than anything else. But racial categorization is not and could not be based upon geography. Population groups that "belong" to different racial groups may be very similar genetically, whereas population groups that "belong" to the same racial group may be relatively dissimilar, genetically speaking.

Secondly, physical differences among racial groups do not appear to reflect genetic differences (Nei & Roychoudhury 1983). Genotypic differences are not reliably mirrored by the differences in phenotype upon which racial group membership is largely based. The physical differences that signify race do not correlate with the genetic differences on which the biological claim for racial categorization appears to rest. Even if genetic variation justified a concept of race, our demarcation of racial groupings based on physical features does not seem to correspond to the underlying genetic differences.

2.2. Social construction of race

Race may be better regarded as a social construction. A century earlier, belief in the biological basis of racial categorization obscured this notion. Now, however, the biological bases of race have been widely questioned (Lewontin et al 1984). From the standpoint of biology, there appear to be no races. Yet, race continues to be among the most meaningful of social categories. From the standpoint of social psychology and psychiatry, race is among the most interesting and important of social phenomenon.

Recent behavioural and social research supports the social-cognitive notion that race is a construct that is based upon observable physical characteristics (such as skin colour) that have acquired socially significant meaning. In addition to physical features, ascribed and other characteristics such as given name, diet and dress may also contribute to categorizations of race. Cultural factors, such as language, religion and nationality, have more often been used in reference to ethnicity – that is, groups of people who share a common heritage, such as various European immigrant groups in the United States (Bobo 2001).

Historically, physical appearance has been the identifiable, surface characteristic on which racial categorization has been based. Physical features such as complexion, hair, lips, nose, and body-type have been central to determining race. The "deeper" properties of race are considered to be comprised not only of a biological essence (such as DNA), but also of psychological and status characteristics as well. Beliefs about those deeper properties constitute the essence of racial categorization. The psychological characteristics of race included factors such as racial sentiments, instinct, affinities, proclivities, and moral character. The social status characteristics include the general (e.g., dominant vs. subordinate) and the specific (e.g., master vs. slave) roles that racial groups often occupy in society relative to one another. Biological conceptions of race often, but not always, underpin beliefs in race-based psychological and social status characteristics.

Although both psychological and social status characteristics may be thought of as the deep properties of race (and therefore as part of the essence of the categories), features of social status (i.e., which roles particular racial groups occupy in society) may be believed to naturally follow form psychological characteristics (Yzerbyt et al 1997). Black African-Caribbeans' often-low status in contemporary times, for example, may be thought to result from an aversion to hard work.

Disparate physical features including hair, complexion and bone structure become understood, through the lens of racial essence, as similar. Some characteristics but not others become salient because they are assumed to signify race. Related to this, surface features such as skin colour and hair texture, according to this view, signify internal qualities of an individual. As suggested by Allport (1954), "[dark] skin implies more than pigmentation, it implies social inferiority". Far from merely contributing to appearance, surface features point toward the unseen moral, psychological, or intellectual properties of race.

2.3. The ambiguity of race

As a social cognitive construct, the meaning of race in the United Kingdom has changed and is likely to continue to change over time with changing socio-political norms, economic patterns and waves of immigration (e.g., the growing acknowledgement of mixed-race origins in the twenty-first century). Population groups and individuals vary in their consistency of reporting race when comparing surveys across time and with each other. For example, because country of birth is recorded on death certificates and in census data, much of the published data in this area has allocated race according to country of birth, a strategy that is clearly inadequate. In addition, many studies have used categories such as Black or South Asian to describe the ethnicity of those studied.

Some people believe self-identification is the only reasonable method to use because it allows people to express their own racial identity. Another alternative is largely to ignore the role of self-perceived ethnicity and to assign racial category according to family origin (Nazroo 2001). Unsurprisingly, perceived racial group and country of family origin have been found to be highly related. Harris (2002) argues that the classification of race is a social process that varies across contexts and observers. To determine an individual's race, people may use one or more ancestry or biological bases, phenotypic or physical characteristics, and cultural bases, such as ideology and language. Obtaining multiple indicators of racial identification would likely provide helpful data to inform racial classification and analysis.

Race should be part of a multi-dimensional construct of social status. Ideally, the construct should include: a) some measure of self-identification; b) a measure of group identity; c) a measure of social distance between the group that the individual belongs to and other groups; d) measures of social mobility; e) socio-economic status; and f) contextual variables of family and community.

2.4. Race and ethnicity as a variable in research

Ethnicity has been used increasingly as a key variable to describe health data, further stimulated by ethnic monitoring in the NHS. Senior and Bhopal identified four fundamental problems with ethnicity in epidemiological research – the difficulties of its measurement; the heterogeneity of the populations under study; the lack of clarity about the purpose of the research; and ethnocentricity affecting the interpretation and usage of the data (1994). They have suggested how the value of ethnicity as an epidemiological variable may be improved: ethnicity should be differentiated from race; ethnicity's complexity and fluidity should be acknowledged; ethnic classifications should be more explicit and their current limitations set out; investigators should recognize the potential influence of their personal values and ethnocentricity upon research an policy-development; socio-economic differences should not be ignored; and the relative importance of environmental, cultural, lifestyle and genetic influences should be factored in to the analyses of difference.

3. Racism

Race has been described earlier as a social-cognitive construct that evolves over time and in which racial categories reflect the person's ancestors' physical features and associated characteristics that have acquired social meaning. Racism may be defined as a belief or doctrine that inherent biological differences among the various human races determine cultural or individual achievement, with a corollary that one's own race is superior and has the right to rule others. When racism, the belief, is applied in practice, it takes forms such as prejudice, discrimination, segregation or subordination. Racism can more narrowly refer to a system of oppression, such as institutional racism. Organizations and institutions that put racism into action discriminate against, and marginalize, a class of people who share a common racial designation. The term racism is usually applied to the dominant group in a society, because it is that group that has the means to oppress others. The term can also apply to any individual or group, regardless of social status or dominance. Racism can be both overt and covert. Individual racism sometimes consists of overt acts by individuals, which can result in violence or the destruction of property. Institutional racism is often more covert and subtle. It often appears within the operation of established and respected forces in the society, and frequently receives less public condemnation than the overt type.

3.1. Racial attitudes

Covert, less obvious aspects of racism are often contained within people's beliefs and attitudes about different races. Although attitudes are more difficult to evidence, it is important to register their presence and attempt to measure them because attitudes may influence behavioural inequity towards different racial groups, and attitudes to racism are often considered no less important than overt acts of racism by the recipients of racial discrimination. There is evidence that negative stereotypes about minority groups are declining. In addition, this apparent increased tolerance extends beyond blacks to other racial and ethnic minority groups as well (American National Election Survey 1995). Despite these trends in the intergroup attitudes of the white majority in the west, there are still reasons for concern. 32% of blacks reported that discrimination is the primary obstacle to achieving equality in the United States (Anderson 1996). Furthermore, despite dramatic improvements in the expressed racial attitudes of whites over time, racial disparities persist. US data shows that gaps between blacks and white Americans in infant mortality, life expectancy, employment, income and poverty have continued to exist; and, in many cases, these disparities have actually increased over the past few decades.

3.2. Aversive racism

Aversive racism represents a prevalent type of modern racial bias which researchers feel is important but often hard to identify (Gaertner et al 1997). In contrast to "old-fashioned" racism, which is expressed directly and openly, aversive racism is a subtle, often unintentional form of bias that characterizes those who possess strong egalitarian values and who believe that they are not prejudiced. Aversive racists are also felt to possess negative racial feelings and beliefs of which they are unaware or that they try to dissociate from their non-prejudiced self-images. The negative feelings that aversive racists have for blacks do not reflect open hostility or hate. Instead, their reactions are found to involve discomfort, uneasiness, disgust, and sometimes fear. That is they are found to regard blacks as "aversive", while, at the same time, they find any suggestion that they might be prejudiced aversive as well.

3.3. Racial microaggressions

An equally subtle yet significant form of racism developed by the US psychiatrist Chester Pierce is the concept of microaggressions (1974). Microaggressions are subtle insults (verbal, nonverbal, and/or visual) directed toward people of colour, often automatically or unconsciously. In and of itself a microaggression may seem harmless, but the cumulative burden of a lifetime of microaggressions can theoretically contribute to raised morbidity and flattened confidence. Little is known about microaggressions, and yet this subtle form of racism is reported as having a dramatic impact on the lives of African Americans. Pierce and his colleagues have defined racial microaggressions as "subtle, stunning, often automatic, and nonverbal exchanges which are 'put downs' of blacks by offenders" (Pierce et al 1978, p. 66). They further maintain that these "offensive mechanisms used against blacks often are innocuous" and that the "cumulative weight of their never-ending burden is the major ingredient in black-white interactions" (p. 66).

3.4. Racial discrimination

A social science definition of racial discrimination may be best used for the purposes of this study. This includes two components: (1) differential treatment on the basis of race that disadvantages a racial group and (2) treatment on the basis of inadequately justified factors other than race that disadvantages a specific racial group (differential effect). Each of these components is based on behaviour or treatment that disadvantages one racial group over another, yet the parts differ on whether the treatment is based on an individual's race or some other factor that results in a different racial outcome.

It is important that research into racial discrimination encompasses categories that include behaviours and processes which are either not explicitly unlawful or not effectively prohibited because of difficulties in measurement or proof. This is in order to capture as true a picture of the experience of racial discrimination for the individual as possible. For example, subtle forms of discrimination which might not be susceptible to legal challenge but fall within this definition include when interviewers of job applicants more frequently adopt behaviours (e.g., interrupting, asking fewer questions, or using a hectoring tone) that result in poor communication and consequently poorer performance by disadvantaged minority ethnic applicants as compared with other applicants. Even though it may be more difficult to prove legally, such subtle discrimination in theory constitutes actionable disparate treatment discrimination.

This definition of racial discrimination is based on behaviours and practices, and as such it differs from a definition that also includes prejudiced attitudes and stereotypical beliefs.

Discriminatory behaviours and practices may arise from prejudice and stereotyping, but prejudice need not result in either differential treatment or effect. Similarly, whereas discriminatory behaviour in many domains is unlawful, prejudiced attitudes and stereotypical beliefs are not.

4. Measuring racial discrimination and its effect upon health

Because discriminatory behaviour can rarely be directly observed, researchers face the challenge of establishing when racial discrimination has actually occurred and whether it explains some portion of a racially disparate outcome. Those who attempt to identify the presence or absence of discrimination typically observe an individual's race (e.g., black) and a particular outcome (e.g., health status) and try to determine whether that outcome would have been different if the person had a different racial origin (e.g., white).

Establishing that racial discrimination did or did not occur requires causal inference. Identifying a racial disparity and determining that an association between race and an outcome remains after adjusting for plausible confounding factors is relatively straightforward. The real difficulty lies in going beyond the identification of an association to the attribution of cause. Ultimately, researchers must rely upon the evaluation of evidence from multiple studies - whilst considering the strength of association, consistency, and plausibility of each study's design and findings – to draw conclusions about causality.

4.1. The challenge of direct measurement of racial discrimination

Legislation passed in the twentieth century both in the UK and the US have made open discrimination on the basis of race or ethnicity illegal, and perpetrators can be prosecuted under both criminal and civil law. Although readily observable acts of discrimination have declined, the persistence of high levels of residential segregation along racial lines and large racial gaps with respect to income, wealth, and other societal outcomes indicate the continued existence of racial discrimination albeit in new forms, that are not as easily identifiable but may be damaging nonetheless (Krieger 2000).

Surveys provide valuable evidence for understanding the extent of discrimination, but they cannot directly measure its occurrence. They tend to measure self-reported attitudes, perceptions or experiences of discrimination which may be unreliable for two main reasons. First, if a discriminatory occurrence is ambiguous, a minority ethnic respondent may misreport its incidence with more subtle forms of discrimination not as easily detected. Secondly, white respondents are often not willing to admit to practising or supporting discriminatory actions, which leads to inaccurate reporting of their true beliefs or attitudes.

There is increasing support for a life-course approach to measuring the effects of discrimination on the individual's outcome with development of theories of cumulative disadvantage over time (Jacobsen et al 2001).Longitudinal studies lend themselves to this approach; they analyze the incidence, causes and consequences of changes in attitudes about race and experiences of racial discrimination at the level of the individual. Their approach is very valuable, although there is a dearth of such work primarily owing to its difficult and costly methods.

4.2. Indirect measurement of health effects of racial discrimination

This approach acknowledges that discrimination may be difficult to measure and thus compares health outcomes of "dominant" and discriminated-against racial groups. An example of this approach is the EMPIRIC (Ethnic Minority Psychiatric Illness Rates) study, which examined common mental disorders and ethnicity in England (Weich et al 2004).

If any obtained differences in outcome cannot be wholly explained by known risk factors (i.e., by statistical adjustment), it may be inferred that the residual difference could be explained by racial discrimination (Krieger et al 1993). It is usually postulated that socio-economic status is the main confounder for such health outcome differences. If a residual difference remains after adjusting for socio-economic status, four alternative explanations may be put forward.

Firstly, socio-economic position has been inadequately measured, which accounts for the residual confounding. Secondly, an intermediary, economically-unrelated variable such as psychological distress has led to the disparity in health outcomes. A third explanation is that unexplained differences are explained by unmeasured factors associated with race and the outcomes have not been accounted for, i.e. unknown confounders (such as culturally-shaped dietary patterns). The final possibility is that of genetic differences between races explaining the residual difference in outcome.

Existing research relying upon indirect strategies to measure the health effects of racial discrimination are able to addressboth the health effects of types of discrimination not readily perceived by the individual (such as the treatment decisions of clinicians), and whether economic disparities can explain the health differences that may occur between racial groups. These methods are not able to measure direct experiences of racial discrimination, nor can they investigate effects related to intensity, duration, or period of exposure to any discrimination.

4.3. The measurement of perceived racism versus objective racism

Research investigating the untoward effects of racism is on the rise. As the empirical literature exploring the associations between racism and health emerges, the development of an equally strong theoretical literature is needed to explain the pathways through which racism may influence health outcomes. Equally, attention should be given to assessments of racism that are reliable and valid.

Although research suggests that perceptions of events as stressful are more predictive of psychological and physiological functioning than objective demands, comparative research exploring the relationship between a person's perceptions an objective demands may provide additional concurrent validity. Further research is also needed to more clearly interpret observed findings with respect to perceived racism. For example, for some people who perceive stimuli as involving racism probably do so because it is less anxiety-provoking than attributing the failure of being say, promoted at work, to personal deficits. Furthermore, some people who do not report perceiving racism probably fail to do so because of denial or as an attempt to avoid the expected psychological distress that would be associated with negotiating an uncontrollable stressor. Accordingly, in addition to assessing the perceptions of racism, the simultaneous measurement of other contributory factors such as attributional style, impression management, self-deception, and affective state would help to delineate the possible mitigating effects of these variables.

Measures used to assess racism should: be reliable and valid for the target groups and subgroups as well as ethnic-gender groups and subgroups being studied; be specific enough to capture the reported multidimensional nature of racism; and be developed with equivalent shorter and longer versions to facilitate use with different study designs.

Notwithstanding this, it is important to note that perceived racism need not be any less significant than objective racism, or an observer-related account of the same racist event. The individual's subjective experience of a putatively racist event is more significant to that individual than some third party account of the same occurrence. Therefore, one might argue, that little may be gained by measuring objective racism rather than perceived racism if it is the latter that holds greater significance and possible predictive ability in terms of prognosis or health outcome.

4.4. Measuring self-reported experiences of racial discrimination and its health effects

A relatively new approach in determining the health effects of racial discrimination is by determining people's direct experiences of discrimination and their relation to health status. The most common outcomes of these studies have been mental health (e.g., depression, psychological distress) and hypertension or blood pressure. The main problem with this approach is a lack of standardization in measuring self-reported experiences in terms of: length, intensity and frequency of exposure; domain of exposure (e.g., global or specific situations); and the targets of discrimination (e.g., individual family members or the family unit as a whole); reactions to racial discrimination.

Empirical studies adopting this approach have tended to focus on the racial attitudes of those who discriminate and used qualitative, in-depth techniques rather than methods that are easily interpretable by epidemiological methods.

There are four factors which may mean people experiencing the same discriminatory "exposure" would report them differently. The notion of "internalized oppression" adopted by some oppressed group-members and a sense of their subordinate status being in some way "deserved", may lead to an under-statement of an actual discriminatory act (Meyer 1995). Secondly, the notion of "social desirability" leads to people shaping their responses according to the perceived status of the interviewer. Thirdly, individuals may exaggerate discriminatory experiences (system-blame) to avoid blaming themselves for failure (Neighbours et al 1996). Finally, the cognitive effects of depressive disorder may lead to overstating or magnifying a discriminatory environmental event.

Researchers have attempted to circumvent the issue of self-presentational biases impairing the self-report of racial discrimination by the use of implicit rather than explicit measures of discrimination. The Implicit Attitudes Test is a computer-measured task which measures response speeds to racially-charged imagery to compute unconscious racism measures rather than through explicit questioning (Greenwald et al 1998). A related approach to avoid such biases would be to incorporate questions to assess identity formation, political consciousness, stigma and internalized oppression.

4.5. Measuring population-level experiences of racial discrimination and their health effects

Racial discrimination measured at a population-level is being increasingly measured in research to see if it relates more closely to population health than individual-level measures of discrimination (Kennedy et al 1997). Although this work is in its infancy, promising measures of population-level indicators of discrimination are: economic segregation of neighbourhoods; occupational segregation of jobs by race/ethnicity and gender (Rothenberg 1988); voting rates and registration of different dominant and subordinate groups; and socio-demographic composition of subsidiary branches of Government, such as the judiciary.

Concerns related to this particular approach to research are that of the aetiological period and the ecological fallacy. With regards to the aetiological period, the issue is making appropriate distinction between the effects of acute and cumulative exposures, and between outcomes with short and longer latency periods. It is harder to infer causality from a potentially aetiological agent when the latency period is longer, the agent far-removed in time, from the outcome. The ecological fallacy centres on whether causal inferences at the population level are valid at the individual level. This fallacy results from confounding introduced through the grouping variable (e.g., city, nation) used to define the group-level dependent and independent variables. It has been suggested that the ecological fallacy could be minimised by population-level measures of discrimination meaningfully combined with individual-level measures through techniques of multi-level analyses (Williams 1997).

5. Racism, physical and mental health

The relationship between racism and both physical and mental health is a complex one. In Figure 1, a framework is provided to understand the relationship between racism and health; the arrows indicate associations. It can be seen that racism is a major societal force that affects health status. At the societal level, racism within medical institutions could affect minority health status through the organisation of medical services. There are large differences in access to medical care and receipt of medical procedures between racial groups in the US (Franks et al 1993; Giles et al 1995), which is likely to affect prognosis and outcome. If racism is so embedded in social and cultural institutions, race-related risk factors and resources such as racial beliefs and racial bias are likely to be important influences upon health.

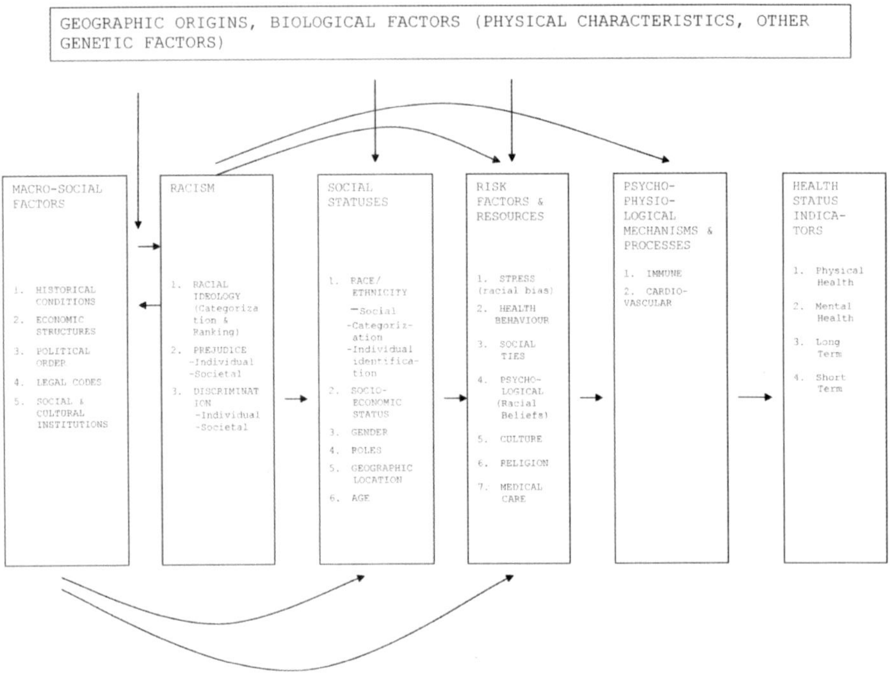

Figure 1. A framework for understanding the relationship between race and health (Williams 1996).

Literature suggests that internalisation of society's negative cultural stereotypes about a racial group by members of that group can lead to worsened health status. African Americans that do so have been shown to have elevated rates of substance misuse and physical and mental illness (Williams & Chung 1995).

Economic institutions are thought to play a powerful role in affecting health status along racial lines. Researchers have argued that there is disproportionate targeting of minority ethnic consumers by the tobacco and alcohol industries leading to over-consumption and worse health (Bryant &Mohai 1992). Residential segregation is an important potential mechanism perpetuating health differences between races. Racism enacted at an institutional level through financial institutions (banks, mortgage lenders) may create and sustain a social status that results in differential housing. And once in place, such segregation restricts employment opportunities, thus socio-economic mobility and the individual's situation worsens. When considering this notion, it is striking that there has been little report of any decline in the level of racial segregation in African Americans over time (Farley & Frye 1994).

Experiences of racial bias at the individual level may have deleterious consequences by acting as a negative stressor (Thoits 1983). The stress literature suggests that the persistence of a difficult situation and its resolution, or lack of it, are important determinants of its adverse impact. To elucidate more clearly the effects of racism as a stressor, there needs to be a greater understanding of the way in which racism combines with other sources and types of stress, as well as the identification of intervening variables that may moderate or mediate the effects of stress on health (coping factors, personality types etc). For example, Lazarus and Folkman (1984) have researched stress in relation to coping and noted that both the subjective evaluation of the seriousness of an event as well as coping responses determine whether a psychological stress response will follow. This may be useful in the development of a model including racism as an environmental stressor.

5.1. Racism and physical health

A recent excellent systematic review of self-reported racism and health is the main source for the information in this section (Paradies 2006). That source reviewed 138 empirical quantitative population-based studies of self-reported racism and health, each study often determining several outcomes and associations. The study designs included were cross-sectional, cohort, experimental and case-control in nature, with the majority (73%) of significant associations determined in cross-sectional studies; this of course limits the inference of causality. However, 12% of the reported significant associations between racism and health outcome were found in longitudinal studies. A variety of ethnic groups were included: African American (most frequent); Asian; Latino; Whites and refugee groups.

The most consistent association found was that self-reported racism had an association with negative mental health outcomes on 72% of occasions. The association was found to be far weaker for physical health outcomes: the association between self-reported racism and worse physical health was only found 36% of the time, with no association found in 63% and a positive association (i.e., with better physical health) in 1% of the research. It is hypothesised that this weaker effect may be due to racism exert a lagged effect upon physical health, mediated by negative mental health outcomes.

The majority of physical health outcome studies examined the relationship between racism and blood pressure (Paradies 2006). 19 out of 79 occasions found self-reported racism was associated with elevated blood pressure, with no association found on 59 occasions, and with a negative association on one occasion. Furthermore, self-reported racism was associated with increased heart rate on five out of ten occasions. A possible pathway through which perceived racism may affect blood pressure is anger (Steffen et al 2003). Perceived racism has been related to higher levels of anger and hostility and large studies have found that African Americans tend to score higher on anger and hostility measures than whites (Scherwitz et al 1991). Paradies' review found a positive association between low infant birth-weight/decreased gestational age and self-reported racism on 15 out of 27 occasions, which may be speculated to be associated with deprivation and poorer access to ante-natal services.

General self-reported health status was identified by Paradies (2006) as a common outcome when measured either as a global measure or through use of the instruments Short Form-12/36. A negative association between health status and self-reported racism was found on 19 out of 45 occasions.

In terms of health-related behaviours, Paradies identified a positive association between racism and increased cigarette smoking on four occasions, increased alcohol misuse on eight out of 14 occasions and increased drug misuse on five out of six occasions (2006). Possibly related to this, results from a national sample found that discrimination was related to an elevated mortality risks over a 13-year follow-up period among African Americans who had self-blaming as opposed to external attributional orientations (LaVeist et al 2001).

5.2. Racism and mental health

Mental health outcomes are the most frequently measured in relation to racism. An alternative theoretical framework to that outlined in Figure 1, linking racism to mental health has multiple, inter-related connections (Turner & Kramer 1995). These connections were divided into the following areas where racism may potentially exert an effect: the definitions of mental health and illness; aetiological theories of mental illness; the evaluation process (assessment and diagnosis); the provision of direct services; the organisation and structure of mental health institutions; and the training of mental health professionals and care providers.

Social class is often cited as a confounder of both ethnicity and poor health status: the inverse relationship between social class and mental illness is consistently reported. This association may be mediated by an increased exposure to, and vulnerability to, social stressors. It has been argued that minority status in itself is a source of stress, independent of social class. A related phenomenon is the "ethnic-density" effect: this is the observation that the incidence of schizophrenia in non-white ethnic minorities is greater when they comprise a smaller proportion of the local population (Boydell et al 2001). Those authors attributed this to a greater vulnerability to social stressors when an individual is a member of a small minority group rather than a larger minority group.

It has been argued that the psychiatric assessment process is undermined by racial biases and ethnocentricity. The argument is that owing to the development of most assessment and measurement tools within Western cultures, this limits their use in different ethnic or cultural groups, leading to a possibility that culturally-acceptable behaviour may be labelled as psychopathology. Cross-cultural clinical assessment is therefore increasingly favoured and researchers have developed a number of approaches to facilitate a more culturally informed assessment and tested these in medical students with success (Chakraborty et al 2009a).

With regards to minority ethnic access to psychiatric services, there is a problem of an inequity of service provision, thought to be linked to racism: minority groups being less likely to receive psychotherapy or counselling than their white counter-parts; and the former being more likely to receive oral or depot-injection pharmaco-therapy and inpatient treatment; more likely to present to psychiatric services via an emergency pathway (the police or Accident and Emergency Departments) rather than through primary care or their families; more likely to be detained under the Mental Health Act; less likely to comply with management plans and remain linked with services (Chakraborty & McKenzie 2002).

Research and training issues are also thought to connect racism to mental ill health in a number of ways. If researchers were to bring racist attitudes, perspectives or values to their scientific enterprise the result could be attribution of inter-ethnic differences to "cultural deficiencies." Secondly, racist research is poorly-conducted research; examples of this kind of poor research are: ignoring the cross-cultural validity of research instruments, neglecting to think about the impact of the ethnicity of the interviewer upon engagement with minority ethnic respondents, under-studying of phenomena in minority ethnic groups with transposition of findings from the dominant ethnic groups, labouring under the assumption that the findings are universally applicable. Similarly, training issues which could be relevant to the service-related inequities between ethnic groups may be the lack of experience acquired by mental health trainees in ethnically-diverse areas, and the relative scarcity of both clinical and academic senior mental health professionals from minority ethnic backgrounds (Turner & Kramer 1995).

Given the ever-expanding presence of minority ethnic groups in the west, the benefits of increasing the minority ethnic mental health workforce would be several: those minority patients whom were thought could benefit from an ethnically-matched therapist would be more likely to access one. Secondly, the increased presence of minority health professionals may be regarded by service-recipients as a clear sign that those services are, in reality, available to them, in turn making help-seeking seem less threatening and more acceptable. Finally, their presence may lead more majority health providers to think of cultural factors as important considerations, with cross-cultural work becoming more mainstream and routine, and less for the sake of "political correctness".

A major and substantial study was a 13-year national panel study from 1979 to 1992, which revealed complex relationships between the experiences and perceptions of racism and the physical and mental health status of a sample of 623 African Americans (Jackson et al 1996). It found that reports of negative racial encounters over the 13-year period were weakly predictive of poor subjective well-being in 1992. A more general measure of racial beliefs – perceiving that whites want to keep blacks down – was found to be related to poorer physical health in 1979-80, better physical health in 1992, and predicted increased psychological distress, as well as lower subjective well-being in 1992. The authors concluded that cumulative perceptions of racism resulted in poorer mental health but, surprisingly better physical health. The latter finding could have been due to those respondents who perceive whites as wanting to keep them down being more vigilant when it comes to their own physical health; hence the better outcome.

Returning to Paradies' review of the extant empirical evidence for associations between mental ill health outcomes and self-reported racism (2006), improved mental health was almost never found to be associated with increased racism. On 40 out of 62 occasions a positive association was found between self-reported racism and psychological/emotional distress, with no association on 21 occasions.

Depressive symptoms or frank depressive disorder were positively associated with racism on 39 from 52 occasions (Paradies 2006). Several models have explained this phenomenon, with the common pathway often identifying racial stress as both a vulnerability factor and a stressful life event. Community-based studies have found a higher prevalence of depression in minority ethnic groups than in the dominant population (Lloyd 1998; Shaw et al 1999).

Obsessional and compulsive symptoms were found to be associated with self-reported racism on five out of five occasions in different studies; however, it could be that this positive finding is artefactual and in fact due to improved recall of racist (as well as other) events in those with an obsessive tendency. Somatisation was found to have a positive association with self-reported racism on five out of five occasions (Paradies 2006). Anxiety symptoms were found to be positively associated with racism on 15 out of 22 occasions. Several stress models describe a relationship between threatening events and the onset of anxiety symptoms. Racial discrimination was found to be the crucial factor associated with high levels of anxiety in non-white immigrants to New Zealand (Pernice& Brook 1996).

Stress was found by Paradies to be associated positively with self-reported racism on 13 out of 22 occasions (2006). Psychiatric symptomatology following a racist threat or attack has been conceptualised by some researchers as a form of post-traumatic stress disorder – PTSD (Dassori & Silva 1998). Loo has described PTSD following race-related verbal and physical assaults, racial stigmatisation and the cumulative effect of racism as a trauma in an Asian group (1994). Other symptoms common to PTSD such as poor concentration, hyper-vigilance, avoidance and autonomic arousal have also been described following experiences of racism.

There is a dearth of empirical evidence considering the association between racism and psychosis. No studies were found by Paradies (2006), although a recent cross-sectional survey found an increased risk of psychosis in UK minority groups after adjusting for gender, age and socio-economic status (Karlsen et al 2005). This study (EMPIRIC) consisted of a multivariate analysis of quantitative, cross-sectional data from a nationally-representative community sample of people aged between 16 and 74 years from the largest minority ethnic groups in England: those of Caribbean, Indian, Pakistani, Bangladeshi, an Irish origin. The researchers found that the experience of interpersonal racism and perceiving racism in the wider society each have independent effects on the risk of common mental disorder and psychosis, even after adjustment.

From the same dataset, authors examined perceived discrimination and its association with common mental disorders among workers in the United Kingdom (Bhui et al 2003). Discrimination was measured as reports of insults; unfair treatment at work; or job denial stemming from race, religion or language. The risk of mental disorders was found to be highest among ethnic minority individuals reporting unfair treatment and racism insults. The overall greatest risks were observed among Black Caribbeans exposed to unfair treatment at work and Indian, Bangladeshi, and Irish individuals reporting insults.

Furthermore, the EMPIRIC dataset permitted the examination of the examination between racism and mental illness in minority ethnic groups, using social support as a moderating factor (Chakraborty et al 2010). Social support was quantified as both the number of relatives as well as their geographical proximity to the individual. When quantified in either way, social support did not moderate the size of the association between perceived discrimination and mental illness. The finding that this association was not reduced by the supposedly "buffering" effect of familial social support, suggests that racism has a strong and pronounced effect.

A population-based incidence and case-control study of first-episode psychosis (Aetiology and Ethnicity in Schizophrenia and Other Psychoses (ÆSOP)) examined the cross-sectional association between ethnicity and psychosis and whether this was mediated by perceptions of disadvantage (Cooper et al 2008). The Black ethnic groups were found to have a higher incidence of psychosis. After controlling for unemployment, the association of ethnicity with psychosis was attenuated by perceptions of disadvantage. This suggests that perceived disadvantage is at least partly associated with the excess of psychosis among Black people living in the UK.

A second group has carried out a series of studies in the Netherlands, looking at the association between discrimination and the incidence of psychotic disorders. The first paper reports upon the incidence of psychotic disorders over seven years in The Hague, a city with a large and diverse minority ethnic population (Veling et al 2007). They found a dose-response relationship between discrimination and age- and gender-adjusted incidence rate ratios of both schizophrenic and all psychotic disorders in ethnic minority groups, suggesting that perceived discrimination might contribute to the increased risk of schizophrenia.

In their second paper, the group describes a case-control study of first-episode schizophrenia investigating whether perceived discrimination at the individual level is a risk factor for schizophrenia (Veling et al 2008). Cases reported somewhat higher rates of perceived discrimination in the year prior to illness onset than their siblings and the general-hospital controls, but these differences were not statistically significant. Therefore they concluded that perceived discrimination at the individual level was not a risk factor for schizophrenia in these data, although they concede that the relationship between racial discrimination and psychosis may vary with the aspect of discrimination that is studied, and may also depend upon the social context in which discrimination takes place.

An earlier UK study reported raised incidences of schizophrenia in all minority ethnic groups presenting to psychiatric services within a deprived, inner-city setting (King et al 1994). Racism has been attributed as a cause of illness by psychotic patients but the study was cross-sectional in nature, limiting an assumption about causality (Chakraborty et al 2009b).

Another study found that black and minority ethnic patients with psychotic illnesses reported no more life events than their white British counterparts, but they were more likely to attribute them to racism, potentially disinclining the minority patients from using services they perceive to be racist (Gilvarry et al 1999). Societal racism has been mooted as a cause of increased risk of schizophrenia in Black populations in the UK; and institutional racism, life events and chronic stress may also be associated with an increased risk of developing psychosis (Perera et al 1991).

Perceived racism (measured by the Perceived Racism Scale – McNeilly et al 1996) has been examined for its predictive effects upon paranoia among African Americans (Combs et al 2006). In a population of African American college students, Combs and colleagues found that perceived racism was highly significantly correlated with both cultural mistrust and with non-clinical paranoia, even following adjustment.

A prospective study from the Netherlands examined people with no history of psychosis at baseline and at three-year follow-up (Janssen et al 2003). It found that baseline perceived discrimination was associated in a dose-response fashion, with delusional ideation at follow-up, irrespective of ethnicity and after adjustment. Both this and the Combs et al study suggest that perceived racism/ discrimination are correlated with both sub-clinical paranoia and frank delusional ideation.

An American study examined racial differences among male outpatients with severe mental illness on therapeutic support, mental health service utilization, and service satisfaction (Tsai et al 2012). A total of 530 participants (289 White, 179 Black, and 62 of another race) across three large mental health centers (two state funded and one federally funded) in Connecticut were examined cross-sectionally. No racial differences were found in therapeutic support, and there were essentially no racial differences in service satisfaction, suggesting there are few racial differences in the reported quality of mental health care and service utilization among male outpatients with severe mental illness.

Race appears to play a significant role as a determinant of health in the UK and US. The study of racism and health is in relative infancy (Chakraborty & McKenzie 2002). The persistence of racial inequalities in health need to be understood in light of the persistence of racialised social structures that appear to affect health status in multiple ways. It may be suggested that the self-reported racism is a neglected determinant of health in research and this, in itself, may contribute to the racial disparities in health outcome.

6. Ethnic inequalities in UK mental health care

Inequitable variation in the use of British health care services between ethnic groups has been a matter of concern for British policy-makers and the Government alike. It has been reviewed that mental health services are unappealing to some ethnic groups, who complain of more coercive treatment as and adverse experiences (Cochrane and Sashidharan 1996) and these experiences have been recently more systematically reviewed (Bhui et al 2003). The UK Government's Department of Health has recognized that there is a problem of race inequality regarding the provision, management and outcome of mental health services and addressed the issue of race and mental health care in the National Health Service in two documents: "Inside Outside: Improving mental health services for black and minority ethnic communities in England" (DoH 2003) and "Delivering race equality in mental health care" (DoH 2005).

6.1. Ethnic differences in experience, adherence and pathways to care

Bhui and colleagues recently conducted a thorough systematic review of UK studies published between 1983 and 2000, which compared access and use of mental health services by different ethnic groups (2003). They suggested that Black people are over-represented among in-patients and that Asian patients use in-patient facilities less often than White patients. Also, there is some evidence for variations in pathways to specialist mental health care, with Black people traversing more complex routes. Variation in primary care assessments or primary care involvement could explain some of those ethnic pathway-differences to specialist services but the primary care literature was found to be limited. The authors end by deeming a future priority as the measurement of discrimination as a potential explanatory factor for some of these differences.

More recently, the Aetiology and Ethnicity in Schizophrenia and Other Psychoses (ÆSOP) study sought to investigate the relationship between ethnicity and pathways to mental health services in two UK centres in a large cohort of patients with a first episode of psychosis (Morgan et al 2005a). African-Caribbean patients were significantly more likely to be compulsorily admitted than White British patients, as were Black African patients. In a companion study, the ÆSOP group investigated the pathways to mental health care and ethnicity in a sample of patients with a first episode of psychosis drawn from two UK centres (Morgan et al 2005b). They found that compared with White British patients, general practitioner referral was less frequent for both African-Caribbean and Black African patients and referral by a criminal justice agency was more common. With the exception of criminal justice referrals for Black African patients, these findings remained significant after adjusting for potential confounders. This suggested to the authors that factors operate during a first episode of psychosis to increase the risk that the pathway to care for Black patients will involve non-health professionals.

Linked to pathways to mental health care, the patient's experience of treatment within services is significant. There is limited research-work examining the effects of ethnicity upon adherence with psychotropic medication. One US study compared psychotropic adherence rates in monolingual-Hispanics (mostly Puerto Ricans), bilingual-Hispanics, and African-Americans as compared with Caucasians in 122 subjects recruited from a community mental health center (Diaz et al 2005). After controlling for possible confounding factors monolingual-Hispanics and African-Americans had lower medication adherence rates than Caucasians.

A second US study of Texan Medicaid claims retrieved for patients diagnosed with either schizophrenia or schizoaffective disorder assessed the association between ethnicity or medication and days' use of the medication in the year following initiation (Opolka et al 2003). It found that African-American and Mexican-American patients were significantly less adherent than White patients, even after controlling for potential confounding factors.

The net result for Black patients of more aversive pathways to care, greater compulsory admissions and poorer medication adherence, unsurprisingly, seems to lead both to increased mutual distrust from both patients and care-providers, as well as a more costly experience for Black patients through mental health services.The finding that Black people are often reluctant to engage with mainstream mental health services with delays in seeking help, seems to create new risks, such as police involvement or use of the Mental Health Act, which leads to disproportionately high rates of hospital inpatient admission, compulsory admission, admission to intensive care and secure services and use of seclusion and restraint in all types of hospital. Such patterns of service-use are negatively experienced and associated with poor outcomes, as measured by relapse and readmission. In turn, these adverse consequences reinforce mistrust of mainstream services that is the initial cause of delayed engagement.

The report "Breaking the Circles of Fear" (Sainsbury Centre for Mental Health 2002) looked into the relationship between African and Caribbean people and mental health services. It confirmed previous quantitative findings in relation to the over-representation of African and Caribbean people in services. It also highlighted: high concentrations of African and Caribbean people within inpatient, acute and secure treatment settings; limited involvement of primary care and a lack of community-based crisis care; people coming into contact with services via the criminal justice system; poor levels of engagement and satisfaction; questionable attributions of risk to Black service users; high levels of fear among Black service users of both mental health professionals and of statutory services; a related high level of fear among mental health professionals in relation to the risks posed by Black service users; and alienation and lack of involvement of Black carers.

6.2. Institutional racism and mental health

Institutional racism may be defined as "the collective failure ofan organization to provide an appropriate and professional serviceto people because of their colour, culture, or ethnic origin. This can be seen or detected in processes, attitudes, and behaviourthat amount to discrimination through unwitting prejudice, ignorance, thoughtlessness, and racist stereotyping which disadvantagespeople in ethnic minority groups" (MacPherson 1999). The concept has been applied to psychiatry and will be discussed later but prior to this and related to it, has been the debate of the provision and delivery of services to minority ethnic groups and to best suit their mental health needs.

The fairly consistent findings reported in the previous section have suggested certain themes of mental health care in relation to the Black British population: that of increased coercion, more aversive pathways to care, leading to greater mistrust, sooner disengagement from services with poorer service-related outcome and greater rates of readmission. These themes have prompted the charge of either a prejudicial or discriminatory mental health system when it comes to care provision for minority ethnic groups, and the need for a suitable solution if the is indeed the case.

The charge of whether or not UK psychiatric services are institutionally racist has also been recently hotly debated in the literature (Singh and Burns 2006; McKenzie and Bhui 2007). A focus of the debate has been the Healthcare Commission's report of the findings of the "Count me in" one-day census of NHS hospitals, private mental health hospitals and learning disability units (Healthcare Commission 2006). The survey of 32,023 inpatients reported that 21% of patients were from black and minority ethnic groups, although they represent only 7% of the population. Rates of admission were lower than average in the white British, Indian, and Chinese groups, but three or more times higher than average in black African, black Caribbean, and white and black Caribbean mixed groups. Not only were people in these three groups more likely to be admitted to hospital, but also those in hospital were 19-39% more likely to be admitted involuntarily. Once in hospital, people who defined themselves as black Caribbean had the longest stay.

Singh and Burns state that these findings do not necessarily prove institutional racism, and that the scientific evidence to support this charge is inconclusive (2006). They argue that the increased rate of psychotic disorder in UK second-generation African-Caribbeans is not a specific phenomenon, rather a common experience of migrants in a new country. They argue that the more aversive care pathways of African-Caribbeans through the mental health system may be better explained by: greater stigma of mental illness within this minority community, and less social support from the immediate family, rather than by psychiatric racism. The racist argument is further undermined, they suggest, by the lower aversive pathways for the south Asian community (which, presumably would also be subject to racism from the system) where the familial support might be stronger. They write that the accusation of racism against the health system can be pernicious, as it sets up distrust in the minority community which may present to services with an expectation of inequitable services leading to their delayed help-seeking further and impeding recovery. It may also undermine staff morale, whom may feel undervalued and blamed as a result of charges of racism.

In response to this, academics have suggested that the above position represents a set of stereotyped responses to charges of racism rather than sound scientific arguments (McKenzie and Bhui 2007). Those inappropriate responses consist of either blaming the individual making the charge of racism; misunderstanding institutional racism as the fault of the individual rather than a systemic failure; requiring proof of intent within a racist action if it is to be truly racist; and finally, ignoring the urgency of the problem by calling for more research rather than suggesting remedial action.

6.3. Epidemiological issues around hospital admission data

The use of psychiatric hospital in-patient admissions statistics to examine ethnic variations in the pattern of mental illness offers both advantages and disadvantages. These statistics present both general challenges as well as those specific to interpreting trends within ethnic groups. On the one hand these data have been available on a national scale and are not likely to be influenced by the research process itself. On the other hand these data suffer from several problems, which means that findings based on them exclusively can be considered only as a starting point in the research process rather than necessarily as a basis for drawing conclusions.

Sashidharan raises problems with epidemiological research in examining the issue of increased diagnosis of schizophrenia in African-Caribbeans in his elegant review, which is still relevant today (1993). He begins by discussing the invoking of a commonality of culture to heterogeneous peoples as misleading: that the categorization of African-Caribbeans as a single cultural group is inappropriately simplistic. He goes on to state that the tradition of epidemiological approaches to cross-cultural comparisons of rates of schizophrenia is often problematic because of vastly different methods used across studies including differing case finding methods, lack of diagnostic criteria and the failure to control for confounding variables such as socio-demographic factors.

6.4. Alternative explanations

There may be other factors than perceived racism, which are predictive of therapeutic engagement in those with schizophrenia and psychosis. These include the following and will be further discussed in the Discussion section: remission of paranoia; impaired insight; involvement with the criminal justice system; recovery style; physical abuse as a child; lack of knowledge regarding consumer rights; difficulties in building an alliance; low neuroticism and high agreeableness (Lecomte et al 2008). It is possible that these factors act alongside that of perceived racism or are in fact either confounders or proxy measures of the relationship between racism and outcome.

7. UK African-Caribbeans with psychosis: A case study

Migration from the Caribbean to the United Kingdom began in the early 1950s. Psychiatric research in Britain over the past three decades has consistently shown elevated rates of schizophrenia among African Caribbean people compared with the indigenous white British population, with Caribbeans typically reported to be three to five times more likely than whites to be admitted to hospital with a first diagnosis of schizophrenia (Chakraborty 2008). These findings have been repeated in studies that have looked at first contact with all forms of treatment, rather than just hospital services (King et al 1994; van Os et al 1996); and the rates of schizophrenia were found to be even higher in the UK-born children of the immigrants (Harrison et al 1988).

Some commentators have not accepted the validity of these data and continue to suggest that a higher incidence remains unproven owing to methodological flaws with the research (Sashidharan 1993). Epidemiological issues are as follows: until the 1991 Census, where a question on ethnic background was asked for the first time, the data on the size of the African Caribbean population in the UK was limited and unreliable, resulting in its possible underestimation and consequent overestimation of morbidity rates. However some have shown that even if the Caribbean population was much larger than initially estimated, the psychosis rate still remains significantly greater than in the white population (van Os et al 1996; Bhugra et al 1997). The incidence rates reported for Caribbeans in their countries of origin however, seem much lower and closer to the rates seen in the white British population in the UK (Mahy et al 1999), although this may only be inferred from certain work where ethnicity was not reported. Therefore, people have sought to explain why there is an elevated rate of psychosis in African Caribbeans in the UK compared with the indigenous population and compared with their counterparts in the Caribbean.

The anthropological argument against applying the Western concept of schizophrenia to people from other cultures has been raised (Fernando 1988). Fernando argues that explanations for differences in rates of schizophrenia are invariably concerned with biological differences between racial groups, whilst failing to consider the socio-political (often racist) context in which the diagnoses are made. He continues that schizophrenia is "over-diagnosed" and this hinges on the nature of a psychiatric diagnosis and the nature of racial bias. Fernando views diagnosis as a hypothesis: no more, no less, but in a psychiatric culture where he perceives racial bias to be active, a correct diagnosis in the psychiatric tradition could still be viewed as a racist one, and therefore inappropriate.

Many non-Western cultures do not regard hallucinations as pathological as they are in the West. This could mean an increased readiness to volunteer hallucinatory experiences by non-Western groups. Indeed, increased hallucinatory behaviour and paranoid experiences have been described by Blacks compared with Whites in both the UK and the US general populations (Sharpley& Peters 1999).

There is a belief that African-Caribbeans diagnosed with schizophrenia experience a more relapsing and remitting illness, with more affective symptoms and social disturbance, but fewer negative symptoms than their white counterparts.McGovern and Cope found greater incidence of atypical psychoses and acute-onset illnesses in UK Caribbean patients, usually associated with a good outcome (1991). McKenzie and colleagues conduced a four-year follow-up study of patients with recent-onset psychosis and found the Caribbean patients spent more time in a recovered state, were less likely to have a continuous illness, although they suffered more compulsory admissions and imprisonments; this may suggest at least an illness with a different outcome if not a different illness entity (1995).

The increased risk of schizophrenia has also been attributed to an underlying genetic susceptibility, obstetric injury, maternal congenital rubella, migration, and cannabis misuse but these theories remain either largely unsubstantiated by the epidemiological evidence or the findings themselves are contradictory.

7.1. Social hypotheses

7.1.1. Urbanicity

There is a clear association between inner-city deprivation and high rates of psychiatric admission in general and schizophrenia in particular. It has been suggested that being born or brought up in the city increases the risk of schizophrenia rather than simply a consequence of social drift or social residue. This increased risk has been linked to stressful life events, isolation, overcrowding, higher crime, and lower socio-economic status. The association may be confounded by the observation that physical risk factors occur more commonly in the city, such as low birth-weight and perinatal infections (Chakraborty 2008). Harrison and colleagues did not find that area of residence alone was capable of explaining the elevated risk of schizophrenia in Caribbeans in UK cities (1988). It could be that African-Caribbean people are exposed to adverse social factors more frequently than their white counterparts, such as stressful life events, lower socio-economic class and unemployment levels (Bhugra et al 1997).

7.1.2. Social disadvantage

Social support systems influence health. The physical structure of communities and social cohesion could either encourage or discourage mutual support, self-esteem, a sense of belonging and enriched social relationships. The level of mutual dependency and positive support that can arise from a community, which has high reciprocity and structured caring, (known as "social capital" [Putnam 1995]) may protect against mental illness.

Researchers have argued that Caribbean community structure is compromised relative to other groups, in terms of more single-parent families, more parental separation and more children raised in foster care or children's homes (Maughan 1989). More people live alone and are imprisoned, leading to a form of social exclusion which may increase a susceptibility to poor health. Indeed, it has been found that the incidence of schizophrenia in non-white ethnic minorities in London is greater when they comprise a smaller proportion of the local population, supporting the "ethnic density" effect (essentially, safety in numbers) as a buffer against psychosis (Boydell et al 2001).

7.2. Pathways to care and within the system

As described earlier, it has been found that African-Caribbean patients with schizophrenia in the UK have more aversive pathways into care, i.e. greater police involvement, less general practitioner involvement and a greater occurrence of compulsory hospital admissions (Davies et al 1996). This appears to be unrelated to the duration of untreated psychosis, occurring in early-onset and more chronic cases alike. It has been thought that African-Caribbean patients may not seek general practitioner help early on in their illness due to embarrassment and shame about stigma, leading to a deterioration in health and the need for more dramatic intervention later on (Owens et al 1991). Young black men are more often perceived as dangerous and threatening, and this too may contribute to increased rates of compulsory admission.

Once within care, black Caribbean patients are more likely to remain in hospital for longer with more frequent admissions (McKenzie et al 1995); are more often treated in secure facilities; are given higher doses of psychotropic medication and larger amounts of depot injections; and receive less psychotherapy than white patients. People of Caribbean origin leave hospital with more untreated symptoms and are less likely to stay engaged with services (Chakraborty 2008).

7.3. The effect of racism

Racism is a plausible explanation for the increased rates of psychosis in UK Caribbeans. Racism compounds the effects of gender and social deprivation (Lillie-Blanton &LaVeist 1996).

In addition, thwarted aspirations have been linked to psychological stress and the persistent, prolonged struggle and failure to overcome difficulties of denied opportunities has been linked to a decrease in psychological well-being and hypertension (James 1994).

Discrimination has been prospectively linked to delusional ideation (Janssen et al 2003) but prospective work examining the association between racism and psychosis is still sparse. It is conceivable that there is an association between racism and lack of adherence as Caribbean psychotic patients are more likely to attribute their problems to racism then mental ill health (Chakraborty et al 2001).

A lack of adherence with treatment is typically associated with a mismatch of explanatory models between doctor and patient (Callan & Littlewood 1998); if the patient is more likely to frame their problems within a framework of racism rather than mental illness, they are less likely to comply with a treatment plan that fails to acknowledge their framework. The perception that services and treatment are discriminatory deters African-Caribbeans from accessing these services.

One could argue that the perception of the African-Caribbean patient's illness experience of the phenomenon known as schizophrenia represents an explanatory map that overlaps with that of a schizophrenic patient from a different culture with both common and distinct elements, with differing emphasis placed on those elements by the illness-sufferer. If greater regard is paced upon the racial elements by the patient and correspondingly less attention is paid to them by the clinician, it becomes understandable why therapeutic alliances fail to form, treatment programmes break down and prognosis and service-related outcomes suffer.

As a result, service-related outcomes, such as poor satisfaction, poor subsequent engagement, compulsory hospitalization and depot medication use, reflect an impaired interaction between the individual and the system of care, which may at least in part be due to the individual perceiving services as racist. A recent US study found that African American men with mild paranoia were less likely to be hospitalized than their white counterparts, suggesting a state of "cultural mistrust" of services by the former group, leading to them delaying help-seeking (Whaley 2004).

In 100 African-Caribbean participants with psychosis, racism was measured at baseline using the Perceived Racism Scale; with adherence, using the Drug Attitudes Inventory and Kemp Scale, and hospital admission-data determined after 12 months (Chakraborty et al 2011; 2009c). We found associations between total perceived racism for the previous year, and everyday-racism for the previous year, with subsequent medication adherence. Shame felt about health-system racism was associated with increased adherence, and powerlessness about it was associated with fewer subsequent hospital bed-days. Finally, health-system racism was associated with both the number of subsequent hospital bed-days, and admission-length. In addition, stratified analyses showed that both baseline adherence and six-month estimated adherence appeared to mediate these effects. In this cohort of African-Caribbean patients with psychosis, perceived racism was a determinant of adherence over 12 months.

Therefore, we proposed a model whereby perceived racism contributes to an individual rejecting mental health services (manifested by the mediating effect of poor adherence) which leads to a poorer outcome, evidenced by a longer hospital stay. Secondly, powerlessness about perceived health-service racism may represent a sense of resignation about the "system", leading paradoxically to greater adherence and better outcome.

8. The first nation experience: A Canadian perspective

The primary and secondary authors have recently migrated to Canada. This affords the opportunity to compare the phenomenon described in the case study cross-culturally namely, in North American indigenous peoples: the First Nation population. The First Nations are the various Aboriginal peoples in Canada having cultures spanning thousands of years, who are neither Inuit nor Métis. The total population is nearly 700,000 people. There are currently over 630 recognized First Nations governments or bands spread across Canada, half of which are in the provinces of Ontario and British Columbia.

Aboriginal people experience a broad range of health issues, and have the poorest health levels in the country. Aboriginal people have shorter life expectancies, experience more violent and accidental deaths, have higher infant mortality rates and suffer from more chronic health conditions (Ontario Aboriginal Health Advocacy Initiative, 2003). Aboriginal people are also more likely to face inadequate nutrition, substandard housing and sanitation conditions, unemployment and poverty, and discrimination and racism; all important factors in maintaining health and wellness.

The First Nation population is distinct from the African-Caribbean comparator, in that the former has not migrated; therefore the potential confound of migration-stress is avoided, as is the potential effect of dislocation from a broader social network which, on some levels, has remained intact.

8.1. Mental health disparities

Socio-economic inequity is associated with higher rates of suicide and mental illness, by exposing individuals to a wide range of stressors, including negative life events, as well as diminishing their hopes and expectations for a positive future with meaningful opportunities for work and life. Rates of mental health problems, such as suicide, depression, and substance abuse, are significantly higher in many Aboriginal communities than in the general population (First Nations Regional Longitudinal Health Survey, 2005).

Thirty percent of First Nations people have felt sad, blue or depressed for two or more weeks. Suicide and self-inflicted injuries are the leading causes of death for First Nations youth and adults up to 44 years of age. (Health Canada, 2003; Kirmayer et al 2007). First Nations youth commit suicide about five to six times more often than non-Aboriginal youth. The suicide rate for First Nations males is 126 per 100,000 compared to 24 per 100,000 for non-Aboriginal males. For First Nations females, the suicide rate is 35 per 100,000 compared to only 5 per 100,000 for non-Aboriginal females (Canadian Institute of Child Health, 2000). Suicide rates for Inuit youth are among the highest in the world, at 11 times the national average. Over a third of all deaths among Aboriginal youth are attributable to suicide. Although the gender difference is smaller than among the non-Aboriginal population, males are more likely to die by suicide, while females make suicidal attempts more often. Suicide is never the result of a single factor, but arises from a complex web of interacting personal and social circumstances. The individual variables that affect suicide in Aboriginal people are no different than those found in other populations and communities, but the prevalence and interrelationships among these factors differ for Aboriginal communities due to their history of colonization, and subsequent interactions with the various institutions of Canadian society.

Alcohol intoxication has been reported to be a major factor contributing to suicide in most studies of First Nation people. The strong association of alcohol intoxication and suicide among First Nations people reflects the high prevalence of substance abuse in many communities with an earlier age of first use (May et al., 2002). A survey of drug use in Manitoba assessed Aboriginal (Indian and Métis residents off-reserve) and non-Aboriginal adolescents over four consecutive years from 1990 to 1993 (Gfellner and Hundleby, 1995). The Aboriginal groups had consistently higher rates of use of marijuana, non-medical tranquilizers, non-medical barbiturates, LSD, PCP, other hallucinogens, and crack cocaine. For both LSD and marijuana, the average rate of usage for Aboriginal adolescents was over three times higher than the corresponding non-Aboriginal rate. This is important to note, as both alcohol and substance misuse are known to interact with mental illness not only as a causal factor, but as a consequence.

However, there are wide variations across Aboriginal communities, with many showing rates lower than the general population. Disaggregating generic figures may shed light on resiliency factors operating in certain Aboriginal communities that guard mental health.

8.2. The legacy of residential schools

An important historical determinant believed to have shaped the mental health of Aboriginal people is the legacy of the residential schools. The Indian Residential School (IRS) system grew out of Canada's missionary experience with various religious organizations, with federal governmental administrative involvement as early as 1874. The schools were located in every province and territory, except Newfoundland, New Brunswick and Prince Edward Island. The children were transported from their homes and families and culture of origin to often distant schools where they were mixed with children from different first Nations traditions. A distinctly Western-cultured learning methodology and belief system was delivered, which determined knowledge acquisition and, indirectly, may have had an impact upon self-esteem. Most residential schools ceased to operate by the mid-1970s; and the last closed in 1996. It is estimated there are 80,000 people alive today who attended residential schools. Although it is not uncommon to hear former students speak about positive experiences in residential school, their stories are often overshadowed by disclosures of abuse, criminal convictions of perpetrators, and the legacy of the IRS system. A research project commissioned by the Aboriginal Healing Foundation found that 75 percent of the case files for a sample of Aboriginal residential school survivors contained mental health information with the most common mental health diagnoses being post-traumatic stress disorder, substance abuse disorder and major depression. (Aboriginal Healing Foundation, 2003).

8.3. Housing

An additional social determinant of mental health may be the problem of housing. In Canada, racial ghettos arose with the formation of First Nations reserves which led to the segregation of people, depriving them of the systemic social supports available. A recent federal evaluation of First Nations housing concluded that the housing shortage on reserves is severe with no immediate sign of improvement (Aboriginal Affairs and Northern Development Canada, 2011). According to the February 2011 report, 35,000 new units would need to be built to meet current demand although the Assembly of First Nations puts the figure closer to 85,000. Housing on reserves appears substandard when compared with housing off reserve: 41.5 per cent of homes on reserves need major repairs, compared with seven per cent in non-aboriginal households outside reserves. Rates of overcrowding are six times greater on reserve than off. In many communities, three generations live under one roof through necessity rather than choice.

The First Nation reserves are very often quite isolated geographically and socially. There often is no employment for young people on the reserve or in the immediate area. The federal allowance or provincial social services is a major source of funding for daily life. At the same time traditional valued social roles such as hunting have been lost. Diversions such as substance abuse have occurred. The absence of social roles and remunerative work on reserves has resulted in some exodus of community members searching for work or meaningful identity, to often inner-city areas where substance use and crime has further undermined their mental health. These features would describe the communities with a high incidence of morbidity. However because of the diversity of the First Nations, some communities are intact, value and preserve their traditions, and have extended families including the elders who pass on the community values, skills, language, belief systems, and identity. These attributes contribute to the community resilience and can support individual health.

Nevertheless, research has shown that inadequate housing and support can lead to deteriorations in mental health, increase risk of suicide, put strain upon family relationships, homelessness and involvement with the criminal justice system, and lead to inappropriate hospitalisation or unnecessarily long stays in hospital (Freeman 2004; Newman 2001; Wong & Solomon 2002).

8.4. First Nations Regional Longitudinal Health Survey

The First Nations Regional Longitudinal Health Survey (RHS) is the only First Nations governed national health survey in Canada (First Nations Information Governance Centre, 2012). In the past, large numbers of First Nations people living on reserve were excluded from major national health surveys such as the National Population Health Survey (NHPS).

Other surveys, which attempted to obtain on-reserve data, did not reach enough communities, and thus, were unable to produce valid statistics at the national or regional level upon the relationships between social determinants and disease prevalence. These pieces of information are crucial to drive effective and responsive policy development to improve the health of First Nations.

The first RHS was in 1997 involving First Nations and Inuit; it was launched to redress the exclusion of First Nations and Inuit from major national health surveys. RHS 1997 is considered to be the pilot survey for the longitudinal RHS. RHS Phase 1 [2002/2003] was designed as a baseline study within a longitudinal survey. Over 22,000 surveys were collected from 238 First Nations communities across Canada. RHS Phase 2 [2008/2010] has been completed, with Phase 3 [2012], finally Phase 4 [2016].

Phase 1 reported upon racism, as well as barriers to health and barriers to accessing health care. Of note, one in ten First Nations adults reported having suicidal thoughts and 50% of those people reported suicide attempts over their lifetime. First Nations youth were found to not access traditional supports or mental health services, despite reporting not feeling emotionally or mentally balanced and not progressing in relation to reducing alcohol and drug abuse. Phase 2 has preliminarily reported upon mental health and substance misuse as well as other areas however, as in Phase 1, there is no quantitative inter-ethnic comparison of mental illness prevalence or service-use.

8.5. The Alberta First Nations Report: A focus on health service use

The closest example of an inter-ethnic comparison and, perhaps a template to compare with our putative model of racism and psychosis in UK Caribbeans, is taken from a 2004 report focussing on health service use in First Nations residents in Alberta (Cardinal et al, 2004). The study reported upon adopted a uniquely bicultural approach, employing both quantitative and qualitative methods to arrive at a holistic understanding of disease and wellness more closely akin to the traditional First Nations' paradigm of illness.

The Alberta Mental Health Board provided information showing that First Nations people had three times more episodes in psychiatric treatment centres than the matched control group (Caucasian Canadians), with the majority of episodes lasting less than one week. However, the control group had more outpatient mental health clinic episodes than did First Nations people. Finally, they found that First Nations people were 2.9 times more likely to be treated in the physician's office for schizophrenia than the control group.

The First Nations findings have striking similarities with the UK Caribbean psychosis trends described earlier: more acute psychiatric inpatient admissions; shorter lengths of stay; lower use of non-emergency, outpatient services; and the greater likelihood of the First Nation patient in the physician's office being treated for psychosis, than their Caucasian counterpart. Overall one could infer that these indicate cultural mistrust in mainstream mental health services with the consequent adverse impact on service-related outcomes. Perhaps a cycle of mistrust is set into motion as before, with the avoidance of outpatient services earlier in an illness; undermining prevention and leading to further deterioration; prompting the compulsion toward emergency treatment through imposed hospital admission; ending in sooner disengagement from this process, exemplified by a shorter admission; in a climate of further distrust. The Albertan authors seem to have recognized the potential for services' mistrust by acknowledging the importance of racism and discrimination upon adverse health outcomes, concluding that culturally-sensitive mental health treatment is required in order to redress these disparities.

9. Conclusion

Research on the impact of racism on adherence and health should pay further attention to the ways in which victims respond to and attempt to manage these negative experiences. More generally, future research should try and identify the health-enhancing resources and cultural strengths that provide protection from at least some of the pathogenic risk factors that may be faced by this group.

Feelings of shame and powerlessness induced by racism from mental health services were found to improve both adherence and reduce hospital admissions; this is a double-edged sword. Those individuals concerned showed improved adherence and outcome, but at what personal detriment to their psyches and feelings of self-worth? It would be interesting to determine the association between such feelings of powerlessness and shame related to health services and the longer-term psychological and social functioning of individuals.

If the experiences of racism are viewed as a significant stressor they, like other stressful life events, could be inquired into and recorded within the psychiatric history-taking process. Indeed, increasing patient-centeredness in African-Americans has been raised as an important strategy to address racial/ethnic disparities in health care (Johnson 2004); which builds on previous research where patient activation has been linked to improved health outcome (Stewart 1995). With common themes emerging in this regard in both UK African-Caribbeans and the Canadian First Nations people, this model could be extended for use in both populations and perhaps, beyond.

Through sensitive and genuine acknowledgement, this could be a way of relieving the sense of disempowerment and shame the patient might have felt about their experiences. Perhaps such a clinical encounter could strengthen the therapeutic relationship through a sense of mutual trust, and hopefully improve the outcome of people in the UK and Canada suffering from the effects of both racism and psychosis.

Author details

Apu Chakraborty, Lance Patrick and Maria Lambri

University College London, UK

References

[1] Aboriginal Affairs and Northern Development Canada(2011). Evaluation of INAC's On-Reserve Housing Support

[2] Aboriginal Healing Foundation(2003). Research Series.

[3] Allport, G. (1954). The nature of prejudice. Reading, MA: Addison-Wesley

[4] American National Election Survey Studies .(1995). Ann Arbor, MI: Interuniversity Consortium for Political and Social Research

[5] Anderson, J. (1996). Black and blue. New Yorker; April 29/May 6 624.

[6] Bhugra, D., Leff, J., Mallet, R., & Der , G. (1997). Incidence and outcome of schizophrenia in whites, African-Caribbeans and Asians in London,. *Psychological Medicine*, 27, 791-798.

[7] Bhui, K., Stansfeld, S., Hull, S., Priebe, S., Mole, F. ., & Feder, G. (2003). Ethnic variations in pathways to an use of specialist mental health services in the UK. Systematic review.B. r J Psychiatry; , 182, 105-16.

[8] Bobo(2001). Racial attitudes and relations at the close of the twentieth century. In America Becoming: Racial Trends and Their Consequences, Vol. I, N. Smel. ser, W. Wilson, & F. Mitchell, eds. Commission on Behavioral and Social Sciences and Education, National Research Council, Washington, DC: National Academy Press

[9] Boydell, J., van Os, J., Mc Kenzie, K., Allardyce, J., Goel, R., Mc Creadie, R., & Murray, R. (2001). Incidence of schizophrenia in ethnic minorities in London: ecological study into interactions with environment.BMJ. Dec 8; , 323(7325), 1336-8.

[10] Bryant, B. ., & Mohai, P. (1992). Race and the Incidence of Environmental Hazards: A Time for Discourse. Boulder, CO: Westview Press.

[11] Callan, A., & Littlewood, R. (1998). Patient satisfaction: ethnic origin or explanatory model? Int J Soc Psychiatry. Spring; , 44(1), 1-11.

[12] Canadian Institute of Child Health (2000)

[13] Cardinal, J. C., Schopflocher, D. P., Svenson, L. W., Morrison, K. B., & Laing, L. (2004). First Nations in Alberta: A Focus on Health Service Use. Edmonton: Alberta Health and Wellness

[14] Cavalli-Sforza, L. (2000). Genes, Peoples, and Languages. New York: North Point Press

[15] Chakraborty, A., King, M., Leavey, G., & Mc Kenzie, K. (2011). Perceived racism, medication adherence, and hospital admission in African-Caribbean patients with psychosis in the United Kingdom". Social Psychiatry & Psychiatric Epidemiology.Sep; , 46(9), 915-23.

[16] Chakraborty, A., Mc Kenzie, K., Hajat, S., & Stansfeld, S. (2010). Racism, Mental Illness and Social Support in the UK".Social Psychiatry & Psychiatric Epidemiology.Dec; , 45(12), 1115-24.

[17] Chakraborty, A., Mc Kenzie, K., Bhui, K., Bhugra, D. . A., Randomised, Control., Trial, . R. C. T., of, Undergraduate., Cross-Cultural, Psychiatry., & Training, . World Cultural Psychiatry Research Review ((2009a). , 4, 65-73.

[18] Chakraborty, A., Mc Kenzie, K., & King, M. (2009b). Discrimination, Ethnicity and Psychosis: a Qualitative Study"; Journal of Ethnicity and Inequalities in Health and Social Care. Ethnicity & Inequalities in Health & Social Care., 2, 18-29.

[19] Chakraborty, A., Mc Kenzie, K., Leavey, G., & King, M. (2009c). Measuring Perceived Racism & Psychosis in African-Caribbean Patients in the Un. ited Kingdom: the Modified Perceived Racism Scale"; Clinical Practice and Epidemiology in Mental Health. 5:10

[20] Chakraborty, A. (2008). Association between perceived racism and medication adherence in patients of Caribbean origin with psychosis.PhD dissertation. University College London

[21] Chakraborty, A., & Mc Kenzie, K. (2002). Does racial discrimination cause mental illness? BJPsych. , 180, 475-77.

[22] Cochrane, R., & Sashidharan, S. (1996). Mental health and ethnic minorities: a review of the literature and implications for services. In Ethnicity and Health. CRD Report 5. York: NHS Centre for Reviews and Dissemination, Social Policy Research Unit, University of York.

[23] Combs, D., Penn, D., Cassisi, J., Michael, C., Wood, T., Wanner, J., & Adams, S. (2006). Perceived racism as a predictor of paranoia among African-Americans. Journal of Black PsychologyFeb. , 32(1), 87-104.

[24] Cooper, C., Morgan, C., Byrne, M., Dazzan, P., Morgan, K., Hutchinson, G., Doody, G., Harrison, G., Leff, J., Jones, P., Ismail, K., Murray, R., Bebbington, P. ., & Fearon, P. (2008). Perceptions of disadvantage, ethnicity and psychosis. The British Journal of Psychiatry; , 192, 185-190.

[25] Crow, J. (2002). Unequal by nature: A geneticist's perspective on human differences. DaedalusWinter):, 81-88.

[26] Dassori, A., & Silva, J. (1998). PTSD and ethnic violence. Psychiatric Services; 49:, 108 EOF.

[27] Davies, S., Thornicroft, G., Leese, M., Higginbotham, A. M., & Phelan, M. (1996). Ethnic differences in the risk of compulsory psychiatric admissions among representative cases of psychosis in Lo. ndon. British Medical Journal, , 312, 533-537.

[28] Department of Health ((2005).) Delivering race equality in mental health care. London: HMSO.

[29] Department of Health(2003). Inside Outside: Improving mental health services for black and minority ethnic communities in England. London: HMSO

[30] Diaz, E., Woods, S., & Rosenheck, R. (2005). Effects of ethnicity on psychotropic medications adherence.Community Ment Health J; , 41(5), 521-37.

[31] Farley, R., & Frye, W. (1994). Changes in the segregation of whites from blacks during the 1980's: Small steps toward a more integrated society. America. n Sociological Review. , 59, 23-45.

[32] Fernando, S. (1988). Race and Culture in Psychiatry. London: Croom Helm.

[33] First Nations Information Governance Centre. (2012). http://www.rhs-ers.ca/node/11.

[34] First Nations Regional Longitudinal Health Survey, 2005

[35] Franks, A., May, D., Wenger, N., Blount, S., & Eaker, E. (1993). Racial differences in the use of invasive coronary procedures after acute myocardial infarctions in Medicare beneficiaries. *Ethnicity & Disease*, 3, 213-20.

[36] Freeman, A., Malone, J., Hunt, G., & (200, . (2004). Astatewide survey of high-support services for people with chronic mental illness: assessment of needs for care, level of functioning and satisfaction, Australian & New Zealand Journal of Psychiatry, 38

[37] Gaertner, S., Dovidio, J., Banker, B., Rust, M., Nier, J., Mottola, G., & Ward, C. (1997). Does racism necessarily mean antiblackness? Aversive racism and pro-whiteness.In M. Fine, L. Powell, L. Weis, & M. Wong (Eds.), Off White (London: Routledge, 167-178.

[38] Gfellner, B.M. and J.D. Hundleby ((1995).). Patterns of drug use among native and white adolescents: -, 1990.

[39] (1993). . Canadian Journal of Public Health ., 86(2), 95-97.

[40] Giles, W., Anda, R., Casper, M., Escobedo, L., & Taylor, H. (1995). Race and sex differences in rates of invasive cardiac procedures in US hospitals: data from the national hospital discharge survey. *Archives of Internal Medicine*, 155, 318-24.

[41] Gilvarry, C., Walsh, E., Samele, C., Hutchinson, G., Mallett, R., Rabe-Hesketh, S., Fahy, T., van Os, J., & Murray, R. (1999). Life events, ethnicity and perceptions of discrimination in patients with severe mental illness. Soc Psychiatry PsychiatrEpidemiol. , 34, 600-8.

[42] Graves JL, Jr(2004). The race myth: Why we pretend race exists in America. New York: Dutton.

[43] Greenwald, A., Mc Ghee, D., & Schwartz, J. (1998). Measuring individual differences in implicit cognition: the implicit association test. J. Personality Social Psychol., , 74, 1464-80.

[44] Harris, D. (2002). Racial classification and the 2000 Census. Unpublished paper prepared for the National Research. Council Panel to Review the 2000 Census, Washington, DC. Institute for Social Research, University of Michigan

[45] Harrison, G., Owens, D., Holton, A., Neilson, D., Boot, A., & (198, . (1988). A prospective study of severe mental disorder in Afro-Caribbean patients. *Psychological Medicine*, 18, 643 EOF-57 EOF.

[46] Health Canada. (2003). A Statistical Profile on the Health of First Nations in Canada for the Year 2000.

[47] Healthcare Commission(2006). Count me in: Results of a national census of inpatients in mental health hospitals and facilities in England and Wales. Commission for Healthcare Audit and Inspection: London

[48] Jackson, J., Brown, T., Williams, D., Torres, M., Sellers, S., & Brown, K. (1996). Racism and the physical and mental health status of African Americans: a thirteen-year national panel study. Ethnicity and Disease. , 6, 109-22.

[49] Jacobsen, J., Olsen, C., Rice, J., Sweetland, S., & Ralph, J. (2001). Educational Achievement and Black-White Inequality. (NCES 2001-061). Washington, DC: National Center for Education Statistics.

[50] James, A. (1994). John Henryism and the health of African-Americans.Culture Medicine and Psychiatry, , 18, 163-182.

[51] Jansssen, I., Hanssen, M., Bak, M., Bijl, R., De Graaf, R., Volleburgh, W., Mc Kenzie, K., & van Os, J. (2003). Discrimination and delusional ideation. Jan; , 182, 71-76.

[52] Johnson, R., Roter, D., Powe, N., & Cooper, L. (2004). Patient race/ethnicity and quality of patient-physician communication during medical visits. *American Journal of Public Health*, 94(12), 2084-90.

[53] Jorde, L., & Wooding, S. (2004). Genetic variation, classification and 'race'.Nature Genetics 36(11 Suppl):S, 28-33.

[54] Karlsen, S., Nazroo, J., Mc Kenzie, K., Bhui, K., & Weich, S. (2005). Racism, psychosis and common mental disorder among ethnic minority groups in England. Psychol Med. 2005 Dec;, 35(12), 1795-803.

[55] Kennedy, B., Kawachi, I., Lochner, K., Jones, C. ., & Prothrow-Stith, D. (1997). Dis)respect and black mortality. Ethn Dis., , 7, 207-14.

[56] King, M., Coker, E., Leavey, G., Hoare, A., & Johnson-Sabine, E. (1994). Incidence of psychotic illness in London: comparison of ethnic groups. BMJ; Oct 29;, 309(6962), 1115-9.

[57] Kirmayer LJ, Brass GM, Holton TL et al(2007). Suicide among Aboriginal people in Canada. Ottawa (ON): Aboriginal Healing Foundation.

[58] Krieger, N., Discrimination, , health, In., Berkman, L., Kawachi, I., (eds, , Social, Epdeimiology., Oxford, Oxford., & University, Press. (2000). 36-75.

[59] Krieger, N., Rowley, D., Herman, A., Avery, B., & Phillips, M. (1993). Racism, sexism, and social class: implications for studies of health, disease, and well-being. Am J Prev Med, Suppl , 6, 82-122.

[60] La Veist, T., Sellers, R., & Neighbors, H. (2001). Perceived racism and self and system blame attribution: consequences for longevity.Ethn Dis.; , 11, 711-21.

[61] Lazarus, R. ., & Folkman, S. (1984). Stress, appraisal and coping. New York: Springer.

[62] Lecomte, T., Spidel, A., Leclerc, C., Mac, Ewan. G., Greaves, C. ., & Bentall, R. (2008). Predictors and profiles of treatment non-adherence and engagement in services problems in early psychosis. Schizophr Res; 102(1-3): , 295 EOF-302 EOF.

[63] Lewontin, R. S., Rose, , & Kamin, L. (1984). Not in our genes: Biology, ideology, and human nature. New York: Pantheon

[64] Lillie-Blanton, M. ., & Laviest, T. (1996). Race, ethnicity, the social environment and health.Social Science and Medicine, , 43, 83-91.

[65] Lloyd, K. (1998). Ethnicity, social inequality and mental illness. BMJ; 316:1763

[66] Loo, C. (1994). Race-related PTSD: the Asian American Vietnam veteran. *Journal of Traumatic Stress*, 7, 637-56.

[67] MacPherson(1999). The Stephen Lawrence Inquiry: report of an inquiry by Sir William MacPherson of Cluny. TSO:London

[68] Mahy, G. E., Mallett, R., Leff, J., et al. (1999). First-contact incidence-rate of schizophrenia on Barbados. British Journal of Psychiatry, , 175, 28-33.

[69] Maughan, B. (1989). Growing up in the inner city. Paediatric and Perinatal Epidemiology, , 3, 195-215.

[70] May, P. A., Van Winkle, N. W., Williams, M. B., Mc Feeley, P. J., De Bruyn, L. M., & Serna, P. (2002). Alcohol and Suicide Death Among American Indians of New Mexico: 1980-1998. Suicide and Life-Threatening Behavior , 32(3), 240-255.

[71] Mayr, E. (2002). The Biology of race and the concept of equality. Daedalus (Winter):, 89-94.

[72] Mc Govern, D., & Cope, R. (1991). Second-generation African-Caribbeans and young whites with a first-admission diagnosis of schizophrenia.Social Psychiatry and Psychiatric Epidemiology, , 26, 95-99.

[73] Mc Kenzie, K. ., & Bhui, K. (2007). Institutional racism in mental health care.BMJ; , 334, 649-650.

[74] Mc Kenzie, K., Van Os, J., Fahy, T., Jones, P., Harvey, I., & Toone, Murray. R. (1995). Psychosis with good prognosis in Afro-Caribbean people now living in the United Kingdom. BMJ Nov. 18; , 311(7016), 1325-8.

[75] Mc Neilly, M., Anderson, N., Armstead, C., Clark, R., Corbett, M., Robinson, E., Pieper, C. ., & Lepisto, E. (1996). The Perceived Racism Scale: a multidimensional assessment of the experience of white racism among African Americans. Ethnicity & DiseaseWinter/Spring. 6(1,2):, 154 EOF-66 EOF.

[76] Meyer, I. (1995). Minority stress and mental health in gay men. J Health SocBehav., , 36, 38-56.

[77] Nazroo, J. (2001). Ethnicity, Class and Health. Policy Studies Institute: London

[78] Nei, M., & Roychoudhury, A. (1983). Genetic relationship and evolution of human races. Evolutionary Biology, , 14, 1-59.

[79] Neighbors, H., Jackson, J., Broman, C., & Thompson, E. (1996). Racism and the mental health of African Americans: the role of self and system blame. Eth Dis., , 6, 167-75.

[80] Newman, S. (2001). Housing and Mental Illness: A Critical Review of the Literature. Washington, DC : The Urban Institute.

[81] Olson, S. (2002). Mapping human history: Discovering the past through our genes. New York: Houghton Mifflin

[82] Omi, M. (2001). The changing meaning of race. In America Becoming: Racial Trends and Their Consequences,. N. Smelser, W. Wilson, & F. Mitchell, eds. Commission on Behavioral and Social Sciences and Education. Washington, DC: National Academy Press, 1

[83] Ontario Aboriginal Health Advocacy Initiative.(2003). Aboriginal Access to Health Care Systems. Ontario Aboriginal Health Advocacy Initiative.

[84] Owens, D., Harrison, G., & Boot, D. (1991). Ethnic factors in voluntary and compulsory admissions. Psychological Medicine, , 21, 185-196.

[85] Paradies, Y. (2006). A systematic review of empirical research on self-reported racism and health. *International Journal of Epidemiology*, 35, 888-901.

[86] Morgan, C., Mallett, R., Hutchinson, G., Bagalkote, H., Morgan, K., Fearon, P., Dazan, P., Boydell, J., Mc Kenzie, K., Harrison, G., Murray, R., Jones, P., Craig, T., & Leff, J. (2005a). Pathways to care and ethnicity. 1: Sample characteristics and compulsory admission. Report from the ÆSOP study.Br J Psychiatry; , 186, 281-289.

[87] Morgan, C., Mallett, R., Bagalkote, H., Morgan, K., Fearon, P., Dazzan, P., Boydell, J., Mc Kenzie, K., Harrison, G., Murray, R., Jones, P., Craig, T., Leff, J. Æ. S. O. P., & Study, Group. (2005b). Pathways to care and ethnicity. 2: Source of referral and help-seeking. Report from the AESOP study.Br J Psychiatry Apr; , 186, 290-96.

[88] Opolka, J., Rascati, K., Brown, C., Barner, J., Johnsrud, , & Gibson, P. (2003). Ethnic differences in use of antipsychotic medication among Texan medicaid clients with schizophrenia.J Clin Psychiatry; , 64(6), 635-9.

[89] Perera, R., Owens, D. ., & Johnstone, E. (1991). Ethnic aspects. A comparison of three matched groups.BJPsych.; , 147, 598-611.

[90] Pernice, R., & Brook, J. (1996). Refugees' and immigrants' mental health: association of demographic and post immigration factors. Journal of Social Psychology; , 136, 511-19.

[91] Pierce, C. (1974). Psychiatric problems of the Black minority.In S. Arieti (Ed.), American handbook of psychiatry (New York: Basic Books., 512-523.

[92] Putnam, R. D. (1995). Bowling alone. America's declining social capital. Journal of. Democracy, , 6, 65-78.

[93] Rothenberg, P. (1988). Racism and sexism: an integrated study. New York: St. Martin's Press.

[94] Sainsbury Centre for Mental Health(2002). Breaking the Circles of Fear: A review of the relationship between mental health services and African and Caribbean communities. London: SCMH

[95] Sashidharan, S. P. (1993). Afro-Caribbeans and schizophrenia: the ethnic vulnerability hypothesis re-examined. *International Review of Psychiatry*, 5, 129-144.

[96] Scherwitz, L., Perkins, L., Chesney, M., & Hughes, G. (1991). Cook-Medley Hostility Scale and subsets: Relationship to demographic and psychosocial characteristics in young adults in the CARDIA study. Psychosom Med.; , 53, 36-49.

[97] Senior, P., & Bhopal, R. (1994). Ethnicity as a variable in epidemiological research. British Medical Journal, , 309, 327-30.

[98] Sharpley, M. S., & Peters, E. (1999). Ethnicity, class and schizotypy.*Social Psychiatry and Psychiatric Epidemiology*. 34, 507-512.

[99] Shaw, C., Creed, F., Tomenson, B., Riste, L., & Cruickshank, . (1999). Prevalence of anxiety and depressive illness and help seeking behaviour in African Caribbeans and white Europeans: two phase general population survey.BMJ; Jan 30; , 318(7179), 302-5.

[100] Singh, S., & Burns, T. (2006). Race and mental health: there is more to race than racism. BMJ; , 333, 648-651.

[101] Steffen, P., Mc Neilly, M., Anderson, N., & Sherwood, A. (2003). Effects of perceived racism and anger inhibition on ambulatory blood pressure in African Americans. Psychosom Med. Sep-Oct; , 65(5), 746-50.

[102] Stewart, M. (1995). Effective physician-patient communication and health outcomes: a review. CMAJ; , 152, 1423-33.

[103] Thoits, P. (1983). Dimensions of life events that influence psychological distress: an evaluation and synthesis of the literature. In H. Kaplan, ed. Psychosocial Research: Trend in Theory and Research. New York: Academic Press. , 33-103.

[104] Tsai, J., Desai, R. A., & Rosenheck, R. A. (2012). Racial Comparison of Therapeutic Support, Service Use, and Satisfaction Among Male Outpatients with Severe Mental Illness. Psychiatr Q. 2012 Apr 3. [Epub ahead of print]

[105] Turner, C., & Kramer, B. (1995). Connections between racism and mental health. In C. Willie, P. Rieker, B. Kramer, B. Brown (eds.) Mental Health, Racism, and Sexism. Taylor & Francis: London

[106] van Os, J., Castle, D. J., Takei, N., Der Murray, G., & , M. (1996). Psychotic illness in ethnic minorities: clarification from the 1991 Census. *Psychological Medicine*, 26, 203-208.

[107] Veling, W., Hoek, H., & Mackenbach, J. (2008). Perceived discrimination and the risk of schizophrenia in ethnic minorities: A case-control study. Soc Psychiatry Psychiatr Epidemiol. Jun 23 [Epub ahead of print]

[108] Veling, W., Selten-P, J., Susser, E., Winfried, L., Mackenbach, J., & Hoek, H. (2007). Discrimination and the incidence of psychotic disorders among the ethnic minorities in The Netherlands. International Journal of Epidemiology; , 36, 761-68.

[109] Weich, S. (1997). Crisis in London's mental health services: empirical evidence was lacking in study. British Medical Journal; 314: 1278

[110] Williams, D. (1997). Race and health: basic questions, emerging directions. Ann Epidemiol, , 7, 322-33.

[111] Whaley, A. (2004). Ethnicity/race, paranoia, and hospitaliza. tion for mental health problems among men. Am J Public Health Jan; , 94(1), 78-81.

[112] Williams, D., & Chung, A. (1995). Racism and health. In: R. Gibson, J. Jackson, eds. Health in Black America. Thousand Oaks, CA: Sage Publications.

[113] Wong, Y. I., & Solomon, P. L. (2002). Community integration of persons with psychiatric disabilities in supportive independent housing: A conceptual model and methodological considerations. Mental Health Services Research , 4(2), 13-28.

[114] Yzerbyt, V., Rocher, S., & Schadron, G. (1997). Stereotypes as explanations. In R. Spears, P. Oakes, N. Ellemers, & S. Hasslam (Eds.), The social psychology of stereotyping in group life (Oxford, UK: Blackwell, 20-50.

[115] Zuckerman, M. ((1990).) Some dubious premises in research and theory on racial differences. American Psychologist, , 45, 1297-1303.

Chapter 8

Somatic Symptom Disorder

Lesley A. Allen and Robert L. Woolfolk

Additional information is available at the end of the chapter

1. Introduction

In the chapter we present our model of treatment for somatic symptom disorder. We begin with a brief history of somatic symptom disorder followed by a discussion of theory and research on it. Finally, we describe our psychosocial treatment for somatic symptom disorder and related disorders, which employs methods from both cognitive behavioral therapy and experiential emotion-focused therapy.

Physical symptoms with uncertain medical explanations are some of the most common presentations in primary care. As many as 25% of visits to primary care physicians are prompted by physical symptoms that lack any clear organic pathology [1]. Although some patients with medically unexplained physical symptoms experience mild and/or transient discomfort, others experience substantial discomfort, distress, and impairment in functioning [2,3]. It is these patients, those with impairing physical symptoms of unknown etiology, who are often refractory to standard medical treatment and overuse medical services [2].

Medicine has long recognized a group of patients with medically unexplained physical symptoms (MUPS) and excessive health concerns. Originally theorized to be caused by a wandering uterus that produced discomfort and pain, MUPS were first described by ancient Egyptians and first labeled hysteria by the ancient Greeks.

It was not until 1980 and the publication of DSM-III that the terms somatization and somatoform were introduced for physical symptoms that were medically unexplained [4]. According to DSM-III somatization disorder was characterized by "recurrent and multiple somatic complaints of several years' duration for which medical attention had been sought but which are apparently not due to any physical disorder" [4]. Also in that volume the diagnostic category of somatoform disorders was created and subsumed somatization disorder, conversion disorder, psychogenic pain disorder, hypochondriasis, and a residual category, atypical somatoform disorder for other disturbances with a presentation of MUPS [4]. Conversion disorder was characterized by a "loss or alteration in physical functioning that suggests a physical disorder but which instead is apparently an expression of a psychological conflict or need" [4]. If the medically unexplained symptom was a pain symptom and the symptom was judged to be associated with psychological factors, the diagnosis of psychogenic pain disorder would be indicated. The essential feature of hypochondriasis was a preoccupation with the fear or belief of having a serious disease.

Both DSM-III-R [5] and DSM-IV [6] used similar diagnostic labels and criteria to those used in DSM-III for presentations predominated by MUPS. An additional diagnostic label, undifferentiated somatoform disorder, was introduced in DSM-III-R and retained in DSM-IV for cases of MUPS but that did not meet all the criteria of somatization disorder. This less severe form of somatization, undifferentiated somatoform disorder, was characterized by one or more MUPS that lasted for at least 6 months [5,6].

Somatic symptom disorder is a new diagnostic label proposed for DSM-5 [7]. The diagnostic criteria for somatic symptom disorder are distressing and chronic somatic symptoms and associated dysfunctional thoughts, feelings, and/or behaviors (Table 1). In contrast to earlier editions of DSM, DSM-5 has shifted from emphasizing the functional status of somatic symptoms (i.e., that symptoms be medically unexplained) to the maladaptive thoughts, feelings, and behaviors related to somatic symptoms. According to DSM-5's Somatic Symptom Disorders Work Group, unlike the criteria for somatization disorder and other somatoform disorders described in earlier editions of DSM, the criteria for somatic symptom disorder require the presence of specific characteristics rather than the absence of characteristics (i.e., evidence of organic basis) and are more reliably determined [7]. Research has shown significant variability among physicians in their tendency to rate symptoms as medically unexplained [8]. Also, patient reports of the functional status of symptoms are unreliable [9]. Thus, the diagnosis no longer requires evidence that symptoms are medically unexplained. In addition to eliminating the assessment of the organic basis of the symptoms, the Somatic Symptom Disorders Work Group has proposed a new, less controversial label for somatically-focused presentations [7]. It seems the diagnoses of somatization and somatoform disorder carried pejorative connotations [10].

A. Somatic Symptoms: One or more somatic symptoms that are distressing and/or result in significant disruption in daily life.
B. Excessive thoughts, feelings, and behaviors related to these somatic symptoms or associated health concerns: At least one of the following must be present.
1. Disproportionate and persistent thoughts about the seriousness of one's symptoms
2. Persistently high level of anxiety about health or symptoms
3. Excessive time and energy devoted to these symptoms or health concerns
C. Chronicity: Although any one symptom may not be continuously present, the state of being symptomatic is persistent (typically "/> 6 months).

Table 1. Proposed DSM-5 Diagnostic Criteria for Somatic Symptom Disorder

2. Epidemiological findings and clinical characteristics

Although there is no published research on DSM-5's somatic symptom disorder, research on some of the older diagnostic categories is likely to apply. Distressing physical symptoms are common in medical clinics. As many as 20% of primary care patients have MUPS [11-13]. Epidemiological research has shown patients with MUPS to be more likely to be female, non-white, and less educated than patients with medically explained symptoms [13-15]. Findings on ethnicity have been less consistent across studies. In the Epidemiological Catchment Area project, examining psychiatric complaints in the general population at five sites in the United States, Hispanics were no more likely to meet criteria for somatization disorder than were non-Hispanics [15]. The World Health Organization study, conducted in primary care clinics in 14 different countries, revealed a higher incidence of somatization in Latin American countries than in the United States [13]. (Note that the terms medically unexplained symptoms (MUPS) and somatization will be used interchangeably in the remainder of this chapter. The term somatization disorder is reserved for cases meeting the full criteria for somatization disorder as outlined in DSM-III, DSM-III-R, or DSM-IV.)

Patients with MUPS often engage in dysfunctional illness behavior. When standard diagnostic evaluations fail to uncover organic pathology, patients may seek additional medical procedures, often from several different physicians. When symptoms continue unresolved, patients may switch physicians and/or treatment approaches. Patients may even subject themselves to unnecessary hospitalizations and surgeries, which introduce the risk of iatrogenic illness [16]. Patients with multiple medically unexplained symptoms have been shown to overuse and misuse health care services [2,17,18].

MUPS may not only prompt excessive use of medical procedures, they may also affect patients' workplaces and households. Patients who are excessively focused on their somatic symptoms may withdraw from both productive and pleasurable activities because of discomfort, fatigue, and/or fears of exacerbating their symptoms. High levels of functional impairment have been associated with somatization [13,18-20].

Comorbid psychopathology is common in patients with MUPS. Ongoing physical discomfort can be demoralizing, anxiety-provoking, and frustrating. Approximately 50% of patient with multiple MUPS meet DSM criteria for an Axis I disorder, most often depression and/or anxiety [19,21]. Also, overall severity of psychological distress, defined as the number of psychological symptoms reported, correlates positively with the number of functional somatic symptoms reported [3,21].

A growing body of research indicates certain cognitive styles may be associated with somatization. Barksy suggested patients with unexplained physical symptoms have a tendency to amplify somatosensory information; that is, they are hypersensitive to bodily sensations which are experienced as intense, noxious, and disturbing [22]. Other researchers have shown that patients with MUPS form negative cognitive appraisals of their physical sensations, thinking catastrophically about their symptoms [23] and/or overestimating the medical severity of symptoms after a medical evaluation [24]. Research demonstrating that memories and expectations of physical symptomatology prime future symptomatology [25] is likely to apply to somatizers.

Two personality styles have also been associated with somatization. Patients with MUPS tend to score high on scales of neuroticism and negative affect [26]. Alexithymia, defined as having difficulty identifying and describing one's emotions, is common in somatization [27-29]. Thus, we see somatization

patients as individuals who may be emotionally and physically hyper-reactive while having insufficient insight into their emotional and physical sensations.

3. Biopsychosocial model

The biopsychosocial model of illness, proposed by George Engel [30], suggests that illness is a complex entity involving the interaction of biological, psychological, and social factors. A biopsychosocial conceptualization of somatic symptom disorder emphasizes the interaction among biology, cognition, emotion, behavior, and environment [31,32].

There is a growing body of research that supports key features of the biopsychosocial model of somatic symptom disorder. Genetic and early environmental factors may predispose individuals to experiencing somatic symptomatology [33]. Patients presenting with multiple somatic symptoms have higher levels of physiological arousal and are less likely to habituate to a stressful task than control subjects [34]. These predisposing factors may be compounded by the dysfunctional attentional and cognitive tendencies described in the previous section. The more attention one focuses upon his or her body, the more likely one is to report somatic symptoms [35,36].

Dysfunctional cognitions may elicit negative emotions or be elicited by negative emotions [37]. This cognition-emotion cycle may interact in a complex fashion with maladaptive behaviors. For example, thoughts of possible illness give rise to feelings of anxiety, dysphoria, and frustration, which are likely to generate and maintain physiological arousal and physical symptomatology. Intending to prevent injury or exacerbation of symptoms, these patients typically withdraw from their normal activities [2,3]. Such time away from activities provides opportunities for additional attention to be focused upon one's physical health. Furthermore, patients suffering from these physical symptoms, distorted cognitions, and negative affect may seek repeated contact with physicians and request medical tests. Pain catastrophizing has been associated with medical utilization and disability [38]. Physicians, in turn, attempting to conduct thorough evaluations and avoid malpractice suits, may encourage somatizing behavior by ordering unnecessary diagnostic procedures. Chronic medical testing may ingrain patients in the "sick role" and reinforce somatizers' maladaptive belief that any physical symptom indicates organic pathology. Also, unnecessary medical procedures, if implemented, may result in iatrogenic illness.

A biopsychosocial model of medically unexplained symptoms leads to specific psychosocial treatment strategies that include behavioral, cognitive, and interpersonal interventions.

Relaxation training may be employed to teach patients to use progressive muscle relaxation and/or diaphragmatic breathing to reduce physiologic arousal. Behavioral activation/activity regulation promotes increases in pleasurable and meaningful activities to modify the tendency of these patients to withdraw from important aspects of their lives. Also, activity pacing is taught so that patients will increase their activity levels gradually without exhausting or injuring themselves. The cognitive restructuring component aims to help patients combat dysfunctional cognitive tendencies. Communication skills, especially assertiveness training, are taught to address the social disability that has been reported by somatizers [39]. Finally, patients' environments are examined for factors that reinforce their physical symptoms. Those factors are targeted for change. In some treatment protocols the patient's spouse/partner is invited to participate in treatment sessions. Given the important role that spouses play in reinforcing patients' expression of pain and pain behavior [40], spousal behaviors that reinforce patients' symptoms may be modified.

4. Treatment outcome research

The financial costs and associated suffering and disability of somatization make it a public health concern. Given that many patients with MUPS fail to respond to standard medical care, alternative treatments have been developed. Although different psychosocial interventions have been used to treat somatization, some administered by primary physicians/clinicians and others administered by mental health providers, most approaches that have been examined in randomized controlled clinical trials have been theoretically grounded in the biopsychosocial model described above. Cognitive behavioral therapy (CBT) is the form of psychotherapy most often examined. Also, a number of different approaches to retraining primary care physicians or integrating CBT into primary care have been investigated.

4.1. Psychotherapy

The first published randomized controlled trials on CBT for somatization included patients presenting with relatively mild levels of somatization, patients presenting with at least one psychosomatic symptom. The treatment protocols included identifying and restructuring dysfunctional cognitions, encouraging patients to reengage in avoided activities, problem-solving, and relaxation training [41,42]. In the first study patients treated with 6 to 16 sessions of individually-administered CBT showed significantly greater improvement in their psychosomatic complaints than did patients treated with standard medical care [41]. The other study found an 8-session group CBT superior to a waiting-list control condition in reducing physical symptoms and hypochondriacal beliefs [42]. In both studies improvements were observed after treatment as well as six months later [41,42]. Both of these studies were conducted in primary care offices, the setting where somatization is most likely to be seen.

Two more recently published randomized controlled trials examined the efficacy of CBT for somatization with patients presenting with more severe somatization than the earlier trials. One study enrolled patients with at least four somatization symptoms [43]. The other trial enrolled participants who complained of five or more unexplained physical symptoms [44]. In both studies patients were identified and treated with CBT in primary care. Treatment protocols were similar to Lidbeck's [42] and Speckens et al., [41] with the addition of involving the patient's spouse or other family member in treatment [43,44]. Spouses are included to provide additional information regarding patients' functioning, to facilitate patients' engagement in and compliance with treatment, and to help reduce reinforcement of illness behavior. Findings from both trials show individual CBT coincided with greater reductions in somatic complaints than did standard medical care [43,44]. CBT was associated with a reduction in the number of physician visits in one study [44].

Our researcher team published a randomized controlled trial on the efficacy of an emotionally-focused cognitive behavioral intervention, affective cognitive behavioral therapy (ACBT) for some of the most severely disturbed patients with somatization [45]. In the study 84 patients meeting DSM-IV criteria for somatization disorder were randomly assigned to one of two conditions: [1] standard medical care or [2] a 10-session manualized individually-administered ACBT in combination with standard medical care. The treatment protocol included some of the usual components of CBT for somatization, i.e., relaxation training, activity regulation, cognitive restructuring, and interpersonal communication as well as facilitation of emotional awareness. Although the elicitation and exploration of affect is an approach rarely used in CBT, we have found this component to be a powerful clinical tool with patients who cannot or do not willingly access and experience emotion. We describe our treatment in the following sections and elsewhere in more detail [46]. Participants' symptomatology and functioning were assessed with clinician-administered instruments, self-report questionnaires, and medical records before randomization as well as 3 months, 9 months, and 15 months after randomization. Just after the completion of treatment as well as one year later, i.e., at the 15-month follow-up assessment, patients who received ACBT experienced a greater reduction in somatization and functional impairment. Substantially more participants who received ACBT than the control treatment were rated as either "very much improved" or "much improved" by a clinician who was blind to participants' treatment condition (40% vs. 5%, respectively). Also, for the 68% of the sample for whom complete medical records were reviewed, ACBT was associated with a reduction in health care costs and physician visits [45]. Thus, the study suggests ACBT can result in long-term improvements in symptomatology, functioning, and health care utilization of the most severely disturbed somatizing patients.

4.2. Primary care interventions

Given the prevalence of MUPS in primary care [1,11,12], much research has centered on primary care physicians' behavior. Smith and colleagues sent a psychiatric consultation letter to patients' primary care physicians, describing somatization disorder and providing recommendations to guide primary care [47]. The recommendations to physicians were straightforward: (a) to schedule somatizers' appointments every 4 to 6 weeks instead of as needed appointments, (b) to conduct a physical examination in the organ system or body part relevant to the presenting complaint, (c) to avoid diagnostic procedures and surgeries unless clearly indicated by underlying somatic pathology, and (d) to avoid making disparaging statements, such as "your symptoms are all in your head." Patients whose primary physicians had received the consultation letter experienced better health outcomes, such as physical functioning and cost of medical care, than those whose physicians had not received the letter. The results were replicated in three additional studies, one study using patients meeting criteria for full somatization disorder [48] and two studies using patients with more moderate levels of somatization [49,50].

Some investigators have attempted to train primary care physicians to better detect somatization and to incorporate cognitive and behavioral techniques into their treatment of these patients. Five groups of investigators have reported controlled clinical trials on the effects of such physician training [51-55]. The two studies providing the most extensive physician training (20-25 hours) resulted in no association between physician training and patients' symptomatology, functioning, or quality of life [51,55]. Three other studies found less intensive physician training programs, 12 hours [52] or 1 day [54] or six hours [53] to coincide with no clear improvement in somatization symptomatology; however, Rief and colleagues did find their training to result in fewer health care visits for the 6 months subsequent to training [54].

One other study examined the effect of training primary care clinicians to identify and treat somatization using a biopsychosocial model [56]. This study involved the most intensive such training programs studied, one entailing 84 hours over 10 weeks. Nurse practitioners were trained to provide a year-long 12-session multidimensional intervention in primary care that incorporated biopsychosocial conceptualizations, behavioral recommendations, and medication management of somatization. Patients who received treatment from these trained nurses reported modest improvements on self-report scales of mental health such as mood and energy and physical functioning. A post hoc analysis was interpreted by the study's investigators as suggesting improvements were attributable to more frequent and appropriate use of antidepressant medication among patients of nurses who received the training [56].

Some researchers have studied the effects of a collaborative care model of treatment, in which mental health professionals work together with medical practitioners in the primary care setting [57,58]. The one study investigating the efficacy of such a model for the treatment of somatization had psychiatrists provide primary care physicians and their staff with training on the diagnosis and treatment of somatization and comorbid psychopathology [59]. Also, the psychiatrist provided case-specific consultations to primary physicians regarding referrals for CBT and/or psychiatric treatment [59]. A control comparison treatment included the same training for primary care physicians and their staff by the psychiatrist without the case-specific consultation. Six months after randomization, participants whose primary care physician received psychiatric consultation reported a greater reduction in somatic symptoms and in health care visits [59].

In all, the literature on the treatment of somatization supports the use of 6-16 sessions of CBT or ACBT administered by a mental health professional. A recent meta-analysis indicated CBT is modestly effective in reducing somatization symptomatology and minimally effective improving physical functioning [60]. To date there is no evidence that CBT reduces health care services when the cost of CBT itself is considered. Researchers have just begun to develop and examine the effectiveness of true collaboration of cognitive behavioral therapist and primary care clinician and integration of their services.

How, why, what aspects of CBT and ACBT works is unknown. We have very little data on the mechanisms by which efficacious psychosocial treatments may have their impact upon somatization. These approaches are multi-faceted and have not been disassembled into discrete components and those constituents systematically assessed. Nevertheless, CBT and ACBT are likely the treatments of choice by default in that no other intervention has demonstrated efficacy.

5. Rationale for an emotionally-focused CBT

In our treatment for somatization we have made systematic and explicit an emphasis on emotional exploration, differentiation, and expression. This therapeutic activity has long been a staple of humanistic and psychoanalytic therapies and is coming to be emphasized by newer approaches that grow out of the cognitive-behavioral tradition. Traditional cognitive approaches were based on a cognitive-appraisal theory of emotion [61,62] in which dysfunctional cognitions were thought to generate aversive affects. Although this view was modified to be more bidirectional and causally reciprocal by Teasdale [37], much CBT has been directed to the reduction of aversive affect, largely through the modification of cognition that was assumed to be the source. Some approaches that have developed within the CBT framework have begun to change this emphasis upon active control of emotion. Clinical work by such investigators as Marsha Linehan and Stephen Hayes has placed emphasis on experiencing, tolerating, and accepting unpleasant emotion, rather than seeking its elimination [63,64]. Recent formulations of generalized anxiety disorder (GAD) suggest that the function of this disorder's primary symptom, i.e., worry, may be to avoid, control, or attenuate emotional experience [65,66]. The authors of these recent formulations of GAD also advocate experiential and acceptance approaches as a means of reducing worry. Samoilov and Goldfried's critique of standard CBT approaches suggests more emphasis upon the elicitation of affect in therapy sessions may produce more effective treatment [67]. The arguments of the revisionist theorists cited above frequently draw from basic work in cognitive neuroscience, work that suggests there are complex, manifold, and partially independent levels of cognitive and affective storage and processing [68,69]. These "experiential" cognitive-behavioral treatments combine training aimed at either emotional exploration or emotional regulation. In an analysis of the perennial tensions between these two valid goals of therapy, Westen describes the broad and difficult therapeutic dilemmas relating the circumstances under which therapy should attempt to assist patients in accessing and exploring affective states or, alternatively, in eliminating those states [70]. He argues that traditional CBT approaches have erred in the direction of attempts to control emotions and failed to address adequately the implicit, tacit, irrational, nonverbal, and emotional aspects of existence.

Experimental research and clinical experience with somatization patients suggest these patients may be particularly well-suited to an emotionally-focused CBT. Investigators seeking to identify cognitive and affective characteristics of somatizing patients have found these patients to experience high rates of negative affect and to be less aware of and less able to describe thoughts and feelings than are other psychiatric patients [27-29]. Other authorities have discussed the "hysterical" emotional styles of these patients [71,72]. Our own impression is that whereas some somatizers manifest attenuated emotional processing and obliviousness to affect, others seem to have exaggerated emotional reactions. Some patients display each style, at different times. Contemporary theory in cognitive neuroscience suggests that emotional processing provides an important source of information about one's reactions to one's environment [68,69]. Incomplete or distorted emotional processing, in a sense, deprives individuals of data that is important to effective problem-solving. Poor understanding of the emotional domain also may result in unresolved negative affective states, and a prolongation of the physiological arousal that accompanies negative affect. Clinicians often report that the affect of somatizers seems incongruent with eliciting circumstances, being either disproportionately flat or exaggerated. Both clinical impressions and the research literature suggest that somatizers fail to integrate and/or express fully their cognitive and affective responses to their environment. Using standard CBT to challenge cognitions that are disconnected from affective experiences seems misguided and unproductive. Thus, we have aimed to design a treatment that helps patients access, process, and accept their implicit cognitive and affective responses.

6. Components of ACBT

The components of treatment are relaxation training, behavioral management, cognitive restructuring, emotion identification, emotion regulation, and interpersonal skills training. Given that somatization patients typically seek relief from their physical ailments, not from emotional distress, they begin treatment more willing to learn behavioral skills than to explore emotional issues. The first sessions are skill-focused (i.e., training patients in relaxation and behavioral management). These initial sessions are designed to provide reductions in discomfort, to introduce patients to the potential benefits of psychotherapy, and to establish a therapeutic alliance in a fashion that is consistent with patients' tastes, proclivities, and expectations. The second phase of treatment is a cognitive-emotional elicitation/regulation module intended to enhance patients' understanding of their thoughts and feelings so that they can interact more effectively with their environments. The third phase of treatment aims to enhance interpersonal functioning and to confront and alter the "sick role."

The individual treatment begins with training in relaxation [73,74]. Emphasis is placed on incorporating relaxation into daily life, before and during stressful situations, and in response to feelings of physical discomfort. Relaxation serves a number of functions in the treatment of somatization. It may interrupt the muscle tension-pain cycle found in chronic pain patients [75]. It may reduce generalized physiological arousal or physiological reactivity [76]. Finally, cognitive benefits may result from patients' observations that they are not completely helpless victims of their symptoms, but instead have some control over them [76].

Once patients begin using one form of relaxation, training in behavioral management begins. This module of treatment aims to increase gradually patients' vocational, social, and self-care activities and to improve patients' mood and physical robustness. Also, sleep hygiene and stimulus control techniques are taught, as needed. The acquisition of these skills may also contribute to each patient's sense of self-efficacy in various areas and reduce feelings of powerlessness.

The cognitive-emotional elicitation/regulation module aims to help patients differentiate and understand their thoughts and feelings so that they can interact more effectively with their environments. The atmosphere of these sessions is more psychotherapeutic and less psycho-educational than that of the earlier sessions. Cognitive and emotion-focused strategies [77,78] in this module are integrated and individualized using case-based formulations [79]. Patients begin by monitoring their thoughts and emotions associated with changes in their physical symptoms. Experiential techniques, such as focusing [80] and techniques from Gestalt therapy [81], are used to assist patients in attending to, identifying, labeling, accepting, and expressing their thoughts and emotions. In our experience, somatization patients typically are disinclined to focus intensively on their emotional experiences. However, these patients are willing to explore emotions co-occurring with their physical symptoms and to try to make sense of those emotions by examining associated thoughts and behaviors. Once a patient's unique patterns of cognitive and emotional tendencies are identified, a semi-standardized, case-based formulation is used to guide the treatment. Emotional elicitation may be emphasized to help assimilate previously disowned or disavowed cognitive and/or emotional experiences. For example, if it is agreed that the patient inhibits feelings anger, portions of treatment sessions and homework may be devoted to facilitating the introspection, identification, labeling, and, perhaps, the expression of anger. Alternatively, emotional regulation strategies, including relaxation, distraction, cognitive restructuring, may be implemented for dysfunctional, destructive, exaggerated, or uncontrollable emotions. Determining which emotions, for a given individual in a given situation, need to be sought or amplified and which need to be examined through the lens of associated cognition or attenuated is a task that is central to the integration of cognitive and emotion-focused methods.

Cognitive interventions are based upon cognitive treatment programs for stress management [82] and pain management [83]. Cognitive errors characteristic of this population, such as thinking catastrophically about somatic symptoms, are addressed with cognitive restructuring techniques. Distraction is taught in order to reduce excessive attention paid to their physical sensations. Also, patients explore the function that the "sick role" plays in their social world. Specifically, they examine whether they derive secondary gains from their physical symptoms and disability. Treatment helps patients develop alternative strategies for attaining those gains derived from the sick role.

7. Therapeutic techniques

The therapeutic posture we assume with patients and the rationale for treatment that we present to them are among the most important elements of our therapy. Our attitude toward patients is empathic and interested. We begin by asking patients about their physical symptoms and about the impact those symptoms have upon their lives. Our questions about the particular nature of the symptoms, such as the types of pain (e.g., stabbing, pounding, burning, aching) and the situations in which symptoms typically occur, provide therapists with important information while concurrently validating patients' discomfort. Patients' beliefs about their physical symptoms and past coping techniques are also explored. Throughout this discussion and throughout the entire treatment, the therapist strives to acknowledge the physical symptoms and the distress associated with them. The therapist's efforts to validate the patient's discomfort and distress are critical to the development of therapeutic rapport. Because patients presenting with somatization symptoms are so accustomed to being discounted or dismissed by their healthcare providers, patients often become more willing to engage in treatment after they feel understood by the therapist.

After communicating a considered appreciation of the patient's difficulties, the therapist describes the treatment's rationale. A biopsychosocial model of physical symptoms is proposed. Here, the therapist's stance is empathic and non-confrontational. For patients who attribute their symptoms to an unknown biological mechanism or to toxic aspects of the physical environment, the therapist suggests that even if symptoms are caused by some organic pathology or by environmental agents, stress is likely to exacerbate them. In this way, the therapist aims to expand and to create variations in patients' explanations of their symptoms, but is careful not to contradict patients' beliefs directly. Faulty beliefs about symptoms are more effectively challenged in future sessions after some trust and credibility have been established.

The treatment is described as stress management. The rationale presented is that because stress is likely to aggravate physical symptoms, the reduction of stress is likely to alleviate physical discomfort. Many patients are open to this idea and, indeed, some already believe that stress might have a physical impact upon their bodily sensations or indeed may have played a role in their underlying but unknown pathology. Most somatizing patients, however, would not accept the notion that their physical symptoms are entirely a "direct" product of stress. Therefore, it is important that therapists clarify that stress is only one factor contributing to patients' physical discomfort. The avowed aim of this treatment is, by limiting the adverse influence of stress, to give patients control over the aspects of their illness that can be controlled.

Virtually all patients diagnosed with somatization syndromes have had extensive, unsatisfying, and futile encounters with the healthcare system. Typically, our intervention is the latest in a long line of treatments, all of which have been failures. Given that their expectations are low, our patients must be motivated to come to therapy, despite minimal initial hope of success. Our patients tell us that what keeps them coming back is the opportunity to be treated by someone who cares about them and who makes a respectful effort to understand what their lives are like.

In ACBT we place a great emphasis on psychotherapy as a caring encounter. We emphasize this to a greater degree than do many expositions of cognitive behavior therapy, a treatment that usually is associated with a didactic therapist-patient relationship, absent the emotional intensity of older more traditional forms of psychotherapy, such as psychoanalysis or client-centered therapy. While it is true that in ACBT the therapist functions as a teacher and a trainer, she also is a confidant and a helper who must earn the patient's trust through being truthful, caring, and empathic. The kind of caring encounter that is based on genuine and sincerely felt compassion is essential to being effective with the patients we see. They have, in many cases, not been treated with kindness nor with courtesy. In the areas of civility and sympathy, our therapy often proves to be a corrective emotional experience. Caring and empathy are not, in themselves, sufficient to produce change in our patients, but they can be important elements in a restored sense of confidence in the healthcare system and in the resolution to attempt to cope with what can be great discomfort and disability.

7.1. Relaxation

We typically teach diaphragmatic breathing for the first month of treatment and an abbreviated progressive muscle relaxation (PMR) for the second month of treatment. Diaphragmatic breathing can be used in concert with PMR. We subscribe to the view that relaxation training is most effective when it enables the trainee to learn how to relax on any given occasion and throughout the day, as opposed to extended sessions occurring once or twice per day during scheduled times when an especially deep state of lowered arousal is achieved.

The therapist introduces diaphragmatic breathing and explains that the long-term goal is for the patient to breathe abdominally as much as possible. However, regular abdominal breathing takes time to establish if it is a departure from the patient's typical practice. Over the course of treatment, the patient is asked to practice breathing abdominally between sessions and to report back on her progress. Eventually, breathing abdominally may coincide with reductions in tension and discomfort, though the patient should be warned not to be disappointed if she initially experiences little significant relief.

The crucial challenge in relaxation training is helping patients use the techniques on a regular basis. The considerable amount of therapy time used to describe, practice, and effectively implement relaxation techniques indicates the importance we place on using them. Even though training in relaxation is often completed by the eighth week of treatment, we continue to inquire into patients' use of relaxation throughout our work with them. Some patients learn to use both abbreviated PMR and abdominal breathing, either in combination or separately. Others have a strong preference for one method or the other. We attempt to train patients in two forms of relaxation and to allow the patient to decide ultimately which to employ. At this point the research literature cannot demonstrate that any form of systematic relaxation will be superior to others for a given individual [76]. What is clear, however, is that relaxation is beneficial only if it is utilized.

7.2. Behavioral management

Behavioral methods are largely based upon the principles of classical and operant conditioning. Existing pathogenic contingencies of reinforcement are replaced with salutary ones. For example, patients learn to connect with friends and family by engaging with them in pleasurable activities instead of interacting with them through activities focused on the patients' physical discomfort. Exercise assignments are designed to be pleasurable and commensurate with patients' physical capacities, so that exercise may eventually be reinforced by inherent natural contingencies. Overall, the acquisition of a broader repertory of activities also may serve to enhance each patient's self-efficacy in multiple areas and reduce feelings of infirmity and powerlessness.

Activity pacing is an important topic to address when discussing the initiation of a new activity. Our clinical experience and some research suggest that some, if not many, somatization patients have perfectionistic tendencies driving them to over-achieve [84,85]. Our sense is that many of these patients may have difficulty moderating their activity levels; they over-function at times and under-function at other times. Of course, by the time they reach a psychotherapist's office, they are under-functioning in important areas of their lives. Nevertheless, once they have been convinced to undertake an activity, they may be inclined to "overdo" it. Given the possibility that somatization patients may over-function or strive for perfection in therapy, the therapist emphasizes the importance of making small changes in a specific behavior at first and subsequently instituting gradual increases in that activity over the course of therapy. Other ways in which activity pacing is incorporated into therapy is by persuading patients to take frequent breaks in the midst of their daily routines.

To increase the likelihood that behavioral changes become a permanent part of patients' lives, they are discussed throughout treatment. The therapist monitors all changed behaviors every week of treatment.

Many patients with somatization syndromes report significant sleep disturbance [86]. Failure to receive adequate restorative sleep is a contributory factor in exacerbating many psychiatric disorders. In somatizers, almost invariably, sleep loss is correlated with a worsening of symptoms. We now believe that treating insomnia early and aggressively is a key to successful treatment of somatization.

Many of our patients, especially those not working outside their homes, engage in problematic sleep practices that may increase the likelihood of insomnia, such as taking naps during the day, keeping erratic sleep schedules, and watching television in bed. To combat poor sleep habits, we provide patients with brief psychoeducational training in sleep hygiene and stimulus control techniques [87].

7.3. Identifying thoughts and feelings

The cognitive-emotional elicitation/regulation components of treatment aim to help patients differentiate and understand their thoughts and feelings so that they can interact more effectively with their environments. The atmosphere of sessions devoted to this enterprise is more psychotherapeutic and less psychoeducational than that of the earlier sessions that are focused upon relaxation training and making behavioral changes.

Patients begin this phase of treatment by monitoring their thoughts and emotions that are associated with changes in their physical symptoms. Experiential techniques, such as focusing [80] and techniques from Gestalt therapy [81], are used to assist patients in attending to, identifying, labeling, accepting, and expressing their thoughts and emotions. In our experience, somatization patients typically are disinclined to focus intensively on their emotional experiences. However, these patients often are willing to explore emotions co-occurring with their physical symptoms and to try to make sense of those emotions by examining the associated thoughts and behaviors.

Symptom monitoring forms are introduced to help patients focus their attention on thoughts and feelings between sessions. These forms are analogous to dysfunctional thought records used with depressed patients [88]. Our symptom monitoring forms require patients to describe two specific moments each day: 1) when their physical symptoms are relatively severe and 2) when their physical symptoms are relatively less severe and they are experiencing greater relative comfort. Because the goal here is to increase patients' awareness rather than to assess symptom severity, it is not critical that the patient write about "the most uncomfortable" or "the least uncomfortable" period of the day. We aim for a record of a representative "physically uncomfortable" and "physically less uncomfortable" episodes. Ideally, these entries will be made as proximate to the time of occurrence as possible at a time each day when patients experienced noteworthy discomfort or the absence of discomfort. On days without significant variation in physical discomfort, patients' instructions are to choose, retrospectively, episodes of relative comfort and discomfort. At the moment of recording, patients note the time of day, the physical symptoms experienced, the environmental circumstances, and thoughts and emotions concurrent with the physical symptoms. The monitoring forms can be used to detect patterns in symptoms and in the relationships among symptoms, thoughts, and emotions.

An initial task is to teach patients to distinguish between physical sensations and emotions as well as to differentiate thoughts from emotions. For example, if a patient says that her physical sensations included anxiety, the therapist might reply, "I would consider anxiety an emotion, not a physical sensation. So, let's put that in the emotion column. But, sometimes people have physical sensations that accompany anxiety. Did you feel anything in your body, any physical sensation, at that time that coincided with the anxiety?" Similarly, if a patient says that she felt stupid, the therapist should 1) label this experience as that of the evaluative cognition that "I am stupid," 2) distinguish cognition and emotion, and 3) question the patient about the emotion that coincided with that cognition. Also, emphasis is placed upon learning to differentiate among emotions. (Patients are asked to use specific emotion terms such as "sad," "worried," or "annoyed," instead of more nebulous emotion terms such as "stressed," "bad," or "upset.")

Many patients presenting with somatization struggle with the self-awareness activities because of difficulties in identifying and differentiating among their thoughts and feelings. Whatever the cause of this difficulty (e.g., alexithymia, repressive coping), our efforts focus on enhancing awareness and acceptance of thoughts and feelings. Many patients find that recognizing and expressing thoughts and/or feelings may be the most difficult component of treatment. Nevertheless, these initial skills must be mastered before cognitive restructuring techniques can be taught. Disputing cognitions is futile unless one can identify one's thoughts and feelings. The heightening of patients' self-awareness is facilitated by therapists' refraining from disputing cognitions until a thorough investigation of emotions and their companion cognitions has been conducted. We want patients to be able to experience and communicate emotions during a session. This work in session is extended to the patient's life outside of therapy via homework assignments that call upon the patient to identify and record emotions, as well as associated physical symptoms and thoughts.

7.4. Cognitive restructuring

An important component of treatment is to help patients examine their cognitive tendencies. After reviewing a few weeks of a patient's symptom monitoring forms, the therapist will have a sense of the patient's typical dysfunctional thinking patterns. Typical cognitive errors that we have observed include perfectionistic thoughts, catastrophic thoughts (about physical symptoms as well as other life events), overestimating the possibility of negative outcomes, "should" statements, and dichotomous thinking. Our sense is that at the core of these errors is a global negative perception of self as being inadequate or unlovable. Although many patients may not acknowledge seeing themselves as inadequate or unlovable, especially a brief episode of treatment, thoughts about being weak, vulnerable, undesirable, unattractive, or helpless may not be far from the surface when the "meaning" of a thought is explored. Once these kinds of dysfunctional beliefs are identified, we employ cognitive restructuring techniques [88].

7.5. Addressing illness behavior

In hopes of interrupting the dysfunctional pattern of physical symptoms prompting physician visits that fail to alleviate or even exacerbate those symptoms, the therapist helps the patient learn to reconsider the thoughts fueling illness behavior. Our patients often make comments like, "there must be something wrong with me that my doctor hasn't found." If such a belief is sound, the rational response is to seek additional diagnostic procedures. However, such beliefs may be assailable. Patients are encouraged to look at the evidence either supporting or undermining that belief. Questions like, "What makes you think there is something medically wrong with you?" or "What evidence is there that the doctor has missed something?" are followed by "What evidence is there that you may not have a serious medical problem?" Also, patients are questioned about the advantages and disadvantages of having another diagnostic procedure. They are asked what would convince them that they are not suffering from the illness they fear. The grounds for the falsification of beliefs are explored extensively to demonstrate that one can never be 100% certain of perfect health. In addition to challenging patients' beliefs associated with illness behavior, the therapist constructs behavioral experiments in which patients test the consequences of avoiding (or, at least, delaying) physician visits. Symptom monitoring forms are used to assess the impact of modifying this aspect of illness behavior. If patients can delay a physician visit long enough, the somatization symptom that initially prompted the intent to seek medical treatment may subside.

The goal of the sick role discussion is to provide patients with some insight into any secondary gain they might derive while experiencing pain or discomfort and to examine the possibility that illness behavior has become habitual. Having identified the secondary gain, the therapist and patient collaborate to find alternative methods for attaining the sick role's benefits. For example, if the patient's spouse is especially nurturing when the patient is in pain, we help the patient ask directly for more attention and affection.

Examining the sick role's benefits is a sensitive issue because family, friends, and physicians may have accused the patient of faking, imagining, or exaggerating his symptoms. Thus, the therapist is careful not to imply that the patient is choosing to experience his symptoms. The discussion will be fruitless if the patient becomes defensive. Because of the sensitivity of this topic, we typically defer its discussion until the third month of treatment.

To avoid raising the patient's defenses initially, the discussion begins by focusing on the patient's perceptions of other people who have been ill, other people whom the patient knows or has known well. The therapist asks who, in the patient's family and social circle, had health problems during the patient's childhood (or during the patient's adulthood, if no one had health problems during the patient's childhood). In our clinical experience, as in Craig et al.'s research [89], many patients meeting criteria for a somatoform disorder report having observed illness during childhood in either a family member or a close friend. The patient is asked to describe the individual who was ill and to talk about the ways in which that person's life was affected by illness or physical discomfort. Specifically, the therapist asks about the sick person's missed opportunities and missed experiences and how others responded to the person. Next, the therapist inquires into "the silver lining" that being unhealthy may have had for the sick person. "Were there any benefits of being unhealthy for that individual?" If the patient believes there were no benefits, the therapist may ask specifically about each of the following possible benefits: receiving special attention or nurture, avoiding undesirable activities, avoiding arguments, gaining a special role in the family, or diminishing one's own expectations for oneself. Usually the patient will acknowledge that the ill individual experienced some benefits from his or her illness.

Having discussed another person's experiences with illness, the therapist shifts the discussion to the impact of illness upon the patient's life. The therapist begins with inquiries into the patient's experience of illness as a child: "How did others respond to you when you were sick or in pain as a child?" "Were you taken to the doctor or did you miss school when you were sick?" "Did you receive special attention or treatment when you were sick?" Afterwards, questions focus on the impact of illness during the patient's adult life: "In previous sessions we discussed the many disadvantages of your health problems these days, are there any advantages to being sick?"

Although almost all of our patients have acknowledged that some benefits accrue from "being sick," therapists often feel anxious during this discussion. It may seem likely that explicit discussion with the patient about the sick role will undermine the therapeutic relationship. But in our experience, no patient has withdrawn prematurely from treatment after discussing the sick role. Although the topic is a sensitive one, it can be productively examined.

Often the discussion of the sick role begins to provide a rationale for assertiveness training as it may reveal deficits in the patient's assertiveness. If the patient is deriving substantial attention or nurture through being sick, he also may be deficient in the ability to ask directly for attention and nurture. Patients who avoid undesirable activities by being sick may have difficulty setting limits on others. One advantage of the sick role is that people can be rewarded without having to ask directly for what they want. The sick role tends to undermine assertiveness and to provide few opportunities to hone skills of self-assertion, except perhaps in interactions with healthcare providers.

If the patient acknowledges that the sick role has become "second nature" to him, we may borrow a technique of fixed-role therapy [90] and have our patient attempt to play the part of a "healthy person" in one or more activities. One method is to ask the patient to find a role-model who is not impaired and to imitate that person's behavior. Another is to have the patient ask the question, "What would a healthy person do in this situation?" and then to act out the answer. Occasionally, as much psychological research has shown, changes in attitudes and emotions will follow changes in behavior rather than preceding them. Expanding the range of the patient's behavior, before the patient feels "healthy enough," can be effective, if the approach is used judiciously. How much to push somatizers to extend themselves is a matter of clinical judgment. Good therapeutic decisions in this area tend to optimize treatment outcomes.

7.6. Assertiveness

At this point in treatment, the therapist will have assessed for deficits in the patient's assertiveness. Some patients effectively assert themselves and have their needs met in some, but not all, situations. Some patients can assert themselves only in regard to certain kinds of needs. Other patients can assert their needs when they are aware of them, but may not always be aware of what those needs might be. Other patients have pervasive, trait-like deficits in assertiveness across virtually all areas of their lives. In our experience, all somatization patients have difficulty expressing their thoughts and feelings assertively in, at least, some situations.

The therapist begins by defining assertiveness and explaining the rationale for helping the patient act more assertively in some situations. We define assertiveness as an open and honest expression of one's thoughts and feelings that avoids blaming or attacking others. Much of ACBT treatment, up to this point, has provided the groundwork for becoming assertive. For example, the self-awareness exercises and symptom monitoring forms direct the patient to pay attention to her thoughts and feelings. Stage 1 of acting assertively involves identifying thoughts and feelings. Stage 2, valuing one's thoughts and feelings, is implicit in and fostered by some of the behavioral techniques. By taking time to relax and to engage in pleasurable activities, patients are, in effect, affirming the value and legitimacy of taking care of themselves.

Before introducing stage 3 of assertiveness, patients may need additional work on stages 1 and 2. Specifically, patients might be asked to track their thoughts and feelings when interacting with others between therapy sessions. (At this point in treatment, unassertive individuals often can identify their thoughts and feelings when they are alone. Yet, they may have difficulty being self-aware while interacting with others, especially others who are accustomed to or expect them to be unassertive.) A homework assignment might be to ask, "What do I think and feel?" during various interactions with others. For patients who continue to have trouble valuing their thoughts and feelings, the therapist should use the technique from fixed-role therapy [89]. Patients are directed to role-play in the outside world, to behave as they would if they really did think their own feelings and needs were important. Through this device, assertive behavior, with a tone of conviction, can be practiced and its often successful results can be witnessed by the patient. Occasionally patients will adopt and assimilate features of this more assertive persona.

Stage 3 of assertiveness involves communicating one's thoughts, feelings, desires, and needs with "I statements". The therapist suggests the patient use the following statement as a model, "I feel __________, when you __________." An example of content in this form is, "I felt worried when you didn't call to tell me you'd be late coming home from work last night." By making such a statement, this individual is taking responsibility for her feelings as opposed to blaming others (e.g., "You're so selfish not to have called"). Also, the statement is indisputable since it is an expression of the patient's emotional reaction. The result is that the person being spoken to is somewhat less likely to react defensively than if attacked or explicitly criticized; the person addressed also may be less likely to attempt to refute the assertion itself.

7.7. Sessions with spouse or significant other

The goals of including the significant other (domestic partner spouse) in treatment are to obtain additional information about the patient, to gain the significant other's support for the treatment, and to alter behaviors of the significant other that may reinforce the patient's symptoms or illness behavior. We view this aspect of the treatment to be so valuable that, even when working within our 10-session treatment format, we ask the patient's significant other to join us for 1 to 3 of those 10 sessions.

We typically invite the significant other to participate in a conjoint session within the first month of treatment. The rationale for meeting together with the patient and significant other is to encourage an open dialogue. In our experience, the therapeutic relationship is not always strong enough to tolerate a therapist's meeting separately with a significant other, as some patients readily become suspicious that "behind my back" others are minimizing their degree of discomfort. And, although we would like to begin deriving the benefits of including the significant other in treatment as soon as possible, for logistical reasons we typically delay the first conjoint session until we have had some time to develop rapport with the patient. We find the third or forth session works well as an initial conjoint session.

The focus of the conjoint session(s) includes discussions about the rationale for a "stress management" treatment and about how such a treatment could be maximally helpful to the patient. The therapist asks the significant other to comment on the impact of stress upon the patient's physical symptoms. Also, the impact of the patient's physical symptoms on the patient's and significant other's lives is examined. Here we aim to elicit information and to suggest that the significant other's involvement in treatment may benefit both parties. Reducing the likelihood that the significant other will undermine the treatment is critical.

After clarifying the treatment's rationale, the therapist attempts to determine whether the significant relationship has been impaired by the patient's illness. Somatizers' tendencies to withdraw from activities may not only diminish pleasure in their own lives, but also in their significant others' lives. When a patient foregoes couple's activities, such as eating at restaurants, going to movie theaters, dancing, or hiking, the domestic partner and their relationship may suffer. The patient and significant other are asked to think about activities they once and might, yet again, enjoy together. Afterwards, the couple and therapist collaborate to develop a plan for increasing pleasurable conjoint activities. Reengaging in these activities may increase satisfaction with the relationship as well as reduce the patient's focus upon her symptoms.

A subsidiary aim of the conjoint sessions is to address the couple's communication about the patient's physical symptoms. Initially the therapist asks the couple to describe a few recent discussions about the patient's physical symptoms. Both members of the couple are asked to describe what each said about the symptoms and what each thought and felt at that time. Afterwards, the therapist summarizes and reflects upon the couple's communication about the patient's symptoms. Suggestions for alternative modes of interacting, that are less likely to reinforce illness behavior, are provided.

8. Conclusions

Somatic symptom disorder and related disorders are distressing, disabling, and costly disorders. Although the treatment of somatization and of somatic symptom disorder is in its infancy, there is sufficient evidence to believe CBT and ACBT have therapeutic value. Given the research conducted to date, we recommend CBT and ACBT as the treatments of choice for these disorders. A manualized 10-session version of our treatment [51] has been tested and found effective with patients diagnosed with very severe as well as more moderate levels of somatization [52, 53].

Author details

Lesley A. Allen and Robert L. Woolfolk*

*Address all correspondence to: woolfolk@princeton.edu

Department of Psychology, Princeton University, Princeton, NJ, USA

References

[1] Gureje O, Simon GE. The natural history of somatization in primary care. Psychol Med 1999;29:669-676.

[2] Smith GR, Monson RA, Ray DC. Patients with multiple unexplained symptoms: their characteristics, functional health, and health care utilization. Arch Intern Med 1986;146:69-72.

[3] Katon W, Lin E, Von Korff M, Russo J, Lipscomb P, Bush T. Somatization: a spectrum of severity. Am J Psychiatry 1991;148:34-40.

[4] American Psychiatric Association. Diagnostic and statistical manual of mental disorders (3rded.). Washington, DC: Author; 1980.

[5] American Psychiatric Association. Diagnostic and statistical manual of mental disorders (3rd ed., rev.). Washington, DC: Author; 1987.

[6] American Psychiatric Association. Diagnostic and statistical manual of mental disorders (4th ed.). Washington, DC: Author, 1994.

[7] American Psychiatric Association. DSM-5 Development. Available at: http://www.dsm5.org/proposedrevision/Pages/SomaticSymptomDisorders.aspx. (accessed 30 July 2012).

[8] Rief W, Rojas G. Stability of somatoform symptoms – Implications for classification. Psychosom Med 2007;69:864-869.

[9] Simon GE, Gureje O. Stability of somatization disorder and somatization symptoms among primary care patients. Arch Gen Psychiatry 1999;56:90-95.

[10] Stone J, Wojcik W, Durrance D, Carson A, Lewis S, MacKenzie L, Warlow C, & Sharpe M. What should we say to patients with symptoms unexplained by disease? The "number needed to offend." British Medical Journal 2002;325:1449–1450

[11] Escobar JI, Waitzkin H, Silver RC, Gara M, Holman A. Abridged somatization: a study in primary care. Psychosom Med 1998;60:466-472.

[12] Gureje O, Simon GE, Ustun T, Goldberg DP. Somatization in cross-cultural perspective: a World Health Organization study in primary care. American Journal of Psychiatry 1997;154:989-995.

[13] Kirmayer LJ, Robbins JM. Three forms of somatization in primary care: prevalence, co-occurrence, and sociodemographic characteristics. Journal of Nervous and Mental Disease 1991;179:647-655.

[14] Escobar JI, Rubio-Stipec M, Canino G, Karno M. Somatic symptom index (SSI): a new and abridged somatization construct. Prevalence and epidemiological correlates in two large community samples. Journal of Nervous and Mental Disease 1989;177:140-146.

[15] Robins LN, Regier D. Psychiatric disorders in America: the epidemiological catchment area study. New York: Free Press, 1991.

[16] Fink P. Surgery and medical treatment in persistent somatizing patients. Journal of Psychosomatic Research 1992;36:439-447.

[17] Barsky AJ, Orav EJ, Bates DW. Somatization increases medical utilization and costs independent of psychiatric and medical comorbidity. Arch Gen Psychiatry. 2005;62:903-910.

[18] Escobar JI, Golding JM, Hough RL, Karno M, Burnam MA, Wells KB. Somatization in the community: relationship to disability and use of services. American Journal of Public Health 1987;77:837-840.

[19] Allen LA, Gara MA, Escobar JI, Waitzkin H, Cohen-Silver R. Somatization: a debilitating síndrome in primary care. Psychosomatics 2001;42:63-67.

[20] Jackson JL, Kroenke K. Prevalence, impact, and prognosis of multisomatoform disorder in primary care: a 5-year follow-up study. Psychosomatic Medicine 2008;70:430-434.

[21] Simon GE, VonKorff M. Somatization and psychiatric disorder in the NIMH Epidemiological Catchment Area Study. American Journal of Psychiatry 1991;148:1494-1500.

[22] Barsky AJ. Amplification, somatization, and the somatoform disorders. Psychosomatics. 1992;33:28-34.

[23] Rief W, Hiller W, Margraf J. Cognitive aspects of hypochondriasis and the somatization syndrome. J Abnorm Psychol. 1998;107:587-595.

[24] Rief W, Heitmu°ller AM, Reisberg K, Ru°ddel H. Why reassurance fails in patients with unexplained symptoms – an experimental investigation of remembered probablilities. PLoS Medicine 2006;3:e269.

[25] Rief W, Broadbent E. Explaining medically unexplained symptoms – models and mechanisms. Clinical Psychology Review 2007;7:821-841.

[26] Noyes R, Langbehn DR, Happel RL, Stout LR, Muller BA, Longley SL. Personality dysfunction among somatizing patients. Psychosomatics 2001;42:320-329.

[27] Deary IJ, Scott S, Wilson JA. Neuroticism, alexithymia, and medically unexplained symptoms. Personality and Individual Differences 1997;22:551-564.

[28] Mattila AK, Kronholm E, Jula A, Salminen J, Koivisto AM, Mielonen RL, Joukamaa M. Alexithymia and somatization in general population. Psychosomatic Medicine 2008;70:716-722.

[29] Kirmayer LJ, Robbins JM. Patients who somatize in primary care: a longitudinal study of cognitve and social characteristics. Psychological Medicine 1996;26:937-951.

[30] Engel GL. The need for a new medical model: a challenge for biomedicine. Science 1977;196:129-136.

[31] Brown R. Psychological mechanisms of medically unexplained symptoms: an integrative conceptual model. Psychological Bulletin 2004;130:793-812.

[32] Sharpe M, Peveler R, Mayou R. The psychological treatment of patients with functional somatic symptoms: a practical guide. Journal of Psychosomatic Research 1992;36:515-529.

[33] Rief W, Hennings A, Riemer S, Euteneuer F. Psychobiological differences between depression and somatization. Journal of Psychosomatic Research 2010; 68:495-502.

[34] Rief W, Shaw R, Fichter MM. Elevated levels of psychophysiological arousal and cortisol in patients with somatization syndrome. Psychosomatic Medicine 1998;60:198-203.

[35] Pennebaker JW. The psychology of physical symptoms. New York: Springer; 1982.

[36] Schmidt AJM, Wolfs-Takens DJ, Oosterlaan J, van den Hout MA. Psychological mechanisms in hypochondriasis: attention-induced physical symptoms without sensory stimulation. Psychotherapy and Psychosomatics 1994;61:117-120.

[37] Teasdale JD. Negative thinking in depression: cause, effect or reciprocal relationship? Advances in Behavior Research and Therapy 1983;5:3-25.

[38] Severeijns R, Vlaeyen JWS, van den Hout MA. Pain catastrophizing is associated with health indices in musculoskeletal pain: a cross-sectional study in the Dutch community. Health Psychology 2004;23:49-57.

[39] Zoccolillo M, Cloninger CR. Somatization disorder: psychologic symptoms, social disability, and diagnosis. Comprehensive Psychiatry 1986;27:65-73.

[40] Snelling J. The role of the family in relation to chronic pain: review of the literature. Advances in Nursing 1990;15:771-776.

[41] Speckens AEM, van Hemert AM, Spinhoven P, Hawton KE, Bolk JH, Rooijmans GM. Cognitive behavioural therapy for medically unexplained physical symptoms: a randomised controlled trial. British Medical Journal 1995;311:1328-1332.

[42] Lidbeck J. Group therapy for somatization disorders in general practice: effectiveness of a short cognitive-behavioural treatment model. Acta Psychiatr Scand 1997;96:14-24.

[43] Escobar JI, Gara MA, Diaz-Martinez AM, et al. Effectiveness of a time-limited cognitive behavior therapy type intervention among primary care patients with medically unexplained symptoms. Annals of Family Medicine 2007;5:328-335.

[44] Sumathipala A, Hewege S, Hanwella R, Mann AH. Randomized controlled trial of cognitive behaviour therapy for repeated consultations for medically unexplained complaints: a feasibility study in Sri Lanka. Psychological Medicine 2000;30:747-757.

[45] Allen LA, Woolfolk RL, Escobar JI, Gara MA, Hamer RM. Cognitive-behavioral therapy for somatization disorder: a randomized controlled trial. Archives of Internal Medicine 2006;166:1512-1518.

[46] Woolfolk RL, Allen LA. Treating somatization: a cognitive-behavioral approach. New York: Guilford Press, 2006.

[47] Smith GR, Monson RA, Ray DC. Psychiatric consultation letter in somatization disorder. New England Journal of Medicine 1986;314:1407-1413.

[48] Rost K, Kashner TM, Smith GR. Effectiveness of psychiatric intervention with somatization disorder patients: improved outcomes at reduced costs. General Hospital Psychiatry 1994;16:381-387.

[49] Dickinson WP, Dickinson LM, deGruy FV, Main DS, Candib LM, Rost, K. A randomized clinical trial of a care recommendation letter intervention for somatization in primary care. Annals of Family Medicine 2003;1:228-235.

[50] Smith GR, Rost K, Kashner M. A trial of the effect of a standardized psychiatric consultation on health outcomes and costs in somatizing patients. Archives of General Psychiatry 1995;52:238-243.

[51] Arnold IA, de Waal MW, Eekhof JA, Assendelft WJ, Spinhoven P, van Hemert AM. Medically unexplained physical symptoms in primary care: a controlled study on the effectiveness of cognitive-behavioral treatment by the family physician. Psychosomatics 2009;50:515-524.

[52] Larisch A, Schweickhardt A, Wirsching M, Fritzsche K. Psychosocial interventions for somatizing patients by the general practitioner: A randomized controlled trial. Journal of Psychosomatic Research 2004;57:507–514.

[53] Morriss R, Dowrick C, Salmon P, Peters S, Dunn G, Rogers A, Lewis B, Charles-Jones H, Hogg J, Clifford R, Rigby C, Gask L. Cluster randomised controlled trial of training practices in reattribution for medically unexplained symptoms. British Journal of Psychiatry 2007;191:536-542.

[54] Rief W, Martin A, Rauh E, Zech T, Bender A. Evaluation of general practitioners' training: How to manage patients with unexplained physical symptoms. Psychosomatics 2006;47:304 –311.

[55] Rosendal M, Olesen F, Fink P, Toft T, Sokolowski I, Bro F. A randomized controlled trial of brief training in the assessment and treatment of somatization in primary care: Effects on patient outcome. General Hospital Psychiatry 2007;29:364 –373.

[56] Smith RC, Lyles JS, Gardiner JC, Sirbu C, Hodges A, Collins C, Dwamena FC, Lein C, Given WC, Given B, Goddeeris J. Primary care clinicians treat patients with medically unexplained symptoms: a randomized controlled trial. Journal of General Internal Medicine 2006;21:671–677.

[57] Katon W, Lin E, Von Korff M, Russo J, Lipscomb P, Bush T. Somatization: A spectrum of severity. American Journal of Psychiatry 1991;148:34-40.

[58] Von Korff M, Gruman J, Schaefer J, Curry SJ, Wagner EH. Collaborative management of chronic illness. Annals of Internal Medicine 1997;127:1097-1102.

[59] Van der Feltz-Cornelis CM, van Oppen P, Ader HJ, van Dyck R. Randomised controlled trial of a collaborative care model with psychiatric consultation for persistent

medically unexplained symptoms in general practice. Psychotherapy and Psychosomatics 2006;75:282-289.

[60] Kleinstäuber M, Witthöft M, Hiller W. Efficacy of short-term psychotherapy for multiple medically unexplained physical symptoms: a meta-analysis. Clinical Psychology Review 2001;31:146-160.

[61] Arnold MB. Emotion and personality. New York: Columbia University Press; 1960.

[62] Lazarus RS. Psychological stress and the coping process. New York: McGraw-Hill; 1966.

[63] Linehan MM. Cognitive-behavioral treatment of borderline personality disorder. New York: Guilford; 1993.

[64] Hayes SC, Strosahl KD, Wilson KG. Acceptance and commitment therapy: an experiential approach to behavior change. New York: Guilford; 1999.

[65] Roemer L, Orsillo SM. Expanding our conceptualization of and treatment for generalized anxiety disorder: integrating mindfulness/acceptance-based approaches with existing cognitive-behavioral models. Clinical Psychology: Science and Practice 2002;9:54-68.

[66] Mennin DS, Heimberg RG, Turk CL, Fresco DM. Applying an emotion regulation framework to integrative approaches to generalized anxiety disorder. Clinical Psychology: Science and Practice 2002;9:85-90.

[67] Samoilov A, Goldfried MR. Role of emotion in cognitive-behavior therapy. Clinical Psychology: Science and Practice 2000;7:373-385.

[68] Izard CE. Four systems for emotion activation cognitive and noncognitive processes. Psychological Review 1993;100:68-90.

[69] LeDoux JE. Emotion: clues from the brain. Annual Review of Psychology 1995;46:209-235.

[70] Westen D. Commentary: implicit and emotional processes in cognitive-behavior therapy. Clinical Psychology: Science and Practice 2000;7:386-390.

[71] Kirmayer LJ, Robbins JM, Paris J. Somatoform disorders: personality and the social matrix of somatic distress. Journal of Abnormal Psychology 1994;103:125-136.

[72] Kaminsky MJ, Slavney PR. Hysterical and obsessional features in patients with Briquet's syndrome (somatization disorder). Psychological Medicine 1983;13:111-120.

[73] Bernstein DA, Carlson CR, Schmidt JE. Progressive relaxation: Abbreviated methods. In PM Lehrer, RL Woolfolk, WE. Sime (Eds.), Principles and practice of stress management (3rd ed., pp. 88-122). New York: Guilford; 2007.

[74] Fried, R. The role of respiration in stress and stress control: Toward a theory of stress as a hypoxic phenomenon. In PM Lehrer, RL Woolfolk (Eds.), Principles and practice of stress management (2nd ed., pp. 301-331). New York: Guilford; 1993.

[75] Linton SJ. Chronic back pain: integrating psychological and physical therapy: an overview. Behavioral Medicine 1994;20:101-104.

[76] Lehrer PM, Woolfolk RL. Research on clinical issues in stress management. In PM Lehrer, RL Woolfolk (Eds.), Principles and practice of stress management (3rd ed., pp. 703-721). New York: Guilford; 2007.

[77] Kennedy-Moore E, Watson JC. Expressing Emotion. New York: Guilford, 1999.

[78] Greenberg LS. Emotion-focused therapy. Washington, D.C.: American Psychological Association, 2001.

[79] Persons JB. Cognitive therapy in practice: a case formulation approach. New York: W. W. Norton, 1989.

[80] Gendlin ET. Focusing. New York: Bantam, 1981.

[81] Perls F. The gestalt approach and eyewitness to therapy. Palo Alto, CA: Science and Behavior Books, 1973.

[82] Beck AT. Cognitive approaches to stress. In: Lehrer PM, Woolfolk RL, editors. Principles and Practice of Stress Management. 2nd edition. New York: Guilford, 1993:333-372.

[83] Philips HC, Rachman S. The Psychological Management of Chronic Pain: A Treatment Manual. 2nd edition. New York: Springer Publishing Co., 1996.

[84] Surawy C, Hackmann A, Hawton K, Sharpe M. Chronic fatigue syndrome: a cognitive approach. Behaviour Research and Therapy. 1995;33:535-544.

[85] Ware NC. Society, mind and body in chronic fatigue syndrome: an anthropological view. In: Bock GR, Whelan G, editors. Chronic Fatigue Syndrome. Chichester, England: Wiley; 1993;62-82.

[86] Affleck G, Urrows S, Tennen H, Higgins P. Sequential daily relations of sleep, pain intensity, and attention to pain among women with fibromyalgia. Pain, 1996;68:363-368.

[87] Morin CM. Insomnia: psychological assessment and management. New York: Guilford Press; 1993.

[88] Beck AT, Rush AJ, Shaw BF, Emery G. Cognitive therapy of depression. New York: Guilford Press; 1979.

[89] Craig TKJ, Cox AD, Klein K. Intergenerational transmission of somatization behaviour: A study of chronic somatizers and their children. Psychological Medicine 2002:32;805-816.

[90] Kelly GA. The psychology of personal constructs. New York: Norton, 1955.

Chapter 9

The Bond We Share: Experiences of Caring for a Person with Mental and Physical Health Conditions

Sharon Lawn, Jeannette Walsh, Anne Barbara,
Margaret Springgay and Patricia Sutton

Additional information is available at the end of the chapter

1. Introduction

The purpose of this chapter is to improve service providers' understanding of how to work with, include and understand the experience and expertise of mental health carers. This information is useful for service providers in clinical mental health, psychosocial rehabilitation across government and non-government, and primary health care settings, and also for managers of services, to help determine training offered to their employees. It may also be useful for carers and carer support organisations, as well as for those who teach undergraduate and postgraduate health professional students.

After reading this chapter, readers will be able to:

- Understand the significant impact of caring for a person with a mental & physical health conditions, from the carer's perspective, and their day-to-day experience of caring;
- Understand how carers can contribute as positive partners with health care providers, in supporting people with mental and physical health conditions;
- Critically analyse and reflect on their practice knowledge, skills and attitudes, in particular, their consideration of carers' input to enhance the clinical and psychosocial outcomes for people with mental and physical health conditions;
- Recognise strategies within their own practice that engage and support carers.

A review of the international and Australian research on mental health carers' experiences of caring for a loved one with mental illness provides a background to the issues. This is followed by a report on the results of a large study conducted in South Australia in 2010, with mental health carers, to explore and examine the issues in more depth.

Family carers are people who provide unpaid support to family members and friends who have a disability, mental illness, chronic physical health condition, terminal illness or who are frail aged. Within an overall population of 22.5 million, Australia has almost 2.6 million family carers. Almost half of all carers have a disability themselves [1-3].

Mental illnesses account for 27% of disability costs in Australia and 60% of disability costs for 25 to 40 years olds. Mental illness often requires long term support and management by the person, informal carers and health systems, posing significant burdens on health and wellbeing for individuals, families and communities [4-6]. The extent and complexity of these burdens on people with mental illness and their carers is not well understood, in particular, the complexities of managing physical health, lifestyle risk factors, and mental health [7]. As the population ages and the incidence of disability and chronic illness increases [8], the role of these carers will become increasingly apparent and the impacts of caring increasingly felt. This is compounded by major policy changes, in Australia and in many other countries, focused on shorter hospital stays and a shift from institutional care to greater care in the community [9]. In Australia, carers contribute substantially to the national economy through unpaid care, yet they are amongst the poorest, most disadvantaged people in our community [10]. In 2005, the productivity loss of this care was estimated at approximately $4.9 billion; a substantial comparison to the $30.5 billion provided for formal aged and disability care services in Australia [11]. Carers spend around 40 hours a week providing care [1]. For carers of someone with a mental illness in Australia, the average time spent providing care is around 104 hours per week [12]. Family carers are usually at the centre of community mental health care, providing the bulk of support and assistance with little or no specialised training [10]. Similar figures have been found in the United Kingdom with 5.8 million carers, of which many are mental health carers [13-15]. In the United Stated, there are 65.7 million carers of which 7% or nearly 0.5 million are mental health carers (not including Alzheimers or dementia) [16]. Outcomes for people with mental illness are therefore highly dependent upon the quality of in-home support. Yet there have been few community-based support services put in place in Australia, or in other countries, to aid the shift to deinstitutionalisation of care for people with mental illness [8]. These phenomena are not isolated to the Australian context [6,17-29].

We do know that mental health carers face unique challenges in their caring role, related to the nature of mental illness itself and that the role entails both positive and negative impacts [30,31]. Tasks of caring such as personal care, involvement in medication monitoring and distribution, support for shopping, household chores such as cleaning and laundry, budgeting and bill paying support are understood as common across caring roles where physical frailty and dependence are evident. Though many mental health carers also undertake such tasks within their caring role, the predictability of these roles does not necessarily apply to mental health caring, especially given mental illness often has marked fluctuations and ever changing impacts on the person with the illness [14, 32-35]. Such fluctuations require mental health carers to navigate their roles within a fine balance of ever-changing need which in turn gives rise to further unique issues for mental health carers that must be understood in order to provide them with effective support in their caring role.

2. Impacts of caring on carers

Caring for someone with a mental illness often comes with enormous personal costs, particularly on the health of carers who experience a broad range of impacts as a result of their caring role [3,36,37]. Research has shown that mothers show the highest level of burden, "because they usually are the key carer and assume the totality of the patient care." (p.722) [38]. Carers have significantly higher levels of depression and stress, and lower levels of subjective wellbeing, self-efficacy and physical health than those without carer responsibilities [9, 39-42]. More than one third of Australian carers experience depression, and being a carer for someone else can be a leading cause of their depression [9]. Similar impacts have been found to affect mental health carers in other countries [21,42-44]. Almost half of all mental health carers' psychological distress is based on difficult personal issues about duty, responsibility, adequacy and guilt [12]. Carers' wellbeing is closely linked to how services respond to individuals and families, partnership orientation, knowledge provision, support and counselling. Individual carer characteristics such as age, family status, employment, education, and language also impact on carer wellbeing [45].

Of significance, carer wellbeing has a direct impact on the recovery rate of the person being cared for [46], with greater use of hospitals and longer hospital stays for those without carer contact [47]. Caring for someone with a mental illness can be difficult because many families, "attempt to care for someone who may Caring for someone with a mental illness can be difficult because many families "attempt to care for someone who may have bouts of acute psychosis; exhibit little motivation for most activities; be self-absorbed much of the time; hardly contribute to the household; and have cognitive difficulties giving rise to forgetfulness, misunderstandings, irritability, frustration, and sometimes outright hostility" (p.1)[48].

A decade of national mental health policies and standards promoting the inclusion of carers, combined with an array of practice reforms and Carer Recognition Acts in many Australian State jurisdictions appear to have had little impact on improving the care and support experiences of carers. Within service systems, carers have reported that they often receive little or no information about their family member's illness and that they are not typically involved in care planning or have their views about the cared for person's needs sought by services [49,50]. This is despite almost two decades of research from which the findings have recommended greater collaboration and partnership with carers [10,51,52]. Carers in other countries have also reported feeling marginalised by services [53]. Carers' role and expert knowledge is often ignored, rejected or seriously undervalued by services, sometimes with detrimental consequences for the person's care, and carer and staff safety [10,50,52,54-56]. Carers report that they are best supported by routine contact and trusting relationships with service providers [57]. Realistic and targeted education and support, appropriate to what families need at particular stages, has also been found to be useful and to improve the health and wellbeing of carers and care recipients [10,58,59].

3. Problem statement

Being a mental health carer is hard work. Carers' health needs are often hidden behind the needs of the person they care for. Building the skills of the mental health, psychosocial rehabilitation and primary health care (PHC) workforce [60,61] is essential for effective support to people with mental health and co-existing physical health conditions, and their family carers. This understanding must go beyond superficial constructions of carer burden and token offers of respite, education and information. Otherwise, there is a danger that service providers will assume that they have understood and addressed carers' needs, and be dismissive of the ongoing and enduring needs that carers have as a consequence of their unique caring role. Policies and programs that understand and address effectively the day-to-day needs and experiences of carers are needed.

The current study supports and builds on the view that 'carer' is an ambivalent term that "fails to do justice to the complexity of interpersonal relationships in the context of mental health problems"(pp.475-476)[34]. Wong uses the term 'chronic stressors' to denote the complex and ongoing nature of the difficulties mental health carers face [29]. Much research on mental health carers has focused on measuring carer burden as a construct in isolation from other processes and impacts associated with the role [62]. Research has also clearly described mental health carers' grief as often prolonged and experienced over the full course of the cared for person's life [63]. Mental health carers have been 'studied' and have provided consultancy to many carer research projects. However, little research has been conducted exclusively by mental health carers, from the carer perspective.

4. Methods

A qualitative design was selected for this study due to the exploratory nature of the study and the need to provide participants with an interview method in which an interpersonal dialogue could take place around potentially highly sensitive and personal information. To achieve this, the study involved focus groups, a large survey and in-depth interviews with mental health carers in South Australia. Results were triangulated and will be discussed comprehensively in the context of how workers in mental health service and primary health care services can work effectively with mental health carers to support the person with mental illness, and help address carers' caring needs.

Ethics approval was granted by the Flinders Clinical Research Ethics Committee. The project was steered by a diverse expert reference group that included mental health carers, representatives from carer organisations and mental health services, and university nursing and social work academics. Across these members, all were mental health carers.

5. Description of the sample and recruitment

Participants were voluntarily recruited through organisational newsletters and communication provided directly by project team members at regular meetings for 12 carer organisations and groups responsible for providing service and/or support to mental health carers across metropolitan and regional South Australia. The researchers were also members of the SA Department of Health Mental Health Unit Carer Advisory Group and have, as their mandate, dedicated and expected links with the field as part of their advocacy and communication roles. Two of the researchers have links across several carer organisations and are heavily involved in training and support group facilitation groups in these organisations. Reference Group members also offered their capacity to link with carer groups. The project team also approached each known carer agency, or support group, and formally invited them to be involved in consultations.We believe that this enabled us to canvass a diverse range of carers. Sampling was therefore purposive for carers and based on convenience of access to a range of carer groups.

5.1. Data collection

In-depth semi-structured interviews were conducted in participants' homes or other confidential and convenient location nominated by participants (only one interview was conducted by phone). Interview topic areas for exploration were informed by extensive literature review prior to commencement of data collection and further established by the expert reference group. Interviews guide questions were as follows:

- Carer role (context, length of time, extent)
- Looking back, experiences of becoming a carer
- Telling their story of being a carer
- Positive aspects /difficult aspects of being a carer
- Impacts on self and others
- Maintaining personal health and wellbeing in the carer role
- Experiences of engagement with services and others as part of the carer role
- What they want workers to understand about their carer role

Interviews were voice-recorded, following consent from participants, and professionally transcribed then checked by the project manager. Extensive notes were also taken to enhance recall of the context of interactions. Carers in regional and rural areas were contacted by phone where indicated. All interviews were performed by the project manager to enhance consistency. Transcripts of interviews were returned to interviewees for checking, verification of data accuracy, and further comments, if they wished to provide them.

Three focus groups were conducted with mental health carers. These were organised to occur within existing mental health carers support groups, and three different types of groups were sought, to ensure a variety of the carer population were canvassed.

Discussions in each focus group were aided by the following question areas, with room for open discussion beyond these areas of interest:

- Positive aspects of being a carer?
- The hardest thing about being a carer?
- Effects of becoming/being a carer on you, your family, and friends?
- What do you do to keep yourself going in your carer role?
- What has been your experience of engagement with mental health and other health services, as part of your carer role?
- What are the most important things that you want workers to understand about you, as a carer?

The first focus group (n=12 carers) was conducted with a Carer Support and Respite Centre Carers Group, that is, carers who had contact with services specifically for support in their caring role. They tended to be carers who were not involved in carer advocacy, and tended to be older carers. The second focus group (n=15 carers) was conducted with an Association of Relatives and Friends of the Mentally Ill (ARAFMI) Mental Health Carers Group. This group contained some longstanding carers and several people new to their caring role, and of all ages. The third focus group (n=12 carers) was conducted with the State Department of Health, Mental Health Unit Carers Advisory Group. This group contained many longstanding carers who were also actively involved in advocacy and committee work throughout the mental health system in South Australia, and national involvement. Data from two of the three focus groups were recorded and professionally transcribed, then checked by the primary researcher. Extensive notes were taken for the third focus group.

A state-wide survey was conducted with electronic and hardcopy surveys distributed through the previously mentioned carers organisations and groups. This included advertising of the survey by the peak state information and support organisation (Carers SA), and the Private Mental Health Consumer and Carer Network Australia (PMHCCN)(open to SA carers only) which both have a regular large electronic and hardcopy mail out of their newsletter to carers. Similar to the focus group guide, the survey contained the following questions:

- What is the best thing about being a carer for someone with mental health and physical health conditions?
- What is the hardest thing about being a care?
- What worries you the most in your role as a carer?
- What effect has being a carer had on you personally?
- What effect has being a carer had on your family and others close to you?

- What are the most important things that you want service providers to understand about your needs and your role?
- Any other comments?

Focus groups and interviews occurred across the same time period and data from each were used to test and generate further question areas for exploration across the interactions with participants. All focus groups and interviews were conducted by the lead author, to ensure consistency. There was no crossover of participation by carers in each method of data collection.

5.2. Data analysis

A thematic analysis of focus group and interview data was undertaken using components of grounded theory [64] within a framework analytic approach [65]. During the first stage of data analysis, the first two authors reviewed the transcripts several times then performed manual open coding, independent of each other. The authors then met to discuss, debate and compare codes as part of inter-rater reliability testing [66] and constructed a detailed codebook/framework to capture key issues and concepts before proceeding with further analysis. Themes were generated as part of constant comparison of the data, using regular meetings between the researchers to discuss the meaning of emerging ideas as interviews proceeded and for accuracy and agreement on codes/categories. The next stage of analysis involved grouping data into broader, conceptual themes based on recurrent patterns occurring across codes. Presentation to and discussion of themes within the expert reference group served as additional verification of face validity for the analysis. An independent expert qualitative researcher checked the themes and subthemes for consistency and logic of presentation prior to them being finalised. Survey data were kept within each clearly structured survey question and a thematic content analysis [67] was performed, with subthemes determined by the researchers, as per the description of methods provided above. In this way, each dataset informed and strengthened the themes found across all methods of data collection (interviews, focus groups, survey).

6. Results

6.1. Demographic details

Sixteen carers were interviewed, including three husband/wife couples caring for adult children. These interview data were treated separately, recognizing that each parent may experience their carer role differently [36]. Carers' experience ranged from seven to more than 50 years. All were caring for someone with serious mental illness that required support from specialist mental health services. Four carers were caring for more than one adult child and one carer had continued to care for her foster son but had also cared for her own son prior to his suicide. Seven carers were sole carers, whilst nine carers had support from their spouses. Carers ranged in age from 20-30 to 80-90 years (median 60-70 years, or at a life-stage when retirement would otherwise be their priority and also when personal physical health problems are likely to emerge if not already present). Of concern, eight carers reported having a diagnosed mental illness and five a diagnosed heart condition. Only two carers did not report having a physical or mental health condition. For many carers, the person lived with them, or very nearby. Fourteen participants where active members of carer support groups or advocacy groups, often in leadership roles with several years of experience at local, state or national level,. Several participants were also carer consultants on local, state or national, mental health sector committees and working parties.

Demographic information for focus group participants was not collected. The number of focus group participants has been reported above. A total of 79 survey responses were received. Demographic information for survey respondents was not collected. However, from an audit of the survey responses, the researchers determined that:

- 56 respondents were carers for adult children (Eight were caring for more than one adult child)
- 16 respondents were carers for their spouse (10 were women caring for their male partner. Six were men caring for their female partner.)
- 6 respondents were caring for their sibling (Four were a sister caring for a brother. Two were a sister caring for a sister.)

As we have no way of knowing the total number of mental health carers within the database for Carers SA and South Australian carers within the PMHCCN database, or whether all blank hardcopy survey forms were distributed, we cannot determine a meaningful response rate. However, we have estimated that the total of 124 mental health carers who participated represent less than 5% of the state's mental health carer population. This statistic is not known, either at state or national level, which is a finding in and of itself (personal communication, Carers Australia).

The combined interview/focus group thematic analysis is provided first; then a summary of the survey results follows. Pseudonyms are used to de-identify all participants and direct quotes are used to exemplify themes.

7. Focus group and interview themes

Participants' comments fell into 9 main themes, many that mirror themes found in the existing research literature, such as the day-to-day experience, burden, grief and loss, obligation, problems with communication of needs with services, personal growth, strained relationships with others, and impacts on their own health and wellbeing [37,40,41,62,63,69,70]. These themes were:

The Experience of Being a Carer

Living with Mental Illness

Cycles of Grief, Trauma, Fear and Vigilance

Communication with Services

The Carer/Mental Health Professional Experiential Divide

Consequences and Trust

The Impact on Relationships

The Impact on Health

How Carers Cope

7.1. The experience of being a carer – 'The burden never ends'

All participants described the impact of being carers on their day-to-day lives, describing a range of burdens that were perceived to be never-ending and which changed many parts of their lives. This often included their capacity to take holidays, maintain careers, maintain friendships and relationships with others, attend to their own health and live a quality life for themselves. Overarching these impacts was the intensity and constancy of the caring role.

(Charlotte and Stanley) We keep going because we have to, there is no option. Who else is going to love her and look after her? There is no realistic option. Until there is a lot better service. Until we die, we're it... We didn't ask for this, we didn't want it, but we're parents, we have no option. We love her so that's it.

(Joan) I'm constantly on alert. I can't go out freely because my husband is suspicious...My son recently called the crisis team without me knowing. My husband blamed me when they arrived at the door unannounced...I had to stay with a relative for two weeks after that because he wouldn't let me back in the house.

Within this constancy, participants also described their role as like 'shifting sand', with them constantly stepping in and out of the caring role as the person's mental health status also shifted constantly, often on a day-by-day basis dependent on what stresses were present in be the person's life at the time. This challenged understood assumptions that workers held, and information carers had been provided about mental illness being episodic. Carers spent each day never completely free of thinking and worrying about the person.

7.2. Living with mental illness – 'Do they think the fairies do all these things?'

All participants believed that service providers had a limited view of what the experience was actually like for the person living with mental illness and their carers. Many carers thought that this was one of the reasons why their views were often dismissed or excluded from decisions about care made by service providers. They compared their life-long knowledge of the person with health professionals who come and go and only see fragments. They also spoke of the over-reliance of service providers on medications to 'fix everything'.

(Gladys talking of the mental health services plans to allow the person to manage their own finances) That's okay as long as they put a plan in place to help him learn how to manage it. But they didn't, they just gave him the money. They just dropped him in it. Do they think the fairies are going to show him how to do it? No they won't. And that's a gap. Like who do they think does these things, and it's usually some carer in the background quietly doing stuff isn't it?

(Elizabeth) If I never went along to any of the appointments with my son, and if they (service providers) went completely on what [son] was telling them... he would never have gotten better and the worker would never have even understood what was going on. We wouldn't have got a service in the first place, despite him being completely psychotic...there's a whole layer that they just don't even see...if they really knew, they would have detained him a 100 times over according to their limited criteria.

7.3. Cycles of grief, trauma, fear and vigilance – 'It just becomes par for the course'

All participants recounted their experience of being a carer as involving some level of grief for the lost potential they saw in their loved one, and trauma which, for several, was ongoing as part of their everyday experience. This has a range of implications for how carers are supported when their relative first becomes unwell, but also for the ongoing health and wellbeing of carers. The level of this trauma was something that these carers felt others didn't and couldn't fully understand. It made their day-to-day experience often feel surreal and their connection with others sometimes distant. Several carers had become accustomed to a level of trauma which they usually concealed from others, as part of their coping within what many said felt like living in two worlds. On the one hand, they maintained their daily routines of family life, social relationships, community relationships or work and other roles as if all was well, so that others who came into contact with these carers perceived this to be so. This often masked significant, regular, distressing events and interactions with the cared for person that required the carer to continually switch back and forth in their vigilance around the person.

(Gladys of her eldest son who suicided 30 years earlier) I just came home from work one day and found him hanging in the backyard, which was pretty ghastly, but if it was his choice, that's his... (Pause, looking into the distance) So that's the way it is.

(Susan) People can say 'Just phone the police or mental health services' but it's the consequences there and then. My husband is twice my size and strong and at 12 o'clock at night when he's saying he wants to shoot all the neighbours and the crisis team is one person on a phone on the other side of the city the consequences are a bit more real...I bear the consequences... [the mental health crisis service] just don't get it...what that actually means, whether you like it or not picking up the pieces, is that the consequences for you can be diabolical and for me - I've got a small child who he was making constant threats to, that he was going to take away with him, and they will be found dead somewhere? The phone crisis worker said to call the police. They came in the middle of the night and took him to ED. I got a call an hour later that he was on his way home. They hadn't detained him despite what had occurred, his history and his recent admission to hospital. They just put it down to alcohol. Even the police were alarmed by this. We were so frightened.

(Clare) When our sons were feeling suicidal, at the time you almost become hardened to it all. The trauma of just the barrage of it just becomes par for the course...and then later on you can crack up afterwards but you have to be strong at the time.

7.4. Communication with services– 'They didn't even ask'

All participants reported that they felt service providers' communication and interaction with them needed improvement. This ranged from service providers just not understanding the extent of carers' input with the person and the nature of their experiences, ignoring and not listening, to actively excluding carers in decisions and dialogue about the person's care and treatment. For many carers, communication was largely one way.

(Sandra) You're a source of information and once they've got the information they don't need you to do anything and they don't need you anymore...You end up being the navigator all the time when the person needs help, and then you're ignored.

These carers strongly believed that they had a unique understanding of the person cared for and therefore much to contribute to what support was needed and how it was developed and delivered. They felt like members of a team of support around the person, but invisible players in that team, in which their input was not realised fully by formal service providers. These carers found this situation frustrating and senseless, given their long-standing relationship with the person, knowledge of them as a 'whole' person and ability to often pick up signs of illness early because they knew the person best.

(Judith) It's the people that know him – you've known him all his life. You can tell, and it's not necessarily anything that they say, it's just a way that they look or a gesture; you just feel it. It's hard explaining that to other people, particularly workers...(Upon trying to alert the worker) His Case Worker said, 'Oh well, he seems alright when he presents to me". And we really felt quite deeply that she hadn't respected our observations.

7.5. The carer/mental health professional experiential divide

All participants believed that service providers had a limited view of what the experience was actually like for the person living with mental illness and their carers. Many carers thought this was why their views were often dismissed or excluded from decisions about care made by service providers. They compared their life-long knowledge of the person with health professionals who come and go and only see fragments. They also spoke of the over-reliance of service providers on medications to 'fix everything'. Unfortunately, all participants reported similar situations where they simply were not listened to and this added to the experience of distress for all concerned, especially the person and their carer. This seemed to be linked to the service providers not understanding or having empathy for the experience of carers, of being removed from the impact of their actions or inactions.

(Ruth) It wasn't until the point of crisis that they took notice of us. And then that was traumatic for us because we had to get the people to come and see him [because he refused to go to them by that point]...and it finally reached a point one night when we could hear him treading up and down...I was shivering in my bed and I said, 'I can't stand it'. The next day I rang them and I said, 'Please come', I really begged, I said, 'Please come and get him'.

(Charlotte and Stanley) They kept on telling us that it was all behaviour...'She is bipolar but really she's just a bad, bad girl; she's nowhere near as ill as you think', until five years ago, she proved to them exactly how ill she was when she burnt down her unit.

7.6. Consequences and trust –'You just don't want to go there'

Participants recounted a number of consequences for them as part of the day-to-day management of risk, especially when the person they cared for was unwell or suicidal. They said this impacted all parts of their lives, usually requiring a number of personal systems in place for emergencies. They felt a clear sense that they were shouldering much of the load and that services could be contributing more. Though several participants reported receiving good support when services worked with them as a team, they also reported some challenges to this process, involving the journey of mental illness itself. The following lengthy examples demonstrate some of the inherent dilemmas in caring for a person with mental illness and consequences for mental health carers:

(Susan) The nature of mental illness is often that the person doesn't recognise when they need help and, when they're highly distressed, and agitated, it's the very last thing they are actually going to do, often. So it needs someone, and it's often the carer, who says "Enough. We have to do something here". And it's a very tricky dilemma to involve police or ambulance or mental health services because you know that is going to be difficult for the person; and you, as the carer, are going to have to face the consequences for that because you often get blamed for things you've not done at all, because the person's either delusional or paranoid, and it's just very emotional. And you spend so much emotional energy giving, so that when the person throws it back at you, it's very difficult...The carer faces the brunt of that [service involvement...I think a lot of carers are put in these sorts of situations that are not always realised by workers...and you almost don't ask for the help when it's needed because you just don't want to go there because it opens up a whole other can of worms that you never intended.

(Jenny) Services often see it as carers just being over-involved, emotional or anxious, but it involves trust also, because there are always consequences for me and the children in engaging with services. With caring for my mum, I always felt isolated from the treatment and involvement with services and like we were just being acted upon rather than in partnership all working together and them utilizing our lived experience and expertise. Because there was no trust in our first five months with the system, it was a fearful system. I didn't want to put my mum through that. She wasn't the same. My experience of that system [mother in hospital] was that my mum just sat on the floor or on the bed the whole time rocking back and forward. I literally had to rip her out of there, then us isolating ourselves as a family. At least she stopped rocking back and forward and found some joy with the children; (pause) but we were all alone. It was a very lonely journey.

7.7. The impact on relationships – 'It certainly made us appreciate who our real friends were'

Participants discussed the impact of caring on their relationships with each other, other family and friends and how they mediated the caring role within their relationships with others. Some carers said that becoming carers for a person with mental illness had brought them closer together, though not without this being a learning process. For others, there were different challenges.

(Yvonne) We had many times when we've thought about splitting up...We didn't agree on everything and that has been the biggest problem.

(Stanley) It certainly made us appreciate who our real friends were because several of them walked away. They were sympathetic but didn't really want to think about mental illness at all. And our other children, although we didn't realise it at the time, but they told us later that we were kind of putting a lot of pressure on them by not giving them a fair share of our time and by kind of putting expectations on them to be the 'normal' ones...I don't think we knew we were doing it except by saying, like, 'Thank God you're okay.'

7.8. The impact on health – 'I'm not allowed to get sick'

All except two of the interview participants reported problems with their physical or mental health as a direct result of their caring role, and its impacts. Of the eight carers who reported having a diagnosed mental health conditions, seven had depression. Five carers reported a diagnosed heart condition; four of these were men. Some carers were now actively looking after their health, whilst others were not. All participants experienced ongoing burden. One carer's description demonstrates the complexity of self-care for carers:

(Sandra) The frustrating thing for me is I'm not allowed to get sick. I'm not allowed to get emotional. I'm not allowed to say how I'm feeling because, although he says that I should do that, when I do that, it actually makes his symptoms worse and it's like he just takes it internally and it becomes this whole other thing which I never intended, and he never expected. It's like they can't give you their empathy, it's like a type of selfishness...So I just don't bother to say anything. It's just easier that way.

7.9. How carers cope – Advocacy, support and 'just getting on with it'

Participants described a range of strategies they use to deal with the impacts of their caring role. This included their views on respite support, carer support groups, support from family and friends, and developing clear limits and boundaries with the person they care for.

Several participants were members of support groups with long experience of being carers, and several had become assertive advocates. They also emphasised the need for carers to look after themselves and seek out support.

(Charlotte) I fall in the deepest of holes and I just want to go to bed and pull the covers over, and that's when Stanley takes over. I just say, 'I can't do this'...And then, as I get better, Stanley might fall into a hole and that's when I would take over... I think we've always talked...There have been times that we've disagreed...but most times it works positively and we counter-balance each other.

(Stanley on service providers and respite support) They think that all we need is respite and therefore...We get away and we'll be right. And it doesn't - it isn't. We've done that - we never did it because we thought it would help, we did it - to shut them up basically...What we've learned is you've got to believe in those feelings that you have. When you feel that something isn't right, then it isn't right. Believe in yourself and then develop the confidence to do something about it.

(John) I really can't do anything much for my sons to be really honest. I can't fix them or anything. All I can do is to stand around and support them a bit. As a result, I drifted and drove myself into advocacy.

(Sandra) Sometimes you get annoyed and sometimes you just resign to it and then other times you just want to wake up and it's not there...And then you sit yourself down and just sort of resign to it and on you go.

Several participants spoke of the importance of adequate accommodation and community support for the person they cared for. One carer, who recounted a period of nine months when health services worked well with each other, the person, and with them as carers, summed it up this way:

(Stanley) We've always said - fix the system so our daughter is taken care of and you'll take care of us.

8. Results – Survey

Each survey question areas is listed, with themes from within each domain described in order (most to least) of the number of respondents whose comments spoke to that theme. However, this does not mean that the more commonly described ideas are necessarily more important to carers than less commonly described ideas. Many comments made across the survey questions were, at times, overwhelmingly powerful and quantifying them is arguably inappropriate. Respondents could provide more than one response to each question.

8.1. The best thing about being a carer

Good Outcomes

Thirty of the 79 participants spoke of good outcomes for the cared for person's health as the best thing about being a carer. This reflected their primary focus and concern for the wellbeing of the person cared for. Good outcomes included the person accepting their mental illness and the need for medication, and keeping a positive attitude, the carer recognising small achievements made by the person, being grateful and enjoying the times when things were going well, carers being pro-active rather than reactive, and effectively providing a safe environment for their loved one.

- Knowing that the person you care about is respected, loved and treated well.
- Seeing them achieve goals no matter how small.
- I have learnt to be really thankful for the times when things are going well. This morning, he's happy. I can tuck that away as a memory for when times may not go so well.

Sharing the experience through connection with others

Fourteen carers stated that sharing their experience with other carers and having a connection with others with similar experiences provided friendship, support and knowledge that they would not have otherwise had. Support groups also provided hope, real empathy and understanding, alleviating their sense of isolation and stigma. For some, support groups gave them a new purpose, role and courage to stand up.

- Finding a support network where friendships and information help to carry the load.
- Knowing I'm not alone; there is a carer support group.
- I have been inspired to become more involved in advocating for those more vulnerable in our community. I have met some extremely brave and inspiring people.

Having Purpose

Ten carers talked about the positive sense of purpose that the caring role provided to them. This included the gratitude received from the person cared for, the sense of making a worthwhile contribution to the person's wellness, keeping the person as safe as possible, and the knowledge that they are cared for.

- To know that you are doing something and helping someone you love.
- It's a good feeling to know they know you'll always be there for them.

Nothing

However, 10 carers' responses reflected the overwhelming sense of burden, grief, struggle and negative impact that the arrival of mental illness can have for some families. These carers were quite clear that there was no best thing about being a carer, despite the immense love and commitment that they expressed for their loved one.

- There's absolutely nothing.
- As I'm caring for my husband who has developed mental illness since I married him, I fail to see that there is a best thing about being a carer.

Love

In contrast, 8 carers' responses showed the immense love they held for the person and the importance of being able to show this. The intensity of these feelings was a mirror image of the adversity and trauma they also described in their responses to other questions.

- I think I can show her that I care about her unconditionally and will be there for her.
- The bond we share. He knows my love for him.
- The journey we have shared has involved some of the worst times of my life. Yet, my love for him is beyond measure because I'm so proud of his courage in spite of this.

Learning

The comments of eight carers reflected their capacity to be resilient and to grow from the experience. They described the best thing for them as finding the resources to educate themselves about mental illnesses, and becoming more accepting and open minded generally, that is, becoming better people for the experience.

- I have educated myself in areas that my friends would not even consider.
- It stretches you to find resources in yourself previously undeveloped.
- It helps me to be more aware of others with disabilities and more accepting. I have learned to be more open minded of others' behaviour.

8.2. The hardest thing about being a carer

Grief in the face of changed lives

Twenty-six of the 79 respondents described the grief and anguish experienced, by now having a family member with mental illness, as the hardest thing about being a carer. This involved seeing their loved one's suffering or having experienced trauma (sometimes whilst in systems of care), coming to terms with the illness and its impact on all of their lives. Some described this as watching a self-destruction process, seeing their loved one living such an isolated lifestyle, experiencing a 'roller coaster' of emotions, and grieving about the person's lost potential for what could have been.

- Seeing my two sons living a very isolated lifestyle, without friends, partners, employment or meaningful activities.
- To watch the suffering of a serious victim of a mental health illness. As family and friends cannot understand the changes in the person that occur as the disease progresses and the anguish they witness. Five or six serious attempts on her own life and time spent at hospital emergency waiting as staff fight to save the life.

Vigilance and never able to relax

Eighteen carers described constant stress, alertness and vigilance that they experience in relation to the person with mental illness as the hardest thing for them about being a carer.

- The stress never leaves me, though it does lessen when she is in a good period, and I dread the phone ringing.
- Not knowing how each day/hour/minute will pan out and trying to steel yourself for whatever happens...Waiting for the next crisis to occur.

Fear

Further to their feelings of vigilance, 14 carers described a fear of not knowing if what they are doing is beneficial for the person, fear for the future when they are dead or cannot care anymore, feeling helpless and hopeless at times, fears about their own capacity to find and maintain employment with the unpredictability of the caring role, fears for their financial security, and fears for the safety of the person and themselves when the person is unwell.

- The guilt I feel when I don't cope and contribute to their misery instead of helping them and the feeling of helplessness.
- Being faced with a son in a very psychotic state, and not knowing what to do about it.

Consequences of system failures / 'The carer is always responsible'

Sixteen carers described the system's failure to provide adequate support to the person as one of the hardest things they have to deal with, explaining it as a major contributor to their enforced vigilance and fears. These system failures included inadequacy of support, difficulties caused by privacy and confidentiality rules, and indifference and neglect of care shown in some situations by service providers. Carers said that they were routinely left to pick up the pieces, frustrated and angry with service providers.

- Having all the responsibility of everything, and that often you personally are seen as the baddie (the one who is pushy).
- There is an apparent indifference displayed to a great degree by 'the system' and the result that carers are left to battle on largely unaided in any meaningful way.

Being heard, understood and included

Twelve carers described their experience of trying to navigate within and express their needs to mental health service providers as the hardest thing about being a carer. This included trying to convince services when the person needed help, a general lack of understanding of carers' perspectives by service providers and, being dismissed, ignored and labelled by services.

- Trying to find a doctor and psychiatrist who are understanding and show empathy and talk to me as a parent.
- Being told by service providers that my 'expectations are too high' regarding their services and supports for my two sons.

Isolation

Eight carers rated their isolation in the caring role as the hardest issue to deal with. This involved physical isolation from supportive others, as relatives and friends distance themselves once the carer became subsumed in their caring role, but also emotional isolation from others as a result of their carer experience.

- The hardest is feeling sometimes that you're the only one, especially when other family members cannot come to terms with the mental illness of the person in question. I feel that they know I will always be the carer, and will leave it all up to me.

- We have no friends any more.

8.3. What worries carers the most in their carer role

Several respondents reiterated issues they found most difficult about their caring role, including never being able to relax. Six respondents mentioned worry about finances, and a further six described worry for the quality of life and future of the person cared for, especially as they observed increasing, insidious physical health problems emerge for the person over time. Fourteen carers expressed their greatest worry being their lack of knowledge of how to best help the person; whether they were doing the right thing. Four carers expressed their main worry as concern for their own physical safety, in particular, their powerless in the face of the person's paranoia where the carer was routinely threatened, blamed and accused by the person. Overwhelmingly, respondents detailed a range of worries that reflected and demonstrated their deep concern for the person's welfare, for the future and for the welfare of others as a consequence of mental illness being present in their lives:

Concern for the person's future when the carer is not there

Thirty-two, or almost half of respondents, cited their main worry as care for the person when the carer was no longer able to provide care.

- I worry about what will happen to my daughter if I die and there's no-one there for her.

- What will happen to my son when I am no longer able to protect him?

Suicide

Eight carers rated fear of the person suiciding as their greatest worry. For some, this was linked to observing the person's poor physical health and quality of life, and grief for what they perceived as the natural order of theirs and their loved one's future.

- Suicide risks with two sons who suffer from depression and anxiety illnesses and have deteriorating physical health. I believe that it is likely that my sons will die before I do.

- Our family member with a mental illness does not live at home, so I worry about suicide, as this has been attempted numerous times in the past.

Fears/Consequences for others

Fourteen carers expressed their main worry being for others as a consequence of the person's mental illness. This ranged from concern for others who were missing out on the carer's attention and time due to the focus on the person's needs, to worry about family members developing mental illness due to their genetic relationship and shared environment with the mentally ill person. Some carers expressed the tension of being stuck in the middle as the primary supporter of the person, and protector, or shield, for other family members.

- I am frightened she will have a manic session and kill some innocent person whilst driving her car.
- Being made aware of and constantly worrying whether it might happen to other members of the family, especially the children. Every now and then I see the signs and it horrifies me. I'm torn between my commitment to the person and trying to make my children's life as normal as possible, which is pretty difficult with a paranoid person in the house.

8.4. Effects of caring on carers personally

Being a carer for a person with a mental illness had many significant potential negative effects on carers but also many significant positive effects for them. For respondents, the effects were often a double-edged sword, and present together for the carer as part of their resignation to the role, and the reality of their circumstances.

Physical health

Twelve carers cited experiencing physical health problems and perceived these as a direct consequence of their carer role. Blood pressure and heart conditions were particularly cited and were linked by carers to the level of worry and vigilance inherent in their carer role.

Mental health

Thirty carers described the negative effects of caring on their own emotional wellbeing and mental health. They described feelings of sadness, grief and loss, difficulty in relaxing, having diagnosed depression and anxiety as a direct result of the accumulative effects of caring,and loss of self-esteem and confidence as a result of isolation within the role. They described doubts about their effectiveness, severe stress, feelings of being emotionally drained, angry and frustrated, feeling powerless, and feeling much of their life was out of their control.

- I feel terribly sad because I have lost my son.
- I suffer with chronic glaucoma, but this discomfort is minimal compared with the sadness and heart break suffered at seeing a grown man who will never reach any satisfaction with his life. This leaves me in a state of endless despair.

Loss of own quality of life

Accumulated pressures inherent in the day-to-day experience of carers had clear negative impacts on their quality of life. Twenty-two carers described this as their inability to look too far ahead, the limits now placed on their social life and leisure time, the inability to travel, and their disconnection from friends and other family due to the burden of caring.

- I've lost my network/social life. I have lost my husband now I live with a stranger. I've gone from being cared for to being a carer. I lost my self-esteem, I feel trapped – frustrated with the system and lonely.
- I'm practically in retirement and my life plans are destroyed.

Loss of career/Financial impacts

Ten carers stated that their caring role had finished their career, whilst others continued to juggle having time off, shifting to part-time work, or to less stressful work. This led to deteriorating financial circumstances and, for some, this meant actual hardship when the cared for person's life was in turmoil due to manic spending or debt.

Finding new purpose

Some carers had effectively turned their frustrations with their role and the systems of care into advocacy for broader mental health reform, and a thirst for more knowledge. Twelve carers clearly articulated the personal growth they experienced because of their caring role.

- It has given me reason to communicate a lot more with others in a similar situation, to learn and be more aware.
- It has totally changed my life; different job, different outlook on life, different attitudes.

8.5. Effects on family and others close to the carer

In response to this question, respondents demonstrated the dichotomy of experiences that are likely present for carers. Some families appeared to pull together, as a consequence of mental illness entering their lives, while other families were torn apart.

Greater cohesion

Twenty-four carers described the experience of caring as bringing them and their family closer together, strengthening relationships between partners, unifying the family around the person, and enabling them to have more meaningful relationships generally.

- More love is shown to my daughter by her beautiful friends and a few of her relations.
- It brought me and my wife closer; supporting each other…We have an exceptional close group of friends who understand.
- Our daughter's illness has united the family.

Greater tension

Equally, 24 carers described the experience as creating unwanted tension within their families and friendship networks, with some withdrawing to cope, and carers isolating themselves from others as a result of their priorities shifting, as the burden of caring is taken up by some and left by others, as differences in understanding emerge, and as family members blame each other and take different paths in their attempts to cope, grieve and variously move on.

- The rest of the family stays away and doesn't even ask how he is. They don't want to know or understand...We're all still grieving.
- They (other family) distance themselves or feel sorry for me. They've no constructive help or support. They try to give advice but don't know anything about the illness, which causes conflict; they judge how I handle things and blame me when things go wrong.
- It demonstrates clearly those who care as opposed to some family members, who see their role as not wanting to know.

Exclusion/Fragmentation of family

Sixteen carers described, in more specific detail, a range of negative impacts that the caring role had on them personally. This was often couched in concern for their relationships with, and concern for, the impacts on other family members, especially children.

- Our other daughter has been affected by thinking she always had to behave well and make up for her sister. She does not have a good relationship with her sister and feels she never really had a sister.
- My immediate family can't cope with being sworn at, so I am the only one at present that my son will relate to and then only on his conditions.
- The other siblings have felt neglected at times and have some resentment.

8.6. Important things for mental health services to understand about carers' needs

Carers had many, often forthright, concerns that they wanted to express to mental health services. These ranged from the need for more understanding of the realities of the caring role, to more inclusion and say in the treatment and care plans for the person cared for, to be listened to and have their views respected more, and to have better services for the person and for carers.

More inclusion, acknowledgement, recognition and listening to carers

Fifty-six of the 79 survey respondents said that they wanted to be acknowledged more for their input and expertise related to the person's needs. They perceived themselves as an untapped resource that was often neglected by services, sometimes with adverse consequences for the person and the carer. They particularly stressed their role in early intervention support for the person and were keen to work collaboratively with service providers. They also saw themselves as a reliable source of information about what was really going on day-to-day for the person, especially when the person's own account or perceptions did not always reflect the facts, according to carers.

- That professionals need to trust what carers say, that we know the person, that this behaviour is out of character, or that the problem is not drug related, but a mental health issue. We need to be listened to. We need to be included. We need to be taken seriously.

We need to be informed; we need to be included in decisions because, as carers, we can help early in the 'flare ups' of the illness.

- I spend all day with him and I know when something is not right.

Better support

Twenty-six carers spoke of the need for more and better support for the person they cared for. Of these, only 4 carers put this directly in the context of their own needs as carers. Most respondents couched their responses as part of the need to improve the person's wellbeing, and that this would directly or indirectly improve their own wellbeing.

- It takes a great deal of effort to get someone to agree to get help, and then the help is not available. I know if my son could have seen someone sooner, he would not have got to such a bad state.

More information and education for carers

Only eight carers made comments about a range of needs related to more information and education for carers. This ranged from where to find support, how to build resilience for themselves and the person they cared for, understanding signs and symptoms of particular mental illness, understanding medications, how to communicate with the person (especially someone with psychosis), and how to communicate with service providers.

Policy-related issues

Only eight carers made mention of broader mental health issues and their policy implications. These issues ranged from moves to address stigma, medication availability, formal carer recognition, accommodation, support funding, and carer payments.

9. Discussion

Being acarer for a person with mental illness can be highly challenging, with many impacts on carers. For participants of this study, impacts were both positive and negative, as others have also found. Several studies have reported recurring themes involving overwhelming feelings of burden on carers' daily lives [7,37,62,70,71]. Looking at the body of comments made here, the selflessness of carers is very apparent. They made little reference to their own physical health and wellbeing, seeming to focus most of their attention and energy on the person cared for. This has implications for neglect of their own needs [39]. Our participants described the caring role as physically and emotionally draining, with many experiencing depression and related physical illness. The strain of caring often caused friction in relationships within the family and loss of friends. Some family units became stronger and shared the support when needed. The high prevalence of chronic illness and risk factors among carers is clearly echoed for this small sample of mental health carers. The prevalence of heart disease, particularly among male participants, warrants further investigation. The incidence of heart disease in female care givers has been studied [72].

These results show that the actual experience and impact of a loved one developing a mental illness cannot be overstated. They mirror many of the fears, dilemmas and concerns highlighted in other international studies [21,35,69,74]. Likewise, other studies have spoken at length about the personal impact on carers in managing day-to-day care of the person and enduring the caring process [14.32-34,37,41]. Of note in our study, these carers were not new to the role, yet they continued to experience significant burden, distress and trauma, suggesting that more needs to be understood about the constantly shifting nature of mental illness and its impact on carers [3,35-37]. These carers also knew a great deal about mental illness. Many were advocates within the system, yet this didn't necessarily shield them from the reality of the experience. The unique nature of mental illness also meant that standard respite support was perceived as virtually useless.

The findings emphasise that, like health service providers, what carers want is improved wellness of the person they care for, and therefore the two groups should be able to work cohesively together for everyone's betterment. Yet, they also confirm that carers often feel excluded and their input not realised, or worse, ignored. Other studies have similarly concluded that carers frequently feel undervalued and marginalized and that the impact of the person's mental illness on the carers themselves has been largely ignored and invisible [10.46,52-57,71,75]. One Belgian study reported that more than one third of carers felt excluded from decision-making by service providers. Coincidentally, this study also found that many carers felt they were best supported by routine contact and trusting relationships with service providers [57]. Trust and understanding were highly valued by our participants.

Another striking feature of the results is what was not mentioned or only mentioned by a small number of participants. One example is the lack of reported need for more information and education. This suggests that there is a significant mismatch between what service providers think carers need and what carers say they need, given that much of the existing focus on support appears to be on 'educating' carers [59]. A large Netherlands study of 19 community-based psycho-educational groups investigating objective and subjective burden concluded that psycho-education, "should concentrate on helping relatives cope with the strain on the relationship with the patient and on improving their ability to cope with the patient's behaviour"(p.375)[76]. Fortune [77] found that coping through seeking emotional support, faith, acceptance and positive reframing of the carer's and the person's situation were associated with less distress, whereas self-blame led to greater levels of distress. Yet, the effectiveness of support groups for mental health carers have shown mixed results [78].

What our study shows is that providing education about mental illness to carers is but one part of providing effective support to them. It has also shown the challenges that mental health carers face regardless of the level and type of support, information and education that they are offered. The findings suggest these challenges go to the very heart of the nature of mental illness itself, with some issues being potentially unresolvable within this unique role. Our study demonstrates that caring for a person with mental illness is a complex role that requires a multifaceted understanding of carer stress and the centrality of the caring role.

10. Limitations

The findings of this study are limited to experiences of mental health carerswithin the Australian context. They suggest that further trans-national research and research exploring gender and relationship differences (child, spouse, parent) in carer experiences would be useful. The purposive sample and its size also pose limits on the generalizability of the findings. As suggested by Hsiao and Van Riper [79], more research is needed to explain why some carers adapt successfully to the carer role, whereas others do not.

11. Conclusions

This study highlights the mental health carer role as never ending and unrelenting, with many impacts on carers. Like Wong, who uses the term 'chronic stressors' to denote the complex and ongoing nature of the difficulties mental health carers face [29], our study confirms this chronicity within the caring role, what we call a 'living grief'. Carers stress that the nature of the illness is so unpredictable at times that there is no room for complacency, especially as they watch the person they care for develop physical illnesses and then the carer then finds themselves caring for someone with a multitude of ailments.

Successful negotiation of the mental health system, early intervention and partnership with service providers have become the key strategic directions for mental health services in Australia, and internationally. Coping, management of the illness, knowledge about illnesses and treatments available are the key mechanisms by which families and people with mental illness can be empowered to navigate the mental health system, to best enhance their wellbeing. Evidence indicates that providing education, support and a family/carer inclusive approach to treatment improves carer wellbeing, has a direct positive impact on the recovery of the care recipient [46,59]. Pivotal to these processes and to the delivery of meaningful support is for service providers to have a clearer understanding of what it is really like to be a mental health carer.

Many of the issues impacting on carers reflect larger problems in providing adequate care to people with mental illness [80,81]. Carers experience significant pressures in their caring role, largely due to their unmet needs for support, information and understanding from health service providers. The experiences of carers are not fully understood and this serves to alienate them from the very supports they need. Moreover, translating an understanding of carers' personal experience of caring into tangible, respectful and meaningful dialogue with service providers, as part of a shared approach to providing support to the person with mental illness, is vital for all concerned.

Acknowledgements

This research, and the Booklet and DVD Resource that arose from it, were funded by the Australian Government Department of Health and Ageing through the Australian Better

Health Initiative: A Joint Australian State and Territory initiative. We wish to acknowledge the important contributions of the many carers and carer organisations that participated in the research. The title of this chapter was inspired by a carer involved in this research.

Author details

Sharon Lawn[1,2*], Jeannette Walsh[2], Anne Barbara[2,3], Margaret Springgay[2] and Patricia Sutton[2]

1 Flinders Human Behaviour and Health Research Unit, Flinders University, Australia

2 Mental Health Carer, Adelaide, Australia

3 Central Adelaide Mental Health Directorate, Adelaide, Australia

4 Mental Illness Fellowship of Australia, Australia

References

[1] Australian Bureau of Statistics (ABS). National health survey (NHS) 2004-2005. Canberra: Australian Government Publications; 2004.

[2] Australian Bureau of Statistics (ABS). A Profile of Carers in Australia, 4448.0. Canberra: Australian Government Publications; 2008.

[3] Carers Australia. Who Cares...? Report on the inquiry into better support for carers. House of Representatives: Standing Committee on Family, Community, Housing and Youth. Canberra: Commonwealth of Australia; 2009.

[4] Awad AG,Voruganti LNP. The burden of schizophrenia on caregivers. Pharmacogenomics 2008;26: 149-162.

[5] Van DorVoort TYG, Goossens PIJ, Van Der Bijl JJ. Burden, coping and needs for support of caregivers for patients with a bipolar disorder: a systematic review. Journal of Psychiatric and Mental Health Nursing 2007;14: 679-687.

[6] Zauszniewski JA, Bekhe, AK,Suresky MJ. Relationship among stress, depressive cognitions, resourcefulness and quality of life in female relatives of seriously mentally ill adults. Issues in Mental Health Nursing 2009;30: 142-150.

[7] Holland KE. Carers' perspectives on caring: A qualitative analysis of open-ended responses to the Carer Health and Wellbeing Index Survey 2007 for Carers Australia. Canberra: Faculty of Communication and International Studies/University of Canberra; 2008.

[8] Australian Institute of Health and Welfare (AIHW). Australia's Welfare, No7 (cat. no. AUS 73). Canberra: AIHW; 2006.

[9] Cummins RA, Hughes J, Tomyn A, Gibson A, Woerner J, Lai L. Special report: The wellbeing of Australians: Carer health and wellbeing. Australian Unity Wellbeing Index Survey 17.1. Melbourne: Australian Centre on Quality of Life/Deakin University; 2007.

[10] Senate Select Committee on Mental Health. A national approach to mental health: From crisis to community. Canberra:Senate Select Committee, Commonwealth of Australia; 2006.

[11] Access Economics. The economic value of informal care. ACT:Carers Australia; 2005.

[12] Mental Health Council of Australia/Carers Association of Australia. Carers of people with mental illness project, Final Report, June 2000. Canberra: Mental Health Council of Australia/Carers Association of Australia, 2000.

[13] Keeley B, Clarke M. Carers Speak Out Project. Report on findings and recommendations. London: Princess Royal Trust for Carers; 2002.

[14] Cormac I,Tihanyi P. Meeting the mental and physical healthcare needs of carers. Advances in Psychiatric Treatment 2006;12: 162-172.

[15] Office of National Statistics. Census 2001. National Report for England and Wales. London: The Stationery Office; 2003.

[16] National Alliance for Caregiving (2009). Caregiving in the U.S. Retrieved November 2, 2010, from http://www.caregiving.org/data/Caregiving_in_the_US_2009_full_report.pdf(accessed 26 July 2012).

[17] Brand U. European perspectives: a carer's view. ActaPsychiatricaScandinavica2001;104: 1-6.

[18] Erlingsson CL, Magnusson L, Hanson E. Family carergivers' health in connection with providing care. Qualitative Health Research 2012; 22: 640-655.

[19] Fujino N, Okamura H. Factors affecting the sense of burden felt by family members caring for patients with mental illness. Archives of Psychiatric Nursing 2009;23: 128-137.

[20] Gutierrez-Maldonado J,Caqueo-Urizar A, Kavanagh DJ. Burden of care and general health in families of patients with schizophrenia. Social Psychiatry and Psychiatric Epidemiology 2005;40: 899-904.

[21] Huang XY, Sun FK. Yen, WJ, Fu, CM. The coping experiences of carers who live with someone with schizophrenia. Journal of Clinical Nursing 2008;17: 817-826.

[22] Joyce J, Leese M, Kuipers E, Szmukler G, Harris T, Staples E. Evaluating a model of caregiving for people with psychosis. Social Psychiatry and Psychiatric Epidemiology 2003;38: 189-195.

[23] LauberC,Eichemberger A, Luginbuhl P, Keller C,Rossler W. (2003) Determinants of burden in caregivers of patient with exacerbating schizophrenia. European Psychiatry 18: 285-289.

[24] Moller T, Gudde CB, Folden GE,Linaker O.M. The experience of caring in relatives to patients with serious mental illness: gender differences, health and functioning. Scandinavian Journal of Caring Sciences 2009;23: 153-160.

[25] Ohaeri J. Caregiver burden and psychotic patients' perceptions of social support in a Nigerian setting. Social Psychiatry & Psychiatric Epidemiology 2001;36:86-93.

[26] Rammohan A,Rao K,Subbakrishna DK. Religious coping and psychological wellbeing in carers of relatives with schizophrenia. ActaPsychiatricaScandinavica 2002;105: 356-362.

[27] Song IY, Chang IY, Shih CY, Lin CY, Yang MJ. Community attitudes towards the mentally ill: the results of a national survey of the Taiwanese population. International Journal of Social Psychiatry 2005;51: 162-176.

[28] Thara R,Srinivasan T. How stigmatizing is schizophrenia in India? International Journal of Social Psychiatry 2000;46: 135-141.

[29] Wong DFK. Stress factors and mental health of carer with relatives suffering from schizophrenia in Hong Kong: implications for culturally sensitive practices. British Journal of Social Work 2000;30: 365-382.

[30] Maskill V, Crowe M, Luty S, Joyce P. Two sides of the same coin: caring for a person with bipolar disorder. Journal of Psychiatric and Mental Health Nursing2010;7, 535-542.

[31] Cassells C, Geront M, Watt E. The impact of incontinence on older spousal caregivers. Journal of Advanced Nursing 2003;42: 607-616.

[32] Schwartz C, Gidron R. Parents of mentally ill adult children living at home: rewards of caregiving. Health and Social Work 2002;27: 45-54.

[33] Magliano L, Fiorill A, de Rosa C, Malangone C, Maj M. Family burden in long-term disease: a comparative study in schizophrenia vs. physical disorders. Social Science and Medicine 2005;61: 313-322.

[34] Ridley J, Hunter S, Rosengard A. Partners in care?: Views and experiences of carers from a cohort study of the early implementation of the Mental Health (Care& Treatment)(Scot) Act 2003. Health and Social Care in the Community 2010; 18: 474-482.

[35] Hirst M. Carer distress: A prospective population-based study. Social Science and Medicine 2005; 61: 697-708.

[36] Pejlert A. Being a parent of an adult son or daughter with severe mental illness receiving professional care: parents' narratives. Health and Social Care in the Community 2001;9(4): 194-204.

[37] Saunders J. Families living with severe mental illness: A literature review. Issues in Mental Health Nursing 2003; 24: 175-198.

[38] Caqueo-Urizar, A. & Gutierrez-Maldonado, J. (2006) Burden of care and general health in families of patients with schizophrenia. Quality of Life Research 2006; 15: 719-724.

[39] Pinquart M, Sorensen S. Correlates of physical health and informal caregivers: A meta-analysis. Journal of Gerontology: Psychological Sciences & Social Sciences 2007;62:126-137.

[40] Singleton N, Aye Maung N, Cowie A, Sparks J, Bumpstead R, Meltzer H. Mental health of carers. Report of a survey by the Social Survey Division of the Office of National Statistics for the Department of Health, UK. London: The Stationery Office; 2002.

[41] Chang KH, Horrocks S. Lived experiences of family caregivers of mentally ill relatives. Journal of Advanced Nursing 2006; 53: 435-443.

[42] Cheffings J. Report of the Princess Royal Trust for Carers. London: Princess Royal Trust for Carers; 2003.

[43] Carers UK. Adding value: carers as drivers of social change. London: Carers UK; 2002.

[44] Sunmin Lee SD, Colditz GA, Berkman LF, Kawachi I.Caregiving and risk of coronery heart disease in U.S. women: a prospective study. American Journal of Preventative Medicine 2003;24: 113-119.

[45] Pagnini D, Carers NSW carers' mental health project stage 2: Action evaluation report. Sydney: Carers NSW; 2005.

[46] Perlick DA, Rosenbeck RA, Clarkin JF, Maciejewski PK, Sirey J, Struening E, Link BG.. Impact of family burden of affective response on clinical outcome among patient with bipolar disorder. Psychiatric Services 2004;55: 1029-1035.

[47] Schofield N, Quinn J, Haddock G, Barrowclough C. Schizophrenia and substance misuse problems: a comparison between patients with and without significant carer contact. Social Psychiatry and Psychiatric Epidemiology 2001;36: 523-528.

[48] Froggat D, Fadden G, Johnson DL, Leggatt M, Shankar R. Families as partners in mental health care: A guidebook for implementing family work. Toronto: World Fellowship for Schizophrenia and Allied Disorders (WFSAD); 2007.

[49] Newbronner E,Hare P. Services to Support Carers of People with Mental Health Problems: Consultation Report. Social Policy Research Unit, University of York, York; 2002.

[50] Mental Health Council of Australia (MHCA). Mental Health Carers Report, November 2010. ACT: MHCA; 2010.

[51] Hervey N, Ramsay R. Carers as partners in care. Advances in Psychiatric Treatment 2004;0: 81-84.

[52] O'Connor B. Wanting to be heard and included: Carers' experiences of hospitals. Health Issues 2007;90: 15-18.

[53] Rethink. Under pressure: the impacts of caring on people supporting family members or friends with mental health problems. Rethink: London; 2003.

[54] Kersten P, McLellan L, George S, Mullee MA, Smith JAE. Needs of carers of severely disabled people: are they identified and met adequately? Health and Social Care in the Community 2001;9: 235-243.

[55] McMahon J, Lawn S. Borderline Personality Disorder - 'Diagnosis of Discrimination': consumers' and carers' experience of care. Adelaide: Private Mental Health Consumer and Carer Network of Australia; 2012.

[56] Pinfold V, Corry P. Who cares? The experiences of mental health carers accessing services and information. Kingston-Upon-Thames: Rethink; 2003.

[57] Jones K, McCrae J, Steffen S. Online survey of carers of people living with schizophrenia: European Federation of Associations of Families of People with Mental Illness. Belgium: Leuven; 2007.

[58] Mottaghipour Y, Bickerton A. The Pyramid of Family Care: A Framework for family involvement with adult mental health services. Australian e-Journal for the Advancement of Mental Health (AeJAMH) 2005; 4. www.auseinet.com/journal/vol4iss3/mottaghipour.pdf(accessed 26 July 2012).

[59] Keller J. Helping families to help their loved ones with a serious mental illness. White Paper for the National Alliance on Mental Health in New York State. New York: National Alliance on Mental Illness/NAMI; 2005.

[60] World Health Organisation. Preparing a health care workforce for the 21st century: The challenge of chronic conditions. WHO: France; 2005.

[61] National Health Priority Action Council (NHPAC). National chronic disease strategy. Australian Government Department of Health and Ageing, Canberra; 2006.

[62] Wynaden D. The experience of caring for a person with a mental illness: A grounded theory study. International Journal of Mental Health Nursing 2007;16, 381-389.

[63] Godress J, Ozgul S, Owen C, Foley-Evans L. Grief experiences of parents whose children suffer from mental illness. Australian and New Zealand Journal of Psychiatry 2004;39, 88-94.

[64] Strauss A, Corbin J. Basics of qualitative research: Grounded theory procedures and techniques. London: Sage; 1990.

[65] Richie J, Spencer L. Qualitative data analysis for applied policy research. In A. Bryman& R. Burgess (Eds), Analysing qualitative data (pp.173-194). New York: Routledge, 1994.

[66] Neuman WL. Social research methods: qualitative and quantitative approaches. 5th Edition. Boston: Pearson Education Inc; 2003.

[67] Burnard P. A method of analysing interview transcripts in qualitative research. Nurse Education Today 1991;11: 461-466.

[68] WuestJ, Hodgins MJ. Reflections on methodological approaches and conceptual contributions in a program of caregiving research: development and testing of Wuest's theory of family care giving. Qualitative Health Research 2011;21, 151-161.

[69] Rees Jones I, Ahmed N, Catty J, McLaren S, Rose D, Wykes T, Burns T. Illness careers and continuity of care in mental health services: A qualitative study of service users and carers. Social Science and Medicine 2009; 69: 632-639.

[70] Reid J, Lloyd C, de Groot L. The psycho-education needs of parents who have an adult son or daughter with a mental illness. Australian e-Journal for the Advancement of Mental Health (AeJAMH) 2005; 4. http://auseinet.flinders.edu.au/journal/vol4iss2/reid.pdf(accessed 26 July 2012).

[71] Sin J, Moone N, Wellman N. Developing services for the carers of young adults with early-onset psychosis: Listening to their experiences and needs. Journal of Psychiatric Mental Health Nursing 2005;12: 589–97.

[72] Chambers M, Ryan A, Connor S. Exploring the emotional support needs and coping strategies of family carers. Journal of Psychiatric& Mental Health Nursing 2001;8: 99-106.

[73] Lee S, Colditz G, Berkman L, Kawachi I. Caregiving and risk of coronary heart disease in US women: A prospective study. American Journal of Preventative Medicine 2003;24: 113-119.

[74] Champlin BE. Being there for another with a serious mental illness. Qualitative Health Research 2009;19: 1525-1535.

[75] Jones K. Addressing the needs of carers during early psychosis. Early Intervention in Psychiatry 2009;3: S22-S26.

[76] Cuijpers P, Stam H. Burnout among relatives of psychiatric patients attending psychoeducational support groups. Psychiatric Services 2000;51: 375-379.

[77] Fortune DG, Smith JV, Garvey K. Perceptions of psychosis, coping, appraisals and psychological distress in the relatives of patients with schizophrenia: an exploration using self-regulation theory. The British Journal of Clinical Psychology 2005;44: 319-331.

[78] Chien WT, Norman A, Thompson DR. Perceived benefits and difficulties experienced in a mutual support group for family carers of people with schizophrenia. Qualitative Health Research 2006;16: 962-981.

[79] Hsiao C, Van Riper M. Research on caregiving in Chinese families living with mental illness: a critical review. Journal of Family Nursing 2010;16: 68-100.

[80] Mental Health Council of Australia (MHCA). Time for service: Solving Australia's mental health crisis. Deakin West, ACT: MCHA; 2006.

[81] Mental Health Council of Australia (MHCA). Adversity and advocacy: The lives and hopes of mental health carers. ACT: MHCA; 2009.

Chapter 10

Parent-Child Attachment, Parental Depression, and Perception of Child Behavioural/Emotional Problems

Lawrence T. Lam

Additional information is available at the end of the chapter

1. Introduction

The issue of whether parents who have experienced symptoms of psychopathology, particularly depression, would be able to provide an accurate report on the behavioural/emotional problems of their children has long been raised. [1] It has been suggested that parental depression plays an important role in their perception of their children's behavioural. [2-7] The early review by Breslau (1988) on the available studies in 1988 found that there was no evidence for any distortion of child behavioural problems using depressed mothers as informants. [1] However, more recent studies have found a positive relationship between parental depression, particularly maternal depression, and report of increased behavioural/emotional problems of their children. For example, in the study by Fergussen et al. on the effect of maternal depression on their ratings of children behaviour found a significant association between their depression and children's conduct disorder and attention deficit behaviour. [3] A recent study by Hall et al. also found that depressive symptoms in mothers contributed significantly to the perception of both internalising and externalising problems of their children when they were asked to report on their children's behaviour [7].

Parent-child relationships, particularly attachment or connectedness between the parent and child, have been reported to have an effect on the behavioural and emotional health of children and adolescents. [8-9] In terms of the parent-child relationship and parental perception of their children's behavioural and emotional problems, it has been noted that few studies have been conducted. [5] The study by Kolko et al. found that low parental acceptance of the child was significantly associated with the difference between parents' and teachers' perception of children's externalising but not internalising behaviour. [10] Another study by Mosley et al. also found that better parent-child relationships in terms of increased involvement also related to a decrease of parental perception on both internalising and externalising behavioural problems. [11] A more recent study by Treulter & Epkins also found that the parent-child relationship, measured as parental involvement and time spent with children, was significantly related to both parents' rating of externalising behaviour. [5] In sum, these studies suggested an overall negative association between parent-child relationships and their perception on children's behavioural/emotional problems such that the better the parent-child relationship, the less the degree of parental perception of children's behavioural/ emotional problems.

The above-mentioned studies have suggested both parental depressive symptoms and parent-child relationships are associated with parent's perception of children's behavioural/ emotional problems. However, the foci of all these studies are on individual variables, either parental depressive symptoms or parent-child relationships, and their associations with parental perception. All of the above-mentioned studies considered only one of the two factors with the exception of the study by Treulter & Epkins. [5] It has been known that parental depression, particularly maternal depression, exerts a significant influence on the parent-child relationship. [12] Therefore, it is logical to consider that there could be an interaction effect of parental depression and parent-child relationship on parent's perception of children's behavioural/emotional problems. A search of the current literature has revealed no related studies on this topic.

The aim of this study is to further examine the relationships between parental depression, parent-child relationship and parental perception of children's behavioural/emotional problems. Of particular interest of the study is the possible interaction effect between parental depression and parent-child relationship, specifically parent-child attachment or connectedness, on the perception of children's behavioural/emotional problems. It is hypothesised that the parent-child relationship acts as an effect modifier in the relationship between parental depression and the perception of children's behavioural/emotional problems in a manner that depressed parents who also have inadequate attachment or connectedness with their children would have a significantly increased rating on their children's behavioural/ emotional problems.

2. Methods

This cross-sectional survey is part of the Guangzhou city primary school students' behavioural problems intervention longitudinal cohort study. The survey serves as the base-line pre-intervention data collected on participating school children and their parents as well as a screening for behavioural problems among children. The cohort study is an on-going study conducted in the YueXiu district, the biggest district of the Guangzhou city in Guangdong Province, since December 2008. Guangdong Province is located in Southern China, and is the most populous province in China of which Guangzhou city is the capital. It is the biggest and most populated city of the Province with an estimated population of nearly 10 million in 2006. Institute ethics approval for the study was granted by the Human Ethics Committee of the Sun Yat-Sen University, GuangZhou, PR China.

The sample was generated from the total student population of grade 4 primary school children within the study district. All students were registered with the Guangzhou city primary school registry. According the latest information from the registry, there were about 8400 grade 4 primary school children enrolled within the study district in 2008. A stratified random sampling method with stratification according to proportions of students in different type of schools: schools run by provincial government, local government, or private schools, were used for sample generation.

The base-line survey was conducted at different schools within the same week. Parents of the selected students from different schools were invited to participate in the longitudinal study via school principals and their teachers, and were encouraged to fill in the baseline self-reported questionnaire designed specifically for the study. Informed consent was sought from each parent by signing a consent form indicating willing participation in the longitudinal study.

The outcome of the study, namely parental perception of child behavioural problems, was assessed using the Child Behavioural Checklist for Ages 6-18 (CBCL/6-18), which was a validated, standardised, and a widely used scale for assessing behavioural problems amongst children and adolescents internationally. [13] Parents were asked to respond to 113 items that described specific behavioural and emotional problems that might occur in children and adolescents. These items were rated by parents on their perception of how true each item described their children now or within the past 6 months using a scale ranging from 0 to 2 (0=not true; 1=somewhat true or sometimes true; 2=very true or often true). The main content of the CBCL/6-18 covers 8 different domains including aggressive behaviour, anxious/depressed, attention problems, rule-breaking behaviour, social problems, somatic complaints, thought problems, and withdrawal. These eight domains are then further summarised into two main clusters of behavioural or emotive problems: internalisation (CBCL-inter) and externalisation (CBCL-exter) problems. A total score was also calculated for each child as an overall summary of the individual's behavioural problems (CBCL-total). Examples of these items included: "Can't concentrate, can't pay attention for long" for attention problems; "Cruel to animals" for aggressive behaviour; and "Unhappy, sad, or depressed" for anxious/depressed emotions. Higher total scores, internalisation, and externalisation scores, indicate a greater severity of behavioural or emotive problems. Ample studies have been conducted on the validity and reliability of the CBCL/6-18 with full information available on the Achenbach System of Empirically Based Assessment (ASEBA) official website [14].

Parental depression was measured using the depression subscale of the Hospital Anxiety and Depression Scale (HADS) which was designed as a self-reported screening instrument for depression. [15] The instrument has been used in many studies and its validity is well proven. [16] The depression subscale consists of 7 items assessing depressive affects. Examples of these items include: "I look forward with enjoyment to things" and "I have lost interest in my appearance". Respondents were asked to respond to questions of how often they had experienced these emotional states in the month prior to the survey. On a Likert scale, responses were rated from 0 to 3 for not at all to all of the time or some equivalent responses with total scores ranging from 0 to 21. Responses were graded in a negative direction in a manner that higher scores represent greater depressive affects. Attachment or connectedness between parent and child was assessed using the Attachment Problems subscale of the Parental Stress Index (PSI). [17] The PSI was designed specifically to evaluate and to diagnose individual parent-child dyads under stress. Of different domains included in the instrument, attachment between parent and child is one "designed to measure the intrinsic investment the parent in the role of parent". [17] It was used to assess the degree of willingness parents would commit and attach in the relationship with their children. Parents were asked to rate how much they agree to a series of statements regarding their relationship with their children on a Likert scale ranging from 0 to 4. Responses were graded in a direction with higher scores indicating greater attachment problems. An example item is "I expected to have closer and warmer feelings for my child than I do and this bothers me". The reliability and validity of the PSI have been demonstrated in many studies [17-19].

Other information collected in the survey included age and sex of the child, respondents' age and sex, parental education levels, occupation, family structure whether intact or divorced, family monthly incomes, and whether the parent suffered any chronic illnesses or hospitalisation. Included in the study were only parents of target children. Other responding relatives, such as grandparents, were excluded.

Data were analysed using the Stata V10.0 statistical software program. [20] Descriptive statistics on the sample including frequencies, percentages, means, standard deviations, and median were presented according to the nature of variables. All CBCL scores were treated as continuous variables. Bivariate analyses were conducted to examine unadjusted relationships between parental depression, attachment problems, demographics, and parental perception of child behavioural problems including the total, internalisation, and externalisation scores. Owing to the fact that CBCL-total, CBCL-inter, and CBCL-exter scores were highly skewed and exhibited problems of over dispersion, it was considered more appropriate to analyse these data with negative binomial regression models. Hence, this analytical technique was applied to all unadjusted and adjusted analyses. Bivariate associations between all variables of interest and parental perception of child behavioural problems were analysed with simple negative binominal regression models and were tested using the Likelihood Ratio Chi-squared tests. All significant variables identified from the bivariate analyses were included in further analyses for the adjusted relationship between parental depression, attachment problems and their perception of their children's behavioural problems. Of particular interest to the study was the interaction effect of parental depression and attachment problems between parent and child, on parental perception of children behavioural problems. Hence, the significance of interaction terms was tested in the final models for CBCL-total, CBCL-inter, and CBCL-exter scores.

3. Results

A total of 1839 parent-child dyads were recruited and provided usable information. This represented 97.1% of the total participants of the longitudinal study. Fifty-six respondents were not parents of the targeted child. The characteristics of children and their parents including parental depression, attachment problems, and parental perception of behavioural problems were summarised in Table 1. In terms of the outcome variables, the mean values of all CBCL scores were larger than their corresponding median values with large standard deviations suggesting all three scores were skewed and had problems of over dispersion.

Variables	Frequency (%) or mean (s.d.), median
Demographics	
Age of the child (years)	Mean=9.5 (0.61), median=9.5
Sex of child	958 (52.2)
Male	876 (47.8)
Female	
Age of parent (years)	Mean=38.7 (4.11), median=38.1
Relation of parent to child	767 (42.7)
Father	1031 (57.3)
Mother	
Family structure	1624 (89.8)
Living with both biological parents	184 (10.2)
Others	
Parent's education level	920 (51.1)
High school or lower	418 (23.2)
Post secondary	462 (25.7)
University or higher	
Parent's occupation	232 (13.1)
Unemployed /retired	465 (26.4)
Farmer/labourer	425 (24.1)
Government official	201 (11.4)
Professional/technical	
Business	
Monthly income (RMB$)*	601 (35.2)
Low	522 (30.5)
Middle	586 (34.3)
High	
Parent having chronic disease or hospitalised	292 (15.9)
Yes	1547 (84.1)
No	

Variables	Frequency (%) or mean (s.d.), median
Parental Stress Index -Attachment Problems scores	Mean=18.4 (3.35), median=18.0
Parental depression HADS depression scores	Mean=4.7 (3.04), median=4.0
CBCL-Total scores	Mean=21.1 (17.66), median=18.0
CBCL Internalisation scores	Mean=5.8 (5.79), median=4.0
CBCL Externalisation scores	Mean=7.9 (7.06), median 6.0
*Low <RMB$3000; middle 3000-4900; high>5000	

Table 1. Description information on the characteristics of children, their parents, parent-child attachment problems, parental depression, and parental perception of child behavioural problems (N=1839)

	Results on association		
Variables	**CBCL total**	**Internalisation**	**Externalisation**
Demographics			
Age of the child	χ^2_1=2.52, p=0.112	χ^2_1=0.49, p=0.485	χ^2_1=3.81, p=0.051
Sex of child	χ^2_1=23.77, p<0.001	χ^2_1=4.50, p=0.034	χ^2_1=50.18, p<0.001
Age of parent	χ^2_1=16.01, p<0.001	χ^2_1=8.09, p=0.0042	χ^2_1=23.69, p<0.001
Relation of parent to child	χ^2_1=1.13, p=0.288	χ^2_1=0.62, p=0.432	χ^2_1=1.14, p=0.216
Family structure	χ^2_1=2.16, p=0.141	χ^2_1=2.50 p=0.114	χ^2_1=1.85, p=0.174
Parent's education level	χ^2_2=5.90, p=0.052	χ^2_2=4.32, p=0.115	χ^2_2=3.95, p=0.139
Parent's occupation	χ^2_4=5.34, p=0.254	χ^2_4=7.21, p=0.125	χ^2_4=3.70, p=0.449
Monthly income	χ^2_2=5.32, p=0.007	χ^2_2=2.67, p=0.263	χ^2_2=7.55, p=0.023
Parent having chronic disease or hospitalised	χ^2_1=22.65, p<0.001	χ^2_1=27.31, p<0.001	χ^2_1=25.36, p<0.001
Parental Stress Index -Attachment Problems scores	χ^2_1=12.13, p<0.001	χ^2_1=19.22, p<0.001	χ^2_1=12.38, p<0.001
Parental depression HADS depression scores	χ^2_1=42.52, p<0.001	χ^2_1=50.62, p<0.001	χ^2_1=28.83, p<0.001

Table 2. Unadjusted associations between child and parent characteristics and parental perception on child behavioural problems: CBCL Total; CBCL-Internalisation: and CBCL-Externalisation

The bivariate relationships between demographics, parental depression, attachment problems and parental perception of child behavioural problems were examined. The results were summarised in Table 2. As shown, among the demographic variables, child's sex, parents' age, monthly income, and parental illness were significantly associated with all three

CBCL scores. Results also suggested the unadjusted association between parental depression and the perception of their children's behavioural problems was highly significant for all CBCL scores (CBCL-total: χ^2_1=42.52, p<0.001; CBCL-inter: χ^2_1=50.62, p<0.001; CBCL-exter: χ^2_1=28.83, p<0.001). This also applied to attachment problems (CBCL-total: χ^2_1=12.13, p<0.001; CBCL-inter: χ^2_1=19.22, p<0.001; CBCL-exter: χ^2_1=12.38, p<0.001).

	Results			
Variables in the final model	β	SE(β)	Z-value	p-value
		CBCL-Total		
Female	-0.21	0.047	-4.45	<0.001
Parent's age	-0.02	0.006	-3.66	<0.001
Parent having chronic disease or hospitalised	0.25	0.062	3.94	<0.001
Attachment problems	0.03	0.007	3.32	0.001
Parental depression	0.05	0.008	5.71	<0.001
		CBCL-Internalisation		
Parent's age	-0.02	0.007	-2.49	0.013
Parent having chronic disease or hospitalised	0.31	0.070	4.50	<0.001
Attachment problems	0.03	0.008	3.97	<0.001
Parental depression	0.06	0.001	5.96	<0.001
		CBCL-Externalisation		
Female	-0.31	0.047	-6.605	<0.001
Parent's age	-0.03	0.006	-4.72	<0.001
Parent having chronic disease or hospitalised	0.24	0.063	3.79	<0.001
Attachment problems	0.03	0.008	3.37	0.001
Parental depression	0.04	0.008	4.25	<0.001

Table 3. Results obtained from the multiple negative binomial regression analyses on CBCL Total, CBCL-Internalisation, and CBCL-Externalisation without interaction terms.

The results obtained from the multiple negative binomial regression analyses were also presented in Table 3 and Table 4. Table 3 presented results on final regression models of CBCL scores, including the total, internalisation, and externalisation, regressing on various study variables with terms of interaction between parental depression and attachment problems included. Results indicated the interaction term in the final model for CBCL-exter was significant (Z=2.19, p=0.029), suggesting that there was a significant interaction effect of parental depression and attachment problems between parent and child on the perception of their children's behavioural problems.

	Results			
Variables in the final model with interaction term	β	SE(β)	Z-value	p-value
		CBCL-Total		
Female	-0.21	0.047	-4.45	<0.001
Parent's age	-0.02	0.006	-3.61	<0.001
Parent having chronic disease or hospitalised	0.25	0.062	3.99	<0.001
Attachment problems	0.04	0.012	3.18	0.001
Parental depression	0.11	0.046	2.41	0.016
Interaction: Attachment*Parental depression	0.01	0.002	1.42	0.155
		CBCL-Internalisation		
Parent's age	-0.02	0.007	-2.45	0.014
Parent having chronic disease or hospitalised	0.32	0.070	4.51	<0.001
Attachment problems	0.04	0.014	2.84	0.004
Parental depression	0.08	0.053	1.54	0.124
Interaction: Attachment*Parental depression	0.01	0.003	0.51	0.611
		CBCL-Externalisation		
Female	-0.34	0.048	-7.01	<0.001
Parent's age	-0.03	0.006	-4.09	<0.001
Parent having chronic disease or hospitalised	0.25	0.063	4.00	<0.001
Attachment problems	0.05	0.013	4.02	<0.001
Parental depression	0.13	0.046	2.90	0.004
Interaction: Attachment*Parental depression	0.01	0.002	2.19	**0.029**

Table 4. Results obtained from the multiple negative binomial regression analyses on CBCL Total, CBCL-Internalisation, and CBCL-Externalisation with interaction terms.

Figure 1 depicted the unadjusted mean scores of externalisation behaviour for different parental depression status by different levels of attachment problems. The figure exhibited a lack of parallelism suggesting an interaction effect between parental depression and parent-child attachment on the CBCL-exter scores. The interaction terms in models for CBCL-total and CBCL-inter were not significant. Table 4 presented results on the final models of CBCL-total and CBCL-inter after removal of the interaction terms. As shown, parental depression and attachment problems between parent and child were significantly related to parental perception of their children's behavioural problems for both the total (depression: Z=5.71, p<0.001: attachment: Z=3.32, p=0.001) and internalisation (depression: Z=5.96, p<0.001: attachment: Z=3.97, p<0.001) scores after adjusting for sex, parental age, and parental illness.

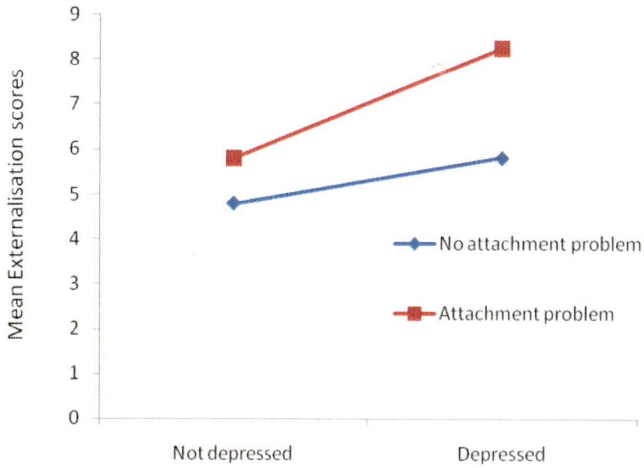

Figure 1. Plot of mean externalisation scores of parental depression status by attachment problems,*Depression status was classified using a cut-off suggested by the HADS author (>7=depressed); Attachment problems was clssified using a cut-off of >15 as suggested by the PSI author.

4. Discussion and conclusion

This study aims to examine the relationship between parental depression, parent-child relationship and parental perception of children's behavioural/emotional problems. Particularly, it aims to test the hypothesis of the interaction effect of parental depression and parent-child attachment on parental perception of children's behavioural/emotional problems. The results provided evidence of a significant interaction effect between parental depression and parent-child attachment problems on parental perception on the externalising of children's problems, but no effects on internalising problems and total problems. The main effects of parental depression and parent-child attachment problems on parental perception of children behavioural/emotional problems were found significant.

Due to the lack of a similar study on the interaction between parental depression and attachment problem and parental perception on children's behavioural/emotional problems, a comparison of results obtained from this study with others reported in literature would be difficult. However, other results obtained from the study are consistent with those obtained in the general literature of parental depression, parent-child relationships and the distortion of parental perception of children's behavioural/emotional problems as highlighted in the introduction section. For example, in the study by Treutler et al, it was found that parental depression and parent-child relationship were both associated with their ratings on internalising behaviours. [5] The results of the current study have rendered further support to this finding. Furthermore, it has shown that parental perception of children's externalising behavioural problems is a function of their own depressive symptomatologies and the attachment to their children.

The results indicated that attachment between parent and child acts as an effect modifier in the relationship between parental depression and their perception of children's externalising behavioural problems. For parents who have a close relationship with their children, it could be considered natural that depression would influence their perception of children's behavioural problems. However, for parents who have experienced attachment problems with their children as well as depression, the alienated relationship with their children tends to enhance their perception of children's behavioural problems to such a degree that is much more than the usual effect brought on by depression alone. In other words, the alienated relationship enhances the effect of depression on parental perception of children's behavioural problems. It is interesting to note that such an interactive effect is observed for externalising behavioural problems, but not for internalising problems. One possible explanation for this phenomenon is that externalising behavioural problems, including aggressive behaviour, rule-breaking, and attention problems, are observable manifestations of childhood problems. Parents can identify these behaviours and perceive them as problematic easily for both depressive and non-depressive parents, with depressive parents labelling them with a greater degree of severity. However, if the parent-child dyad has been experiencing a detrimental relationship, it is likely that the parent would have a heightened sensitivity to the child's observable behavioural problems. This heightening of awareness or sensitivity is further enhanced in a parent who is also experiencing depression. This heightening of awareness may be absent for those less observable behavioural problems such as withdrawal and depression.

The results obtained from this study have a direct clinical implication on the validity of using parents as informants for children's behavioural assessments. As above-mentioned, parental distortion in their report on children's behavioural assessments has long been identified and established as a potential source of error. [7] The results of this study further indicate that parents' perception of their children's behaviour is a function of their own internal state as well as their relationship with their children. The potential for distortion in reporting of child behaviour is great if a single parent is used as the sole informant. Should this aspect be overlooked, systematic biases would result due to distortion errors. This may occur in research as well as in clinical assessment. In fact, it has been advocated that multiple informants, especially non-familial informants, should be used for any childhood behavioural problems in both research and clinical settings. [21-22] If possible, observational tools instead of self-reported instruments should be employed and non-family observers should be used as informants. [23] In the current longitudinal study, children who have been identified with scores higher than the recommended cut-off will be assessed by a child psychiatrist using another clinical assessment tool.

In terms of prevention and early intervention of developmental psychopathology in children, the results of the study can also shed some lights. Tackling attachment problems between parents and their children may provide an inroad to, not only the change of perception of child behavioural problems but also, the actual developmental problems during early childhood and behavioural problems throughout the entire child and adolescence period. A recent study has identified that the quality of interaction between mother and child, particularly in the area of emotion availability of the mother, has a direct bearing on the functioning, behavioural problems, and depressive symptomatologies of the child. [24] In this longitudinal study, it has been found that dysfunctional mother-child relationship and poor attachment at infancy is predictive of developmental and behavioural problems at later years of childhood. [24] However, early intervention program in enhancing attachment between parent and child could have a positive effect in improving the quality of parent-child relationship and reinforcing a secure attachment. [25] This could, in turn, have a direct impact on the on-going development of the child. Furthermore, it could also be possible that the problematic parent-child relationship may have contributed to the depression of the parent. An improvement in parent-child attachment could have an alleviating effect of the parent's depression and, in turn, reinforcing a better relationship with the child and resulting in a better behavioural outcome.

As in all studies, there are strengths and weaknesses in this study. This is a population-based study that includes a random sample of students. The use of a standardised and validated assessment instrument for the outcome measure minimised some measurement biases. The assessments on parental depression, parent-child relationship, and parental perception of children's behavioural problems were concurrent and captured the current status on all these variables, hence minimising biases due to the lapse of time. A potential limitation has been identified in this study. Information on the exposure variables, namely parental depression and attachment problems is obtained via a self-reported questionnaire. Hence this will constitute a report bias in the exposure variables and it would likely present as a differential bias due to depressive parents reporting more severe symptomatologies as well as parent-child relationship problems. To improve the quality of the study, parental depression and parent-child relationships are best to be assessed by multiple informants as well as by observers as suggested by [23].

Author details

Lawrence T. Lam[1,2]

Address all correspondence to: lawrence.lam@nd.edu.au

1 The School of Medicine Sydney, The University of Notre Dame, Sydney, Australia

2 Discipline of Paediatrics and Child Health, Sydney Medical School, The University of Sydney, Australia

References

[1] Breslau, N., Davis, G. C., & Prabucki, K. (1988). Depressed mothers as informants in family history research- are they accurate? *Psychiatry Research*, 24, 345-59.

[2] Richters, J.E. (1992). Depressed mothers as informants about their children: a critical review of the evidence for distortion. *Psychological Bulletin*, 112, 485-99.

[3] Fergussen, D. M., Lynskey, M. T., & Horwood, L. J. (1993). The effect of maternal depression on maternal ratings of child behaviour. *Journal of Abnormal Child Psychology*, 21, 245-69.

[4] Connell, A. M., & Goodman, S. H. (2002). The association between psychopathology in fathers versus mothers and children's internalizing and externalizing behaviour problems: a meta-analysis. *Psychological Bulletin*, 128, 746-73.

[5] Treutler, C. M., & Epkines, C. C. (2003). Are discrepancies among child, mother, and father reports on children's behaviour related to parents' psychological symptoms and aspects of parent-child relationships? *Journal of Abnormal Child Psychology*, 31, 13-27.

[6] Luoma, I., Koivisto, A. M., & Tamminen, T. (2004). Fathers' and mothers' perceptions of their child and maternal depressive symptoms. *Nordic Journal of Psychiatry*, 58, 205-11.

[7] Hall, L. A., Rayens, M. K., & Peden, A. R. (2008). Maternal factors associated with child behaviour. *Journal of Nursing Scholarship*, 40, 124-30.

[8] Ackard, D. M., Neumark-Sztainer, D., Story, M., & Perry, C. (2006). Parent-child connectedness and behavioural and emotional health among adolescents. *American Journal of Preventive Medicine*, 30, 59-66.

[9] Liu, Y.L. (2006). Parental/maternal attachment, peer support, social expectations of peer interaction, and depressive symptoms. *Adolescence*, 41, 705-21.

[10] Kolko, D. J., & Kazdin, A. E. (1993). Emotional/behavioural problems in clinic and nonclinic children: Correspondence among child, parent, and teacher reports. *Journal of Child Psychology and Psychiatry*, 34, 991-1006.

[11] Mosley, J., & Thompson, E. (1995). Fathering behaviour and child outcome: The role of race and poverty. *Marsiglio W. (ed.) Fatherhood: Contemporary theory, research, and social policy. Beverly Hills: Sage*, 148-165.

[12] Burke, L. (2003). The impact of maternal depression on familial relationships. *International Review of Psychiatry*, 15, 243-55.

[13] Achenbach, T.M. Manual for CBCL 6-18 years. *Burlington: ASEBA; 2001.*

[14] Achenbach, TM. (2009). Achenbach System of Empirically Based Assessment. http://www.aseba.org/index.html, (accessed 15 January 2012).

[15] Zigmond, A.S., & Snaith, R.P. (1983). The Hospital Anxiety And Depression Scale. *Acta Psychiatricia Scandinavica*, 67, 361-70.

[16] Bjelland, I., Dahl, A. A., Haug, T. T., & Neckelmann, D. (2002). The validity of the Hospital Anxiety and Depression Scale. An updated literature review. *Journal of Psychosomatic Research*, 52, 69-77.

[17] Abidin, R.R. (1995). Parenting Stress Index (PSI) manual 3rd Edition. *Charlottesville: Pediatric Psychology Press.*

[18] Hutcheson, J., & Black, M. (1996). Psychometric properties of the Parenting Stress Index in a sample of low-income African-American mothers of infants and toddlers. *Early Education Development*, 7, 381-400.

[19] Ostberg, M., Hagekull, B., & Wettergren, S. (1997). A measure of parental stress in mothers with small children, dimensionality, stability, and validity. *Scandinavian Journal of Psychology*, 38, 199-208.

[20] StataCorp. (2007). *Stata Statistical Software: Release 10.0. College Station: StataCorporation.*

[21] Soussingan, R., Tremblay, R. E., Schaal, B., et al. (1992). Behavioural and cognitive characteristics of conduct disordered-hyperactive boys from age 6 to 11: a multiple informant perspective. *Journal of Child Psychology and Psychiatry*, 33, 1333-46.

[22] Kristensen, H. (2001). Multiple informants' report of emotional and behavioural problems in a nation-wide sample of selective mute children and controls. *European Child and Adolescent Psychiatry*, 10, 35-42.

[23] Cunningham, C.E. (2007). A family-centred approach to planning and measuring the outcome of interventions for children with attention-deficit/hyperactivity disorder. *Journal of Pediatric Psychology*, 32, 676-94.

[24] Easterbrooks, M. A., Bureau, J. F., & Lyons-Ruth, K. (2012). Developmental correlates and predictors of emotional availability in mother-child interaction: a longitudinal study from infancy to middle childhood. *Developmental Psychopathology*, 24, 65-78.

[25] Wendland-Carro, J., Piccinini, C.A., & Millar, W.S. (1999). The role of an early intervention on enhancing the quality of mother-infant interaction. *Child Development*, 70, 713-21.

Chapter 11

Working on Adolescent's Motivation to Improve the Outcome Within a Multimodal Treatment

Gatta Michela, Testa C. Paolo, Del Col Lara,
Spoto Andrea, Dal Zotto Lara,
De Sauma Maxim and Battistella Pier Antonio

Additional information is available at the end of the chapter

1. Introduction

What is motivation? From a psychological point of view it is a force, of psychic nature, which makes the individual show certain behaviour. Freud said that each behaviour, also the most strange, always responds to a motivation and the motivation's meaning is often unknown not only by people in contact with the subject but also by the subject himself. If we wanted to contextualise motivation within the alliance relationship, we could consider the last one as an interaction between two poles: one is the therapist the other is the patient, each with his own intrapersonal and interpersonal features, in a specific space defined by the setting, motivation is one of the intrapersonal patient's characteristics. Therapeutic alliance is a strong predictor of outcome in individual psychotherapy across diverse treatment orientations and modalities both with adult patients [14], [26] and adolescents [10], [13]. Patient's motivation, within the working alliance, during therapeutic intervention has been much studied [21], [7], [15], [30], [24], [25], [29], whereas the motivation associated with the diagnostic moment has been given less importance in scientific literature [22], [17]. Close to the theory there is clinical experience related to the centre we work in. Longitudinal studies about adolescents' therapeutic compliance and clinical evolution done within our Services [9], [10], [11] showed most of adolescents did not follow therapeutic suggestion about undergoing psychotherapy after the diagnostic process. Compliant and not compliant adolescents were different because of motivation expressed during the diagnostic process: the most of motivated adolescents started therapy, whereas the most of unmotivated adolescents did not. The clinical evolution resulted in association with adolescents' motivation as well: after six months a clinical improvement was statistically more frequent among motivated than among unmotivated adolescents.

These results and other ones from literature, evidencing that an early alliance has been found to be a better predictor of outcome than alliance averaged across sessions or measured in the middle or late phase of treatment [26], [12], stimulated us to think of and to evaluate, during clinical practice, some strategies to favour adolescent's motivation to follow therapeutic suggestion given at the end of the diagnostic process. For this reason we think of a diagnostic protocol which considers, with psychiatric diagnosis (ICD 10) and clinical evaluation (psychopathological investigation), to pay particular attention to motivational aspects. To do that we referred to the experience of interviewing used at the Brent Centre of Young People of London.

Looking at the literature we can deduce that the word "interviewing" has been introduced quite recently. Few authors discussed this process (interviewing) itself. The idea of "Interviewing" with adolescents at the Brent Centre comes from the belief held by M. Laufer that most adolescents were not able to engage in and make use of long term psychoanalytic psychotherapy without some preparatory work, as theorized by Freud (the development of the "observing Ego"). The word "assessment" wasn't used because it reminded to a psychiatric meaning. When the Centre was founded adolescents could come and "walk-in" for any reason. According to the presenting problem, the clinician provided the connection with the general practitioner (GP), the lawyer or the social worker. The aim was to focus on vulnerable adolescents to work on the accessibility, the potentiality for making therapeutic connections. It was considered to work on a long term base and to involve only trained analysts because it takes time and experience to modify the defenses. The results of the first researches showed that the Centre was working with severe neurotic patients and it was considered extremely important to engage the adolescents in order to offer a preventive help. P. Wilson [32] linked intervention in adolescence to the developmental model conceptualized by Laufer and stressed the importance of making an assessment before starting any kind of intervention: " Whatever the extent of intervention, it should be based on an assessment of his feelings about himself, his body and relation to his parents, and designed to contribute towards facilitating progressive movement and so serve to prevent breakdown and the possibility of mental ill-health in adulthood". From his words, it's possible to consider the interviewing as the preliminary work with the adolescent in which there is an assessment about his way of coping with the adolescence tasks. In 'Adolescence and developmental breakdown' [17] it is again stressed that the application of the developmental model to the assessment of psychopathology in adolescence is fundamental to make further decisions about management and treatment of the adolescent. The word "interviewing" appears in the paper written by C. Bronstein and S. Flanders in 1998 [4]. In it, the emphasis is put to another meaning of this process, linked to psychotherapy. The process that develops in this first contact with the adolescents we call *interviewing*, though it could also be described as *psychotherapeutic consultation*. It is stressed that a mere assessment followed by therapy can't give the adolescent the possibility to understand what therapy means, leading to a further drop out. It means that the aims of interviewing are both to assess the extent and the nature of the patient's disease and to give the adolescent the possibility to express his feelings and fears, to come into touch with anxiety, to make the "unknown" less frightening. Another aim of the interviewing process could be to set up the framework for further treatment, if this is considered necessary. It means dealing with "plans, arrangements, preparation, undertakings" because it can allow the adolescent and his parents to understand better the meaning of further treatment. It is stressed the importance of making the adolescent an active part of the process and of involving him in it. For example the interviewer can use the explanation to make easier the understanding and to involve more the adolescent; the adolescent is made aware of the interviewer's concerns and of severity and implications of his problems in his present and future life. On the other hand the interviewer has to guide the intervention. Any reaction is "within the strict limits set by our specific role" [19] and it is important to avoid collusion, carefully not trying to take sides and allocate blame [18]. It's also part of the process setting up the framework of further treatment, if it's necessary. It means helping the adolescent and the family in understanding the meaning of the therapy but also talking together about practical problems [17].

1.1. The semi-residential adolescent psychopathology service

The study involved patients attending the Daily Service for Adolescents at the Neuropsychiatric Unit for Children and Adolescents in Padua. The main purposes of this service are the care and rehabilitation of adolescents with severe psychopathological disorders (mood disorders, psychotic disorders, antisocial behavior and personality disorders), particularly optimizing their welfare and providing intervention for these young patients through an integrated clinical and pedagogical approach. Various professional figures cooperate on the therapeutic project and this multi-professional team includes a child and adolescent neuropsychiatrist, a psychologist, two educators and a social worker. Adolescents attending the center undergo an initial diagnostic process, leading to a psychiatric diagnosis formulated according to the ICD 10 [33] and the therapeutic project involves attending a day center.

The centre receives adolescents (males and females from 12 to 18 years of age) with various types of psychiatric and behavioral disorder of moderate to severe degree: it has a capacity to treat approximately 25 patients in all and can simultaneously accommodate up to six adolescents, with the ratio of one operator to every two patients.

The adolescents attend from Monday to Friday from 09.00 to 17.00. Access to the structure is based on individual projects prepared by the team, which establishes the number of weekly visits and their duration. The educators can also implement tailored and/or home-based interventions in situations where an adolescent suffers from significant social isolation, and in acute cases requiring temporary hospital stays, acting as companions and providing support while the patient is in hospital. Patients can also be received in emergency situations (moments of acute crisis, or when a "buffer intervention" is needed while a patient is waiting to join a residential community). These latter interventions do not follow the normal enrolment protocol.

The general goals of the service are:

- to optimize the patient care and education measures for adolescents in situations of particular mental illness and at particularly crucial times;
- to support the families in their educational role;

- to construct an integrated clinical and pedagogical project with the various services on different levels and with different institutional roles;
- to improve the social involvement of adolescent in their living environment.

1.1.1. The multidisciplinary team

The multidisciplinary team consists of: a developmental neuropsychiatrist responsible for the service, a psychologist-psychotherapist, two educators, a social worker, a coordinator, and an administrative assistant.

There are also trainee psychologists, trainees on the degree course for professional educators at the Faculties of Education Sciences and Psychology, and physicians training in developmental neuropsychiatry.

The team holds the following meetings:

- a weekly meeting to coordinate their clinical-pedagogical work and program the educational activities;
- a weekly team meeting to discuss the cases;
- periodical meetings with social-sanitary operators and clinicians to report on the cases being treated in the semi-residential setting to discuss the clinical issues, assess the adolescent's progress, and recommend new patients for the treatment;
- a monthly supervisory team meeting with an outside psychiatrist-psychotherapist.

1.2. Protocol for enrolling new patients at the semi-residential center

The phase for assessing and enrolling an adolescent at the semi-residential center for adolescent psychopathologies is completed according to the following protocol.

1. The case is presented to the team operating at the semi-residential service for adolescent psychopathologies by the psychologist or neuropsychiatrist proposing their enrolment at the Neuropsychiatric Unit for Children and Adolescents and a file is prepared for the patient being recommended.
2. The case is discussed and, where applicable, a preliminary period of observation and assessment of the adolescent is decided.
3. A meeting is held with the patient and family to formalize the proposal to start with a preliminary period for the adolescent to get to know the semi-residential service. In addition to patients and their parents, this meeting is also attended by the clinician referring them and an educator.
4. The observation period starts, normally involving four meetings according to the following schedule:
    - the first meeting is for introductions, observations and free activity (playing, computer, exploring spaces);

- the second meeting is when an observation file is completed (a semistructured interview) by a "third party" educator, i.e. an educator who has had the least to do with the adolescent so far, in order to guarantee the utmost neutrality in the administering the assessment tool. Then activities are proposed in small groups to see how the adolescent functions in group situations;
- at the third meeting activities are proposed on the basis of the adolescent's interests emerging from the previous interview;
- the fourth and last meeting is where, in addition to the activities already begun at the third meeting, there is also space for a conversation and exchange of ideas with the adolescent, to provide feedback relating to the previous meetings, the adolescent's mode of participation and greater or lesser willingness to enroll at the semi-residential center.

5. The reference educator completes an initial observation file on the trend of the four meetings.
6. The team assesses the observation period within two weeks after its completion and decides whether to recommend that the adolescent continue with the semi-residential experience or terminate it.
7. The patient and family are informed about the child's progress so far and there is an exchange of ideas relating to the adolescent's and the family's experiences and motivations. If all concerned agree to the semi-residential program, this decision is shared and signed jointly by the family and by the physician referring the case to the team, and these parties agree on a first integrated, tailored therapeutic and educational project, and an initial schedule for the adolescent's attendance at the center.

1.3. The path for taking the patient into care

1.3.1. Formulation of the tailored educational project and schedule of attendance at the semi-residential center

This phase is completed by the working team and the object is to prepare a first project in the light of the findings during the preliminary observation period. A record is made of patients' and their families' demographic details, the motives for enrolment on the program, the internal and external activities conducted, the established goals, the general and specific objectives of the course of therapy, a description of the integrated intervention designed for each adolescent of and the timing for assessing their progress and the project.

Access is always formulated on the basis of a tailored individual project and the adolescent's weekly attendance is constantly monitored. Punctuality and adherence to the agreed frequency of attendance is an important tool for assessing the adolescents' and their families' compliance with the agreed educational project, as well as being a necessary premise for implementing the semi-residential program. For each patient, a schedule is agreed with the family, the specialist and the adolescent concerned, starting from a minimum of two attendances a week (lasting four hours each).

1.3.2. Periodical clinical interviews and progress monitoring

For each patient, there are periodical clinical meetings with their own doctors to monitor their psycho-developmental trends and personal response to the therapy. The parental couple is also followed up with regular meetings with a clinician (neuropsychiatrist or psychologist), possibly with the support of an educator.

This action on the families needs to be supported and empowered to help parents establish a different image of their child from the one they knew before, and make sense of the changes taking place in the child during the period in semi-residential care, as well as providing input on how the parents themselves need to respond to the child on a daily basis. A course of psychotherapy proper for both the adolescents and their parents is often recommended and implemented.

1.3.3. Completion of a file for recording changes and reviewing the therapy

After the first six months of attendance at the semi-residential centre, the educational project is reviewed, and the goals and/or operating methods are expanded and/or diversified, based on a first structured assessment of the adolescent's progress that involves completing and checklist of specific indicators relating to the various areas of intervention (relational, social, autonomy).

1.3.4. Ongoing assessment

The ongoing assessment of the adolescent's progress is based on various methods:

- periodic team discussions,
- periodic meetings with reference clinicians,
- periodic meetings with family,
- periodic meetings with teachers,
- periodic assessment of files completed by the reference educator,
- observation/assessment charts recorded before and after laboratory activities,
- the periodic administration of standardized tests (YSR 11-18) [1] at the baseline, when the patient is taken into care and subsequently every six months,
- the periodic completion by the team of the Global Assessment of Functioning test [31] (at the time of compiling the therapeutic and educational project and subsequently every six months).
- This assessment and constant monitoring procedure enables the ongoing adjustment of the objectives of the integrated individual projects, which is normally done every 3-6 months. The tests can also be used as a tool for pre-and post-assessment of the effects of the intervention at the start and end of a specific laboratory activity to evaluate it efficacy.

1.3.5. Discharge

The end of the course of therapeutic intervention can be decided by various factors. In the most favorable of outcomes, the project may be concluded because the preset goals have been achieved and the adolescents have regained their social contacts and schooling experience, and the course of therapy undertaken can be consolidated.

Attendance at the centre may also be interrupted due to poor compliance on the part of the adolescent and/or the family (with repeated and unjustified failures to attend appointments at the semi-residential centre or meetings with clinicians, or inadequate cooperation). The program may also be stopped by the need to include the patient in a residential community. In each case, the conclusion of the project is confirmed during the course of a final meeting attended by all the parties involved (the adolescent, the family, the reference educator, the psychologist and the neuropsychiatrist).

1.4. Pedagogical activities

The object of the pedagogical activities is to support the adolescents in the course of their development by means of a relationship with the figure of the educator, who serves as an "auxiliary ego" and consequently as a supportive companion. This is achieved by providing a space, which takes practical shape in the rooms at the semi-residential centre, and by designing a project that involves customized objectives and timings.

In experiences of research applied to different educational settings, various functions have been identified on which the educator's action is concentrated. The educator thus has several functions [23], [28]:

- as a mediator between the adolescent and the adult world,
- to provide protection in relation to the adolescent's interior conflicts,
- to accompany the patient on a path towards a normalizing educational context,
- as containment, providing stability and helping the adolescent to manage the dynamics of his/her daily life.

The *general educational goals* of the educational process providing the starting point of an individual educational project tailored to each patient include:

- helping the adolescents to gain awareness of their own sentiments, impulses and behavior;
- helping them to test their abilities in a protected setting and to raise their self-esteem;
- helping them to realistically assess their living environment.

The *activities* in which the psycho-educational process takes shape are designed to achieve the individual objectives of each adolescent's project and rely on fundamental tools, such as providing a setting as a framework in which to enable to the experience of meeting, using the operator's capacity for empathy to create a relationship that can help the adolescent to let their emotional experiences resound inside themselves and thereby increasingly gain control over them, promoting organized behavior patterns, abilities and motivations that can pave the way to satisfactory social relations and an adequate performance in the completion of tasks and the achievement of goals. During their attendance at the center, the adolescents conduct activities designed to develop their personal interests, acquire skills and reinforce their self-esteem. Outings, the preparation of a newspaper, painting, watching films, playing, writing, and dramatizations are activities conducted at the center, individually and in small groups, in the constant presence of the educators. There are also structured laboratories involving pet therapy, horse therapy, art therapy and naturalistic experiences at teaching farms organized in cooperation with other associations, as well as participation in therapeutic winter and summer holiday camps. For many young people, these activities are the only opportunities they have to put themselves to the test away from their usual living environments, to measure themselves against an adventure outside the home, and thereby testing their capacity to manage on their own, to experiment with detachment from the family, to live in groups and share the group's behavioral rules.

Finally, courses are also organized to support the adolescents' formal education in cooperation with their schools. This involves formulating tailored teaching programs and the presence of teachers at the semi-residential centre.

2. Sample

Sample is formed by adolescents who, during a semester, consecutively came to the Neuro-psychiatric Unit for Children and Adolescents in Padua, Italy, requesting a psycho diagnostic evaluation and then were suggested to undergo multimodal intervention at the Daily Service for Adolescents. The main purposes of this service are the care and rehabilitation of adolescents with severe psychopathological disorders (mood disorders, psychotic disorders, antisocial behavior and personality disorders), particularly optimizing their welfare and providing intervention for these young patients through an integrated clinical and pedagogical approach. Various professional figures cooperate on the therapeutic project and this multi-professional team includes a child and adolescent neuropsychiatrist, a psychologist, two educators and a social worker. They are 50 individuals, 33 males (66%) and 17 females (34%), aged 13 to 18 years (mean 15,6 y.). The only exclusion criteria were age below 13, chronic rather than acute psychotic state, QI < 70 and presence of known organic pathology associated with mental disease.

3. Methodology

Neuropsychiatric consultation was articulated into 5 diagnostic interviews with adolescent and his parents, separately. The last session was deputed to communication of psychiatric diagnosis and therapeutic suggestion. We added to this protocol, which was the usual one, another semistructured meeting finalised to the discussion about therapeutic indication. This difference with respect to usual diagnostic protocol (where the diagnostic communication and therapeutic suggestion formed the last meeting with the adolescent) was set up with the aim of giving information about semiresidential treatment (what it is, how it works, what it is useful for) (1) and raising adolescent's questions, doubts, fantasies and anxieties about therapy and to talk about them with the specialist (2); the hypothesis was that giving voice to these issues and receiving information could be useful to create motivation towards multimodal intervention.

Adolescent's motivation was evaluated at the beginning and at the end of the diagnostic process, considering these three elements according to Marcelli and Bracconier [23]:

- Awareness of the disease,
- Worry about his/her own psychological state,
- Self observing and describing capacities.

Recognising and admitting an uneasy state is the first step to deal with it. Being preoccupied with it means to be in touch with anxiety caused by one's own condition and to hinge on this to desire to change. Having the capacity to self observe and describe means to be in touch with one's own inner world and to quite tolerate anxiety coming from conflicts.

An anamnesis schedule collecting data about adolescent's identification, his/her family, psychosocial situation and clinical elements was filled in for each subject.

The psychiatric diagnosis was formulated using ICD 10 [33]. Additionally, we grouped subjects into three categories according to the severity of the psychopathology and pathologic personality organisation as described by Kernberg [16]. Neurotic personality organization is characterized by psychostructural conditions that include: 1) intact reality testing, 2) a consistent sense of self and of other people, and 3) generally rely on mature defense mechanisms when stressed. At the opposite end of the personality organization dimension are severely disorganized personalities, the Psychotic one which is characterized by: 1) severely compromised reality testing, 2) an inconsistent sense of self and others, and 3) utilize immature defenses. Along the middle of this dimension are personalities organized at the borderline level: 1) the syndrome of identity diffusion, 2) the predominance of primitive defensive mechanisms centering around splitting, and 3) maintenance of reality testing.

Data about patient's therapeutic compliance and clinical evolution were collected during a visit of control after nine months by the last diagnostic session. They are based on both what was referred by the patient about subjective perception of health state and on what the specialist verified about psychosocial functioning changes in a nine months period. Clinical evolution was evaluated throughout the Global Assessment Functioning Scale (GAF) [31], which was filled in before and nine months after the beginning of the semiresidential intervention. The GAF is a scale used by the operators to rate a patient's psychosocial functioning and activities, regardless of the nature of their psychiatric disease. It corresponds to Axis V of the DSM IV [2]. The GAF scale comprises 10 levels (further divided into 10 points) and each patient is assigned to a given level on the strength of a scoring system: the higher the score the better the patient's psycho- social functioning. The patients were retested nine months later:

an improvement was considered when the GAF score changed to an upper level, an unvaried situation when the score remained in the same level and an aggravation when the score decreased to an under level with regard to the initial scoring.

Statistical analysis: data analysis considers the variable motivation in relation with gender (male/female); age (13-15 years old, 16-18 years old); educational level of family - valued on parent's education degree (low, middle, high); arrival status (voluntary, by referral); support by parents - evaluated by empathetic capacities towards adolescent, availability to come to the interviews, collaborative capacities about therapeutic project (supportive family, not supportive family); diagnosis (ICD 10); compliance with therapeutic project (in therapy, drop out, therapy never started); nine months follow up (better, unvaried, worse).

The data are expressed as frequencies and percentages. Variables are expressed using nominal and ordinal scales. Cross-tabulations were analyzed using the chi-square test, considering $P<0.05$ as significant. The analyses were performed using SPSS rel. 14.

4. Result and discussion

The sample is formed by 50 individuals, 33 males (66%) and 17 females (34%), aged 13 to 18 years. They were divided in 2 age groups: 13-15 years old (24 subjects, 48%) and 16-18 years old (26 subjects, 52%). 6% attended primary school, 36% secondary school, 56% college and 2% had abandoned school. Gender/age cross tabulation shows that males are younger (61% in age range13-15, 39% in age range16-18) than females (23.5% in age range 13-15, 76.5% in age range 16-18). The family's educational level the adolescents come from, results low in 18%, middle in 62% and high in 20% of cases. Arrival status is by spontaneous request for psychodiagnostic consultation in 40% of cases and by referral in 60% of cases. Diagnosis are summarised in table 1, where comorbility is referred to depressive mood disorder and personality disorder.

Diagnosis (ICD 10)	Frequency(N)	Percent (%)
anxiety disorders	18	36
mood disorders	3	6
psychotic disorders	3	6
personality disorders	10	20
behaviour disorders	8	16
eating disorders	3	6
mental retardation	2	4
comorbility (depression and personality disorder)	3	6
Total	50	100

Table 1. Psychiatric diagnosis according to ICD 10

Adolescent's motivation has been evaluated on the basis of three elements: knowledge of a disease, preoccupation about personal psychological state and self observing and describing capacities. Three categories have been individuated on the basis of this evaluation: motivated adolescents –38%-(who recognise the disease, are worried about it and desire to change it), indifferent adolescents –34%-(who admit and describe the disease, but do not seem worried and tend to minimise their psychological condition) and contrary adolescents 28%-(who arrive to the service obliged by parents, do not recognise a disease and say that it is others' fault if they are there) (graphic 1). The difference between indifferent and contrary categories, considering the psycho-relational way of functioning, is the dimension respectively passive and active which characterizes their resistance to meet the clinician.

The motivation, evaluated at the first interview, shows that less than half of the cases (38%) agrees on diagnostic process. This result suggests that adolescent's motivation to be helped is an aim of an intervention rather than an assumption. This is confirmed by literature [23] and agrees with the result about arrival status which shows that more than 50% of subjects came because they were referred by others rather than coming by themselves and also in this last case, the visit was requested by parents and not by the adolescent. We wanted to determine whether the variable initial motivation was significantly different among groups defined by gender, age, educational level of family and diagnosis. Statistical analysis evidences that diagnosis, gender and educational level influence in some way adolescent's initial motivation. Actually, distribution of initial motivation in adolescents grouped for sex, educational level and diagnosis is not casual, while age doesn't seem affect initial motivation like the other factors (tables 2, 3, 4).

			Initial motivation categories			**Total**
			motivated	**indifferent**	**contrary**	
Gender	male	Count	6	17	10	33
		% within gender	18,18	51,51	30,3	100
		% within motivation	40	80,95	71,42	66
		% of Total	12	34	20	66
	female	Count	9	4	4	17
		% within gender	52,94	23,52	23,52	100
		% within motivation	60	19,04	28,57	34
		% of Total	18	8	8	34
Total		Count	15	21	14	50
		% within gender	30	42	28	100
		% within motivation	100	100	100	100
		% of Total	30	42	28	100
Chi-Square Tests						
	Value	df			Asymp. Sig. (2-sided)	
Pearson Chi-Square	6,794	2	0,033			

Table 2. Crosstab: initial motivation in relation with gender

			Initial motivation categories			Total
			motivated	indifferent	contrary	
family's formal education	low	Count	1	6	2	9
		% within education	11,11	66,66	22,22	100
		% within motivation	6,66	28,57	14,28	18
		% of Total	2	12	4	18
	medium	Count	13	12	6	31
		% within education	41,93	38,7	19,35	100
		% within motivation	86,66	57,14	42,85	62
		% of Total	26	24	12	62
	high	Count	1	3	6	10
		% within education	10	30	60	100
		% within motivation	6,66	14,28	42,85	20
		% of Total	2	6	12	20
Total		Count	15	21	14	50
		% within education	30	42	28	100
		% within motivation	100	100	100	100
		% of Total	30	42	28	100
Chi-Square Tests						
	Value	df		Asymp. Sig. (2-sided)		
Pearson Chi-Square	10,194	4	0,037			

Table 3. Crosstab: initial motivation in relation with family's cultural level

			Initial motivation categories			Total
			motivated	indifferent	contrary	
psychopathological categories	nevrosis	Count	10	7	2	19
		% within diagnosis	52,63	36,84	10,52	100
		% within motivation	66,66	33,33	14,28	38
		% of Total	20	14	4	38
	psychosis	Count		5		5
		% within diagnosis		100		100
		% within motivation		23,8		10

			Initial motivation categories			Total
			motivated	indifferent	contrary	
		% of Total		10		10
	borderline	Count	5	9	12	26
		% within diagnosis	19,23	34,61	46,15	100
		% within motivation	33,33	42,85	85,71	52
		% of Total	10	18	24	52
Total		Count	15	21	14	50
		% within diagnosis	30	42	28	100
		% within motivation	100	100	100	100
		% of Total	30	42	28	100
Chi-Square Tests						
	Value	df		Asymp. Sig. (2-sided)		
Pearson Chi-Square	16,743	4	0,002			

Table 4. Crosstab: initial motivation in relation with diagnostic categories

With respect to gender (table 2 a), motivated are prevalently females, while indifferent and contrary are prevalently males; these differences are statistically significant (p=0.033). This could be explained by the general tendency of females to be more reflexive and capable of insight than males teenagers, added to the fact that in our sample females are older than males and then more mature.

With regard to the educational level of family (table 2b), the most of motivated adolescents come from family with a middle educational level, the most of indifferent come from family with a low educational level, and contrary prevalently come from family with high educational level (p=0.033). Considering initial motivation in relation with nosographic categories, anxiety disorders and eating disorders are the most frequent diagnosis among motivated; acute psychosis, mood disorders and borderline mental retardation (70<QI<85) are more frequent among indifferent; conduct disorders and personality disorders are prevalent among contrary adolescents (p=0.007).

We considered motivation categories in relation to Kernberg's personality organisation categories too. It is interesting to note that the association between motivation categories and personality organisation categories (motivated -nevrosis, indifferent- psychosis and contrary-borderline), as showed in table 2c, reminds about the kind of bond that usually characterises the clinical relationship with the patient according to different psychofunctional level: the neurotic one (patients motivated to get better given their good reality test and a differentiated sense of social tact and sensitivity), borderline one (patients ambivalent and often oppositive towards therapist, given their lack of capacity for a mature empathy with others, and a lack of mature evaluation of other people, who are seen either as idealized, persecutory or devalued persons), psychotic one (patients often not conscious of their diseases, with a rigid relational modalities and then mainly indifferent towards therapy).

The aim of the diagnostic process, and overall aim of the last interview, was to create a relationship with the patient whose objective was to become aware of the disease and to want to change. So we tried to change the situation where the specialist evaluates the patient and at the end delivers a verdict - instead we tried to build a collaborative relation with adolescent where the main objective is to give a sense to the symptoms, to verify where the adolescent had stopped and to make the therapy to be perceived as something useful.

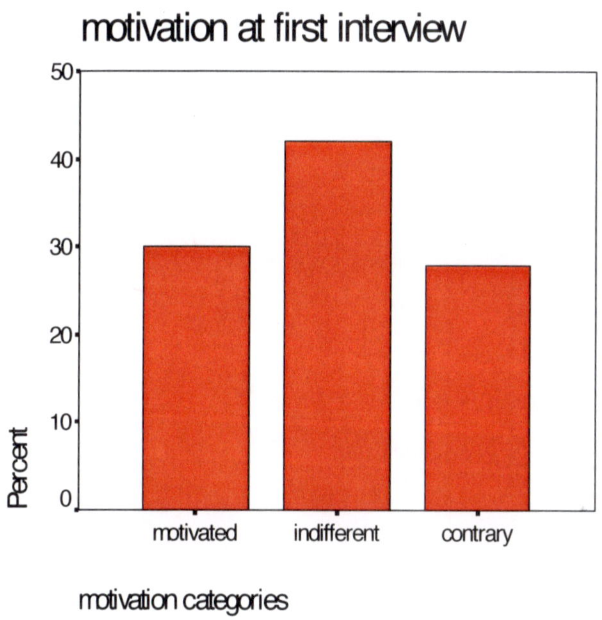

Scheme 1. Motivation at the beginning of the psychodiagnostic process

Adolescent's motivation was evaluated again at the end of the diagnosis process (basing on the same elements). The result was an increase of motivated and a decrease of indifferent and contrary adolescents (scheme 2), without relevant difference regarding gender within the three categories ($p=0.19$). The relation between motivation and diagnosis looses statistical significance too ($p=0.09$), whereas educational level remains significant in regard to adolescent's motivation (X2=11.38 (DF4), $p=0.023$). This result suggests that sociocultural aspects (like educational background) influences thinking capacity more than other more constitutional factors (like gender or psychiatric disorder); moreover, it could make operators inclined to differentiate the way of approaching psychopathology in case of particular cultural conditions, like the realization of more supportive rather than expressive intervention with people coming from a low socio-cultural background. It is interesting to note that the change to a motivated category is bigger among contrary than among indifferent adolescents: actually first halved during the diagnostic process, showing major capacities of mobilization (compare scheme 1 and 2). This could be linked to what was said before about the psychopathological features of these subjects: indifferent who are mainly psychotic organised are characterised by a defending setting and a psychorelational functioning which are less flexible and changeable than the one of contraries who enter mainly the borderline and neurotic psycho structural organisations.

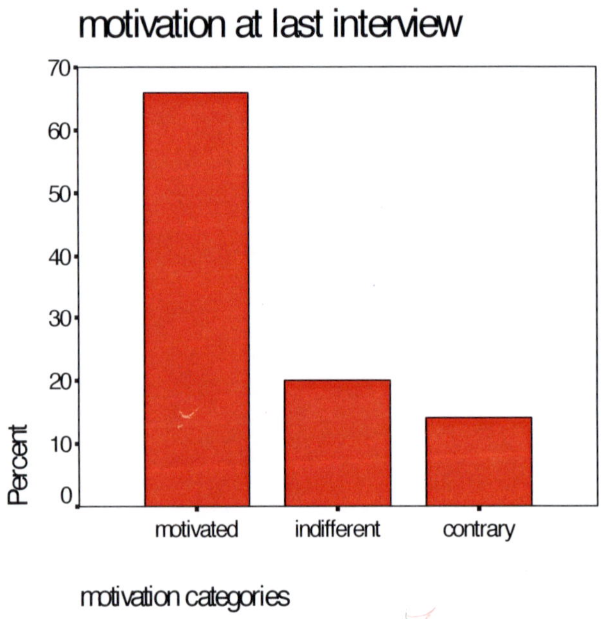

Scheme 2. Motivation at the end of the psychodiagnostic process

Evaluation of adolescents and their family showed, among contrary subjects, high frequency of difficult relationships and conflict with parents. This aspect seems preponderant in influencing the adolescent's feeling towards the specialist and psychological space. It is as if the difficulty with the parents is expressed by the difficulty and refusal in regards to psychiatric consultation, to which the adolescent has been lead by parents rather than coming by him self. In these cases, focusing on problematic relations and working on the relationship with the parental couple in terms of separation/ individuation, seems to favour the use of psychodiagnostic space as one's own rather than as something to be used to attack parents. This was shown by contrary adolescents as major capacity to thinking for them selves, to recognise personal difficulties and to accept help to sort them out. Contrary adolescents, even if more oppositional evidently, are more "malleable" than indifferent adolescents whose defences are rigid and whose emotive distance makes it difficult to establish an emphatic relationship.

A nine months follow up have permitted verification of therapeutic compliance and clinical evolution. 84% of the adolescents are compliant, 8% have dropped out and 8% have never started psychotherapy. 62% of the adolescents have improved, 34% have not varied and 4% have got worse. There are significant statistical differences both in regard to therapeutic compliance and clinical evolution: motivated and indifferent adolescents mainly follow the therapeutic suggestion at the end of the diagnostic procedure, whereas contrary do not even start therapy (p=0.006) (scheme 3). In parallel after nine months motivated get better, indifferent do not vary and contrary adolescents do not vary or get worse (p=0.000) (scheme 4). The evidence of a missed clinical improvement nine months later even if indifferent are compliant for 90%, suggests - and confirms what said before about that - the presence of stronger rigidity of personality structure and defence mechanisms and/or necessity of a longer period to get better in these subjects.

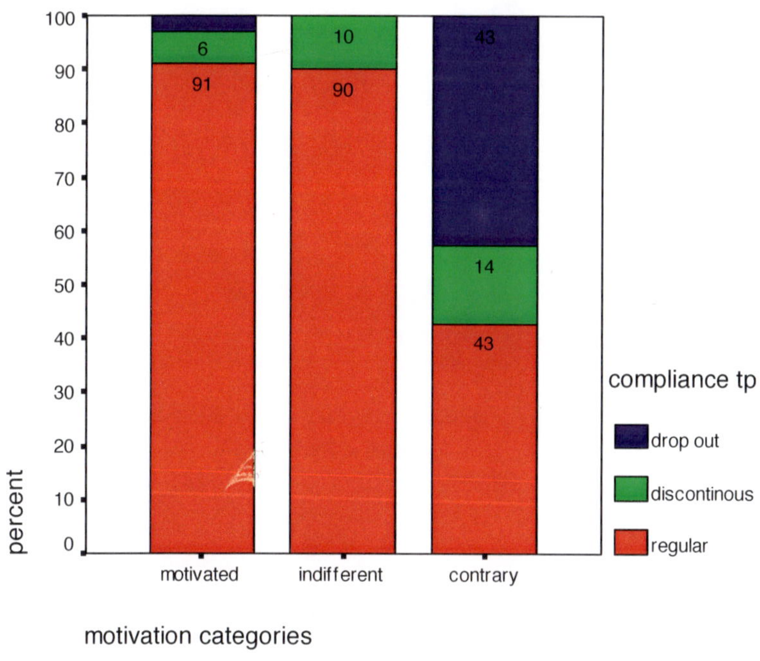

Scheme 3. Motivation in relation with therapeutic compliance after nine months by the beginning of the semiresidential treatment

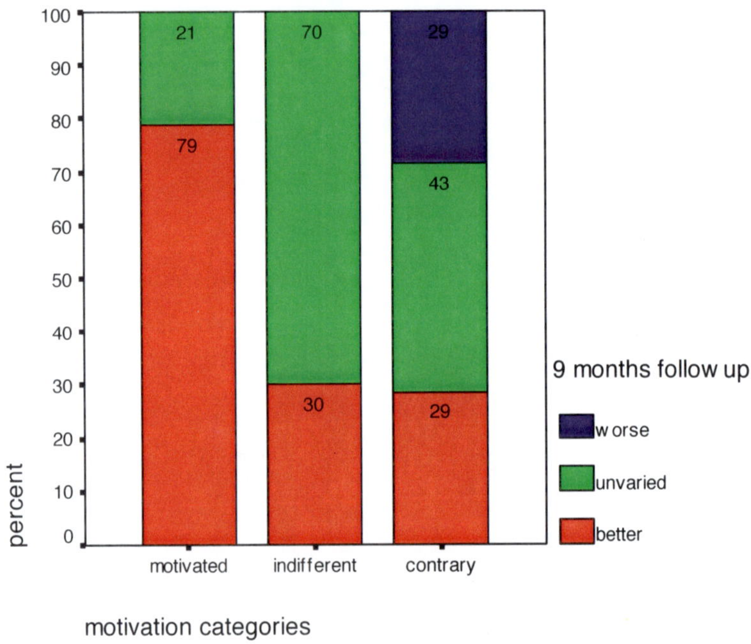

Scheme 4. Motivation in relation with outcome nine month by the beginning of the semiresidential treatment.

This result is relevant because it indicates that adolescent's motivation is linked not only to therapeutic compliance but also to therapeutic efficacy. In fact the elements we considered to define motivation are significant ingredients to build an alliance relationship; this one is an important factor in regard to efficacy of therapeutic process [20], [14], [5], [8],[3].

Significant, statistically only in the latter case, the result about parents' collaboration in regard to therapeutic compliance and clinical evolution: 10% of adolescents do not start multimodal treatment or drop out among supportive families, whereas the percentage becomes 30% among not supportive families. With respect to clinical evolution: nine months later there was a clinical improvement in 73% of cases with supportive families, while the improvement regarding 31% of subjects with not supportive families (p=0.005).

This data seems to indicate that parental support for adolescents is more important to the efficacy of intervention than to compliance, as if adolescent's motivation was fundamental to start treatment, but then the family's support becomes significant as well to get clinically better.

5. Romeo (R), 18 years old: Reports diagnostic interviews by interviewer's words

5.1. First diagnostic session

Yesterday R's mother (Mrs A) phoned to confirm the appointment and asked if it would be possible to speak to me before his son would. Today Mrs A arrived at the Institute on time and the secretary found her screaming asking for someone, from the balcony upstairs on the first floor. Mrs A said she couldn't find anyone immediately upon entering the building and she didn't know where to go. Mrs A asked the secretary if she could speak to me before I saw R (R was waiting into the car). The secretary said she could spend the first 10 minutes with me whilst R was present – then she went to get R.

After I had introduced myself, we entered the room together and R's mother started to speak to me about R. "R has been suffering panic attacks for 4 months, he has got very nervous, he can't sleep, he has a lot of difficulties with his exams, he needs help in facing going to university, panic attacks, girls..." Furthermore she asked for medication to help him to sleep. She was very agitated and I felt R's anxiety rising while she was speaking. After a while I asked her to leave and wait for R. Then I asked R what he thought and he replied that what his mother had said was true, and he started to tell me about his panic attacks. They started since February when he had to do his first exam. He was at home, having a shower; his heart started to beat faster, he couldn't understand what was going on and he went to his mum (who was in the kitchen) to ask for help. I wondered within myself what he was doing or thinking while having a shower. His mum suggested he drink a glass of water but it didn't work. His legs and arms started to tremble and he was not able to control them. So his mum took him to the hospital where he had a lot of tests; everything was all right medically.

The second panic attack came a month later, at home too, nobody was in. R called his dad who went home and took R to the hospital again. Then panic attacks became more frequent: until two weeks ago they were every day. During these two last weeks R has been feeling a bit better (the exams have finished). His General Practitioner (GP) did not prescribe any medication, instead he suggested R come to the Service. I asked him what he thought about that and he answered he preferred not to take medication at that moment. I asked him about University and he told me the choice to go on to study was a very important one. Before he had been working at his stepfather's shop for nearly one year. Now he has to study a lot, he has no more time for friends and recreation. His life consists of going to university then coming back home and so on again, every day. He did not look worried or sad saying this. He doesn't want to give university up "even if it causes my panic attacks". His words made me remember that his mum had said that 'there are guys who are able to study and guys who aren't able to bear the burden and R should understand if he's able or not; he could eventually leave university...'

After about 20 minutes someone knocked on the door, twice. I went to open it and it was R's mum who wanted to tell me she'd wait for R outside, in the car. In the meantime she was trying to look behind me to see R, at the same time, looking at me making a lot of signs with her face and her hands as if to say "is it all right with him?" I closed the door with a gentle smile and went back to my seat feeling annoyed; I looked at R with a questioning glance. He did not say anything about his mum, he did not seem ashamed or embarrassed or annoyed. He seemed to me a bit relieved instead. I asked him more about his parents: R's mum is from South Italy while his father is North Italian. They divorced when R was 6 because his father had an affair. His mum, who now is a housewife, has been living with another man for 10 years. He told me about the first time he'd met his mother's partner, saying that he'd liked him from the start.

R said he gets on very well with both his dad and his stepfather. It seemed to me it was very important for R to tell me that everything is all right with his family. This picture (intrusive and anxious mum, close family, worry about school, not many friends) gave me the image of a little boy, even though I was listening to a tall, broad, handsome man of 18 years. I felt a sort of big gap between his physical appearance and the way in which his mum treated him plus the way in which his symptoms seemed to ask for care. R was very keen to go on with interviews (what struck me was that he spoke about finding a way to face panic attacks rather then a way to rid himself of them). We agreed to see each other next week at the same time.

5.2. Second diagnostic session

R arrived on time, brought by his stepfather who waited for him outside. R had had his hair cut and he was wearing a cap that he did not take off. He started to tell me about his last panic attack that had happened while he was reading an article about a 12 y.o. girl's death. R told me that horror films made him have panic attacks as well. I asked him what he'd felt about the girl's death and he was able to say only that he'd felt strange "how can things like that happen?" Then he told me yesterday he went to his GP who prescribed R some medication (paroxetine) for his shaking. He went on to speak about his panic attacks, how they happen, how he feels and so on, talking very fast and repeating the same things. R links them to the fear of exams, stubbornly, as if he had to convince himself about that.

R said he gets very anxious thinking about his exams. I asked him what he's scared of. He's scared of failing. What could happen if you failed an exam? R answered he wouldn't know what to do. I asked him if it's something to do with him only and he said that he's worried what others could say about him too. He was getting very anxious so I asked him what he was going to do after his graduation. He seemed relieved to change the topic and said he'd like to get a job and a house. I asked him if he would like to live with anyone; he answered it doesn't matter. I asked him about girlfriends: he has never had one and he doesn't care...now he has no time to think of this. He told me he used to speak with his mother about these things, also because she asks him a lot...even if it is not so easy and a bit embarrassing too, he added. I wondered whether he wouldn't find easier to talk to his father about things like this, "between men"...R looked a bit thoughtful then said that yes, probably it'd be easier.

What about friends? He has a few good friends, but now he has no time anymore to go out with them. I asked R what his mum would think about him going to live on his own. R said that it would be difficult for her to accept, but she knows it'll happen one day. He told me he gets on very well with his mum, she's very supportive and that's been very important for R. I asked R if anyone else in his family was suffering panic attacks. He, looking as if he had been discovered of some secret, answered that his mum had had panic attacks too, when she was the same age as R. According to this she used to tell him not to worry because "panic attacks are going to stop spontaneously". He did not look very sure about this. His voice and way of talking made me ask him whether he's worried about his mum. "Yes" he said "because she's worried about me". I took up it looks like a sort of vicious circle and R agreed but he did not add anything else.

R likes music very much; he can play the piano (he had studied in a music school for some years). His dream is to become a musician...I took up he had chosen quite a different subject (computers) and R said it was because after you qualify you can get a job easier.

Towards the end of the session I asked him how he felt and he said with a smile he's feeling much better, he needs to talk to somebody about himself and what's happening "I should have come before". I thought he had been saying only a little of the whole and the way in which he used to speak about his panic attacks (using the most of our sessions talking about them) seemed to me a sort of defense for avoiding different topics or for not telling me something deeper.

R's mother phoned to the service saying that R wasn't very well so he could not come today. He'd phone when he was better. The secretary who answered the phone, told her we would send a new appointment anyway and R's mum said not to do that because R would phone when he felt ready to ask for another appointment.

It was phoned for another appointment.

5.3. Third diagnostic session

R arrived on time, he looked anxious as usual, but smiling. As soon as he sat down he started to say that he feels much better. I asked him what had happened (I was referring to last missed interview) and R told me he had managed to confide in his father about something he had been keeping to himself and that had been really hard to bear. He added it had been easier to speak between men and his father had supported and reassured him, so now he feels really well. Furthermore the day after he had spoken with his dad he managed to speak to his mum as well "so now it's all sorted out". He told me when the first panic attack came he was masturbating under the shower. He felt he had damaged his body, he felt really ashamed and scared at the same time. Until now he has been feeling that something wrong had happened to him, he's been fearing he couldn't masturbate anymore, he's been fearing about what might happen with girls.... Now the truth has come out he feels really better. It's all over. He has no fear anymore; he has not had panic attacks since he managed to talk about it. I asked what his mum had said. She had told R he shouldn't have worried, that's normal, besides the same had happened to his father years ago (!). The mother told him she thought it might be something to do with sex and now he has told her she feels better. R told me he should have spoken before. I commented he'd probably needed a period in order to understand and to face a lot of feelings that had been coming out, not always easy to deal with. He agreed and repeated he had felt really ashamed and guilty. In particular, he had been scared of what his mum could have thought about him. I took up that it was difficult to say such personal things to his mum, especially now that he's growing up, and that growing up could be also be something to feel guilty about. He agreed and said it had been very important to speak to his dad before... because he's a man.

We spoke a bit about girls; R got a bit anxious and it seemed to me he wanted to censor the topic. He repeated he's very well, he wants to go on with University, he's able to go out again and so on. I felt he was censoring interviewing as well so I asked him openly what he had thought about continuing to come here. He seemed relieved by my question and answered that he felt he had received the help he needed and that he was very grateful. I proposed to him to take some time to think about that and to see each other next week again...he seemed more agitated and in trouble, then he repeated his thanks for the help he has received and that he preferred to stop there, because he was really OK and he did not need help anymore.

I took up his anxiety (probably linked to sexuality and body) and his fear in facing it: I told him I thought it would be important for him to have a deeper look inside; I also said that, looking at his anxious state, I could feel that perhaps it was too much for him at that moment and that it was important and right to respect his feelings of being scared by those thoughts and emotions. So I reassured R about the possibility of finding someone to help him here, if and when he decides to ask for further help.

We said goodbye each other.

Six months later, R came and ask for psychotherapy. He was chosen a male therapist for him. The compliance has been good from the beginning.

6. Conclusions

Results of this study suggest that it is possible to work on adolescent's motivation using relational instruments. Data from follow up indicates the importance of preparing the adolescent and his family, since during the diagnosis process, for treatment with the object of fair compliance and clinical evolution. With regard to that this paper suggests that an improvement of interviews, specifically used to discuss therapeutic referral, could be methodologically useful to improve motivation. In conclusion the motivation influences both compliance and clinical evolution, so it is important to pay attention to motivation since the start of the diagnosis process. This study moreover suggests that it is important to work with adolescent's parents too to obtain effective results from the treatment. If we consider that a missed therapy opportunity for psychological disease during the developmental age could become a psychiatric disease in adult age [6], [27], then what mentioned before gains the meaning of prevention too.

Author details

Gatta Michela[1], Testa C. Paolo[2], Del Col Lara[2], Spoto Andrea[3], Dal Zotto Lara[1], De Sauma Maxim[4] and Battistella Pier Antonio[1]

1 Woman and Child Department-University of Padua, Italy

2 Neuropsychiatric Unit of Child and Adolescent - ULSS Padua, Italy

3 Department of General Psychology- University of Padua, Italy

4 Brent Centre For Young People, London, UK

References

[1] Achenbach, T. M, & Rescorla, L. A. Manual for ASEBA School-Age Forms and Profiles. Burlington: University of Vermont, Research Center for Children; (2001).

[2] American Psychiatric AssociationDiagnostic and statistical Manual for Mental Disorders, Axis V. Washington DC: American Psychiatric Association; (1994).

[3] Barber, J. P, et al. Therapeutic alliance as predictor of outcome in treatment of cocaine dependence. Psychotherapy Research (1999)., 9, 54-73.

[4] Bronstein, C, & Flanders, S. The development of a therapeutic space in a first contact with adolescents. Journal of Child Psychotherapy (1998)., 24(1), 5-35.

[5] Castonguay, L. G, et al. Predicting the effect of cognitive therapy for depression: a study of unique and common factors. Cons Clin Psychol (1996)., 64, 497-504.

[6] Ferdinand, R. F, & Verhulst, F. C. Psychopathology from adolescence into young adulthood: an 8 years follow up study. Am J Psychiatry (1995)., 152(11), 1586-1594.

[7] Frieswyk, S. H, et al. Therapeutic Alliance: its place as a process and outcome variable in dynamic psychotherapy research. J Cons Clin Psychol (1986)., 54(1), 32-38.

[8] Gaston, L, et al. Alliance, technique and their interactions in predicting outcome of behavioural, cognitive and brief dynamic therapy. Psychotherapy Research (1998)., 8, 190-209.

[9] Gatta, M, & Giovanatto, C. Condini A. L'attività clinica in un servizio di psicopatologia dell'adolescenza: studio longitudinale ed epidemiologico di una casistica ambulatoriale. Giornale It. Psicopat. Psichiatria Inf. Adolesc. (2003). X(2): 107-120.

[10] Gatta, M, Giovanatto, C, Salviato, C, Testa, P, Acconcia, C, & Condini, A. La relazione di alleanza con l'adolescente: centralità della motivazione. Giornale Italiano di psicopatologia e psichiatria dell'infanzia e dell'adolescenza (2004). XI(2): 197-209.

[11] Gatta, M, Spoto, A, Testa, P, Svanellini, L, Lai, J, Salis, M, De Sauma, M, & Battistella, P. A. Adolescent's insight within the working alliance: A bridge between diagnostic and psychotherapeutic processes. Adolescent Health, Medicine and Therapeutics (2010). , 1, 45-52.

[12] Gatta, M, Spoto, A, Svanellini, L, Lai, J, Testa, C. P, & Battistella, P. A. Alliance with patient and collaboration with parents throughout the psychotherapeutic process with children and adolescents: a pilot study. Giornale Italiano di Psicopatologia (2012). , 18(1), 28-34.

[13] Hintikka, U, Laukkanen, E, Marttunen, M, & Lehtonen, J. Good working alliance and psychotherapy are associated with positive changes in cognitive performance among adolescent psychiatric inpatients. Bull Menninger Clin (2006). , 70(4), 316-35.

[14] Horvath, A. O, & Symonds, B. D. Relation between working alliance and outcome in psychotherapy: a meta-analysis. Journal of Counseling Psychology (1991). , 38, 139-149.

[15] Horvath, A. O, & Luborsky, L. The role of therapeutic alliance in Psychotherapy. J Cons Clin Psychol (1993). , 61, 561-573.

[16] Kernberg, O. F. A Psychoanalytic Theory of Personality Disorders. In John F. Clarkin & Mark F. Lenzenweger (eds.) Major theories of personality disorder. New York: Guilford; (1996).

[17] Laufer, M, & Laufer, M. E. Adolescence and developmental breakdown. New Haven: Yale University Press; (1984).

[18] Laufer, M. The suicidal Adolescent. London: Karnac Books; (1995).

[19] Laufer et al(1997). Adolescent breakdown and beyond. London: Karnac Books; 1997

[20] Luborsky, L. The therapeutic alliance measures as predictors of future benefits of psychotherapy. Paper presented at the annual meeting of the Society for psychotherapy Research, Wintergreen, VA; (1990).

[21] Luborsky, L. The therapeutic alliances as predictors of psychotherapy outcomes: factors explaining the predictive process. In Horvath AO., Greenberg LS. The working alliance: Theory, Research and Practice. New York: John Wiley and Sons; (1994). , 38-55.

[22] Marcelli, D, & Bracconier, A. Adolescence et Psychopathologie. Paris: Masson; (1983).

[23] Marcelli, D, & Bracconier, A. La consultazione terapeutica. In Adolescenza e Psicopatologia, Milano: Masson; (1998). cap. 21, , 505-523.

[24] Marmar, C. R, & Gaston, L. Manual for the California Psychotherapy Alliance Scale-CALPAS. Unpublished Manuscript, S.Francisco: Department of Psychiatry, University of California; (1988).

[25] Marmar, C. R, Weiss, D. S, & Gaston, L. Towards the validation of the California Therapeutic Alliance Rating System. Cons Clin Psychol (1989). , 1, 46-52.

[26] Martin, D. J, Garske, J, Davis, P, & Katherine, M. Relation of the therapeutic alliance with outcome and other variables: a meta-analytic review. J Consult Clin Psychol. (2000). , 68(3), 438-50.

[27] Newman, D. L, et al. Psychiatric disorder in a birth cohort of young adult: prevalence, comorbidity, clinical significance, and new case incidence from ages 11 to 21. J Counsult Clin Psycol (1996). , 64(3), 552-562.

[28] Pani, R, Biolcati, R, & Sagliaschi, S. Psicologia clinica e psicopatologia per l'educazione e la formazione,. Bologna Italy: Il Mulino; (2009).

[29] Piper, W. E, et al. Quality of object relations versus interpersonal functioning as predictors of therapeutic alliance and psychotherapy outcome. Journal of Nervous and Mental Disease (1991). , 179, 432-438.

[30] Ryan, V. L, & Cicchetti, D. V. Predicting quality of alliance in the initial psychotherapy interview. Journal of Nervous and Mental Disease (1985). , 173, 171-125.

[31] Startup, M, Jackson, M. C, & Bendix, S. The current validity of the Global Assesment of Functioning (GAF). British Journal of Clinical Psychology (2002). , 46(1), 126-142.

[32] Wilson, P. A View of intervention in Adolescence. In: Adolescence (1976). Monograph Not published., 6, 27-35.

[33] WHOICD 10, International Classification of Diseases, Geneva: World Health Organization; (1994).

Chapter 12

Current Advances in the Treatment of Major Depression: Shift Towards Receptor Specific Drugs

Ashok Kumar Jainer, Rajkumar Kamatchi,
Marek Marzanski and Bettahalasoor Somashekar

Additional information is available at the end of the chapter

1.Introduction

Depression is one of the most common psychiatric disorders with a life time prevalence of 10% - 20% in the general population and women being at twice the risk of developing depression compared to men (Kessler et al., 2007). Literature suggests that prevalence of depression is higher in patients with chronic illnesses (Katon 2003). It is estimated that around 11%-15% of patients with diabetes, 15%-23% of patients with coronary artery disease, and 9%-31% of stroke patients suffer from depression. The prevalence of depression has been reported even higher among patients with chronic neurological illness such as parkinson's disease (20%-30%) and multiple sclerosis (16%- 30%).

The high prevalence of depression in the general population has an adverse impact on the community and depression affects the patients well being and their productivity in life. It is reported as the third leading cause of disability as measured by disability adjusted life years (DALYs) and is projected to became the second leading cause in 2020 (WHO 2012). Furthermore, the life time risk of suicide in patients diagnosed with depression is as high as 6% (Inskip et al., 1998).Therefore effective treatment of depression is very important to prevent disability.

The management of depressive disorder is challenging for most clinicians. Over the last 50 years, repeated attempts were made to develop a novel antidepressant, with the intention of maximising the efficacy and minimising the side-effect profile. The research has moved from time to time as in the beginning it was focussed on noradrenaline neurotransmission, later on serotonin neurotransmission. In the last decade, it has moved towards dual action and receptor specific agents. In this chapter we review and update the high quality evidence for pharmacotherapies of depressive disorder and highlight the future trends in the development of new promising antidepressants.

2. Evolution of pharmacotherapy for depression

In 1957, the antidepressant property of isoniazid was discovered serendipitously and this has led the pharmacological research to develop drugs which inhibit monoamine oxidase and drugs which block the reuptake of noradrenaline. This resulted in the development of various monoamine oxidase inhibitors (MAOI) and tricyclic antidepressants (TCA) which dominated the treatment of depression for over 30 years, predominantly TCA's. In the 1990's selective serotonin reuptake inhibitors (SSRI) were introduced and quickly they became the first line of treatment for depression. These agents were reported equally efficacious with less side-effects and are safer in overdoses. Over the last decade the research was focussed to enhance the efficacy, accelerate the onset of action and reduce the side- effects. In this regard, many newer agents were introduced with different mechanisms of action and proved very helpful in many aspects. They include noradrenaline reuptake inhibitors (NARI), serotonin and noradrenaline reuptake inhibitors (SNRI), noradrenergic and specific serotonergic antidepressant (NaSSA) and more recently agomelatine.

The combination of SSRI with another newer antidepressant has proved very effective for treatment resistant depression (Blier et al., 2010). RCTs have shown superior effectiveness for combination of antidepressant and psychological intervention (cognitive behavioural therapy) compared to psychotherapy alone (Cuijpers et al., 2009). In addition, studies have confirmed the usefulness of long term antidepressant treatment to prevent further relapses (Nierenberg et al., 2003).

The mechanism of action of currently available antidepressants is mostly monoamine based. Their efficacy is relatively modest and the benefits may be limited by poor tolerability. This has led research to search for antidepressants with different mechanisms of action including multimodal serotonergic agents, triple uptake inhibitors, neurokinin based drugs and glutamate based agents.

3. Monoamine hypothesis of depression

The monoamine hypothesis remains the main aetiological theory of depression. It suggests that depression occurs as a result of an abnormality in the monoamine neurotransmitter system in the brain. The monoamines involved are serotonin, noradrenaline and dopamine.

Numerous abnormalities in the monoamine system have been linked with depressive symptoms in patients suffering major depression. The earliest evidence came from the observation that reserpine causes depletion of monoamines and induces a state similar to depression (Healy & Savage 1998). Studies have reported abnormalities in the metabolism of these neurotransmitters as well as changes in the neuroendocrine measures which are affected by these monoamines. These include decreased plasma tryptophan levels, a precursor of serotonin, noted in untreated depressed patients (Anderson et al., 1990) and low cerebrospinal fluid (CSF) concentrations of 5-hydroxyindoleacetic acid (5-HIAA), the metabolite of serotonin, found in depressed patients who attempted suicide (Brown and Linnoila 1990). Furthermore, depletion of serotonin or noradrenaline in patients who were recovered from their depressive episode made them more vulnerable to relapses (Smith et al., 1997; Berman et al., 1999).

Monoamine theory has been supported by the receptor changes that occur during treatment with antidepressant medications whose main mechanisms of action are to either increase the synaptic levels of monoamines or to have an effect on post-synaptic receptors. Initially due to low levels of neurotransmitters, the post-synaptic receptors become supersensitive. On antidepressant treatment, the levels of neurotransmitters are increased and the receptors go into a persistent activated mode. This may be a cause of delay in the onset of action of antidepressants. During the long term treatment, the alpha- 2 auto receptors in noradrenergic system become desensitized resulting in additional release of noradrenaline from the neurons. Further studies have helped to recognise the different roles of various monoamine receptors and the effects of the drugs acting on these receptors.

The possible pharmacological properties of the antidepressants acting via neurotransmitters on the various receptors are shown in Table 1.

Pharmacological properties	Possible clinical effects
Inhibition of MAO	Alleviation of depression
Inhibition of NA re-uptake	Alleviation of depression
Inhibition of 5HT re-uptake	Alleviation of depression
	Sexual dysfunction, anorexia, gastro-intestinal distress, headache, dizziness
Activation of 5HT1a receptors	Alleviation of depression
Antagonism of 5HT2 receptors	Alleviation of depression, weight gain
Antagonism of 5HT3 receptors	Alleviation of anxiety and psychotic symptoms
Activation of 5HT3 receptors	Nausea/ vomiting
Antagonism at H1 receptors	Potentiation of central depressant drugs, sedation, drowsiness, confusion
Antagonism at muscarnic receptors	Blurred vision, dry mouth, sinus tachycardia, constipation, urinary retention, confusion
Antagonism at alpha 1 receptors	Postural hypotension, dizziness, reflex tachycardia, sedation, drowsiness
Antagonism at alpha 2 receptors	Alleviation of depression

(Adapted from Quasim and Kumar 1999)

Table 1. Possible pharmacological properties of antidepressants.

4. Increasing synaptic levels of monoamines

4.1. Tricyclic Antidepressants (TCA)

Tricyclics increase the levels of monoamine neurotransmitters in the synapse by inhibiting re-uptake of both serotonin and noradrenaline back into the pre-synaptic neurons. They also act on various other receptors including cholinergic and histaminergic receptors which relate to their side-effects. They have cardiac membrane stabilising action which can cause arrthymias and heart blocks. The use of TCAs has declined over time due to poor tolerability and high toxicity in overdoses, particularly cardiac side-effects. Repeated attempts to modify this side-effect has led to the development of Lofepramine, a relatively new TCA which has less cardiac side-effects and seems to be safer in overdose, while its efficacy remains similar to that of other tricyclics. There is good evidence that TCAs are more effective in severe depression, particularly inpatients compared to SSRI's (Geddes et al., 2002) and a small number of TCA's are still used in clinical practice.

4.2. Monoamine Oxidase Inhibitors (Irreversible MAOI)

Traditional MAOIs increase the levels of neurotransmitters by irreversibly blocking monoamine oxidase enzymes in the synapse and the enzyme blockade lasts for two weeks even after stopping MAOI. They block both MAO-A and MAO-B enzymes, not only in the nervous system but also in the gut. As a result, they have a dangerous interaction with tyramine containing foods and sympathomimetic drugs causing a hypertensive crisis. This restricts patients from consuming tyramine containing foods and certain other medications such as cold remedies and cough suppressants.

MAOIs are now used as third line drug in the treatment of depression due to these limitations. They are very useful in patients who do not respond to SSRI and TCA. It is also useful in atypical depression (depression characterised by mood changes, increased sleep and appetite, weight gain and sensitivity to rejection) and in phobic anxiety disorders. A recent review concluded that MAOI, **Phenelzine** remains as the gold standard treatment for atypical depression (Stewart 2007).

4.3. Reversible inhibitor of monoamine oxidase –Type A (RIMA)

These new generation MAOIs are more selective in their action, in that they block only MAO-A not MAO-B enzymes. The inhibition is reversible and it doesn't require the lengthy wash-out periods after stopping them. The efficacy of **Moclobemide,** the only drug currently available in this group, is similar to other MAOIs but with a much reduced possibility of hypertensive crisis. However it causes serotonin syndrome in combination with an SSRI. The therapeutic dose range is between 150-600mgs/day. It is shown to produce rapid and significant improvement in both social functioning and quality of life (Lorinquivst et al., 1994).

5. Selective Serotonin Reuptake Inhibitors (SSRI)

The discovery of SSRIs in 1989 was a turning point in the treatment of depression. It switched the emphasis from noradrenergic to serotonergic system and stimulated research on serotonin receptors. SSRIs are more selective in inhibiting only serotonin reuptake and have no action on histamine, adrenaline and cholinergic receptors. Therefore their tolerability is much better compared to TCAs or MAOIs. They have similar efficacy to older drugs, but better tolerability and safety in overdoses and have become the first line of treatment for depression over the last two decades. There are six drugs available in this group namely **fluoxetine, fluvoxamine, paroxetine, sertraline, citalopram and escitalopram**.

Although these six medications differ in their chemical structure and pharmacokinetics (Van Harten 1993), there are no major differences in their efficacy or side-effect profile (Aguglia et al., 1993). The common side-effects include gastro-intestinal problems, dry mouth, sweating, headache, asthenia and sexual dysfunction such as ejaculatory delay/failure and anorgasmia. SSRIs have fewer drug interactions compared to older drugs and the most important one is with MAOI when concurrent administration may cause serotonin syndrome. Therefore MAOIs and RIMA are contraindicated in combination with SSRIs and there should be a washout period before swapping them.

The safety profile of these drugs was found to be similar (Price et al., 1996) and they do not cause physical dependence. However, abrupt withdrawal or marked reduction in the dose of SSRI may lead to the development of discontinuation symptoms. The common symptoms are dizziness, paraesthesia, tremors, anxiety, nausea and increased heart rate which may last for up to 10 days. Paroxetine causes discontinuation symptoms more often (5.1%) than other SSRIs (0.06- 0.9%).

Escitalopram, the active isomer of citalopram, is a highly selective SSRI and has shown better efficacy in the treatment of severe depression, both in effect size and time of onset of action (Azorin et al., 2004). In a recent multiple-treatment meta-analysis, escitalopram and sertraline have shown the best profile of acceptability and sertraline had the most favourable balance between benefits, tolerability and cost-effectiveness (Cipriani et al., 2009).

6. Serotonin Antagonist and Reuptake Inhibitors (SARI)

Trazodone and nefazodone belong to this group and chemically they are phenylpiperazines. They have dual action on the serotonergic system, as they are potent 5HT2 receptor antagonists and weak reuptake inhibitors. This combination of actions enhances 5HT1a mediated neurotransmission and is thus effective in the treatment of depression.

Trazodone has been available since 1998 but it is used infrequently as antidepressant because of its sedating property. Rather it is been prescribed in lower doses as hypnotic in addition to SSRIs. Sexual side-effects are less frequent but it can cause priapism in some patients. A recent review (Papakostas & Fava 2007) showed that trazodone has efficacy comparable to SSRIs and nefazodone. It is also relatively safe in overdose.

Nefazodone is a derivative of trazodone and is chemically related. It is found to be as effective as TCAs and superior to placebo in daily doses of 200-600mgs (Rickels et al., 1995). Sexual dysfunction was less reported with nefazodone compared with other antidepressants and there were no reports of priapism (Baldwin et al., 1997). It is less sedating than trazodone. However concerns regarding its hepatotoxicity led to withdrawal of nefazodone from the market in most countries.

7. Noradrenaline Reuptake Inhibitors (NARI)

Reboxetine is similar in structure to fluoxetine but it is a relatively selective noradrenaline reuptake inhibitor. Its therapeutic effect is mainly through increasing noradrenaline neurotransmission and it has no interaction with other receptors such as histaminergic, muscarinic or alpha 1, which were responsible for most side-effects associated with TCAs. Therefore reboxetine is useful for patients who could not tolerate tricyclics or who have been treatment resistant to SSRIs.

Reboxetine is equally effective as TCAs in both hospital patients and outpatients (Berzewski et al., 1997; Dubini et al., 1997) and has better efficacy than fluoxetine. It also helps in alleviating anxiety symptoms associated with depression. It has moderately alerting effect and improves the motivation of the patients. The main side-effects are linked to sympathetic overstimulation and include dry mouth, insomnia, sweating, tachycardia, vertigo, urinary hesitancy and impotence. The daily dose range is 4-12mgs.

8. Selective Serotonin and Noradrenaline Reuptake Inhibitors (SNRI)

SNRIs have dual action and inhibit both serotonin and noradrenaline reuptake. They do not act on muscarnic, histaminic or adrenergic receptors. As a result they have more benefits and less side -effects compared to other antidepressants. Venlafaxine, duloxetine and milnacipran belong to this group.

Venlafaxine, a phenylethylamine, inhibits the reuptake of 5HT and NA and at higher doses inhibits the reuptake of dopamine. It has a rapid onset of action and improvement may be noticed within the first week of treatment. This is because of the fast down-regulation of beta receptors induced by venlafaxine, which usually occurs only during long term treatment with other antidepressants (Holliday 1995). Venlafaxine is as effective as imipramine or fluoxetine in doses ranging from 75mgs to 375mgs/day (Guelfi et al., 1995). It is better tolerated compared to TCAs and safer in overdoses. It has less sedative and proconvulsant effects and shows minimal drug interactions. Venlafaxine is also effective in the therapy of treatment resistant depression (Nierenberg et al., 1994).

Desvenlafaxine, a synthetic metabolite of venlafaxine, is a new SNRI available since 2008. Studies have reported that it has short-term efficacy in major depression (Thase et al., 2009) and could improve the social functioning of the patients (Soares et al., 2009).

Duloxetine, another SNRI, is considered as the most potent in this group. It blocks both neurotransmitters equally, whereas venlafaxine has a stronger tendency towards serotonergic system and milnacipran towards noradrenergic system (Nierenberg et al., 1994). A latest review reported that duloxetine is safe and effective in the acute phase treatment of depression at doses of 40-60mgs/day (Mallinckrodt et al., 2006). However it appears to be less effective compared to venlafaxine in both remission and response rates (Vis et al., 2005).

Milnacipran, another drug in this group, is reported to be as effective as TCAs with a 65% response rate and has slightly superior efficacy to SSRIs (Montgomery et al., 1994; Lopes-Ibor et al., 1996). A recent meta-analysis suggested that milnacipran has equal efficacy and tolerability compared to other antidepressants but can be slightly more favourable to TCAs in terms of adverse effects (Nakagawa et al., 2008). Dysuria and headache are the common side-effects.

9. Noradrenergic and Specific Serotonergic Antidepressant (NaSSA)

Mirtazapine and mianserin belong to this group. Mianserin is not used in most countries because of its hepatotoxicity and the risk of neutropenia. Thus mirtazapine is the only agent available in this group.

Mirtazapine has unique pharmacological properties. It increases the release of serotonin and noradrenaline by blocking central alpha 2 auto and heteroreceptors. It has a marginal affinity for alpha 1 receptor and a low affinity for 5HT1a receptor but good affinity for 5HT2 and 5HT3 receptors. The antidepressant effect appears to be a result of increased serotonin and noradrenaline neurotransmission (De Boer & Ruigt 1995). Due to its antihistaminergic action, it acts as a relatively sedative antidepressant although this effect is diminished at higher doses. It also blocks 5HT2 and 5HT3 receptors; therefore the sexual side-effects and nausea are less common compared to SSRIs (Chen et al., 2008).

Mirtazapine has a more rapid onset of action (Thase et al., 2010) and is equally effective as SSRIs (Papakostas et al., 2008). It also showed higher remission rates compared to SSRIs. Its side-effects are relatively mild and transient.

10. Dopamine and Noradrenaline Reuptake Inhibitors (DNRI)

Bupropion is another dual acting agent which inhibits reuptake of dopamine and noradrenaline. It is been used as antidepressant in some countries and in smoking cessation clinics. Its metabolite hydroxybupropion is a potent reuptake inhibitor and it has low receptor blocking effects. It is useful in the treatment of bipolar depression, depression with psychomotor retardation and atypical depression because of its dopamine related activating properties. The main side-effects are caused by dopamine over-stimulation and include nausea, insomnia, agitation, dry mouth, weight loss and psychosis. It also lowers the seizure threshold and fits can occur in 0.5% of patients. In overdoses it leads to hallucinations, tachycardia, seizures and rarely death (Harris et al., 1997; Shrier et al., 2000).

Bupropion was found to be as equally effective and tolerable as SSRIs (Thase et al., 2005). It may be beneficial for patients with symptoms of sleepiness, fatigue, low energy, anhedonia and loss of interest (Papakostas et al., 2006; Nutt et al., 2007).

11. Serotonin reuptake inhibitor and 5HT1a receptor partial agonists

Vilazodone is a relatively new antidepressant which has been available for a year in the United States. It has dual action of inhibiting serotonin reuptake and partial agonism at 5HT1a receptors. It does not cause weight gain and claimed not to cause any sexual side-effects. Nevertheless, compared to other antidepressants, the data regarding its efficacy are limited and more research is required.

12. Melatonin based therapy –Agomelatine

In the last decade, advances in the understanding of the pathophysiology of depression including genetic, neurobiological and neuroimaging studies shifted the focus of research from the monoamines to different theories of depression. One of them assumes that disturbances in the circadian rhythms may play a significant role in the pathogenesis of depression.

The links between circadian disturbances and symptoms of depression such as delay in sleep onset, early morning wakening, fatigue during the day, blunting of normal peaks in subjective energy, mood and alertness are very strong (Germainand Kupfer 2008). Circadian disturbances affect the secretory rhythms of various neuroendocrine hormones such as melatonin, cortisol and noradrenaline. There are also changes in the diurnal variations of core body temperature and plasma cortisol levels. If this internal system desynchronises, the timing of various circadian rhythms is out of phase resulting in depressed mood, sleep changes and impaired neurocognition (Czeisler et al., 2005). Therefore any treatments of depression focusing on circadian rhythm not only restore the sleep-wake cycle but also will have substantial improvements in mood, cognition and day-time fatigue (Hickie & Davenport, 1999).

Melatonin is a hormone naturally secreted by the pineal gland in the body. Its secretion is usually high at night time in normal individuals. It has an important role in the regulation of circadian timing systems by binding to melatonin receptors (MT1 and MT2) in the brain (Weaver 1999). Based on this idea, melatonin based therapies have been developed recently for the treatment of depression.

Agomelatine is a new antidepressant with a unique mechanism of action. It is a selective agonist at MT1 and MT2 receptors and an antagonist at 5HT2b and 5HT2c receptors. It has a rapid absorption rate and peak plasma levels are achieved between 45 and 90min after a single oral dose of 25-50mgs. It has clinically significant antidepressant and anxiolytic effects (de Bodinat et al., 2010; De Beradis et al., 2011). The clinical benefits occur from the combined effects of melatonin and monoamine actions as well as non-circadian processes such as increased production of brain- derived neurotrophic factors (Palzanis et al., 2010). Agomelatine has similar efficacy to SSRIs (Kasper et al., 2010; Hale et al., 2010) and venlafaxine (Kennedy et al., 2008). The common side-effects include nausea, dizziness and headache.

13. Combination treatments for treatment resistant depression

Although the newer antidepressants have better efficacy in the treatment of depression, nearly one third of patients fail to achieve remission. Moreover complete remission is not always possible and partially treated patients are at higher risk of relapse, experience more personal and socioeconomic problems and have poor quality of life. A patient is considered to suffer treatment resistant depression (TRD) if they fail to achieve remission with adequate trials of two different classes of antidepressants. There are few strategies available to tackle treatment resistance including both pharmacological and non-pharmacological therapies.

Combination of two different antidepressants to treat resistant depression has become a common practice. A recent systematic review (Rocha et al., 2012) showed that antidepressant combination was more effective than a single antidepressant in achieving remission. The superior combination was mirtazapine with SSRI. The other effective combinations are mirtazapine and SNRI, SSRI with bupropion, TCA with SSRI and bupropion with venlafaxine or mirtazapine.

Combination of an antidepressant with an antipsychotic is another useful strategy in treating resistant depression. 5HT2a/ 5HT2c antagonist effect of atypical antipsychotics potentiate the efficacy of antidepressants and at times counteract the side-effects of SSRIs. The most useful combination appears to be an SSRI with an atypical antipsychotic (Thase 2002). Weight gain and sedation are the common adverse effects.

The **augmentation** of an antidepressant with lithium, triiodothyronine and omega-3 fatty acids have also been beneficial in some patients. Combinations of pharmacological and non-pharmacological treatments are described in section 14 below.

14. Advances in non-pharmacological treatments of depression

Psychological therapies and physical (non- pharmacological) treatments have been developed and refined in the last few decades. In this section, the evidence of their efficacy in the treatment of depression will be reviewed.

14.1. Psychological interventions

Many psychological interventions have been used in the treatment of depression. These include supportive counselling, cognitive – behavioural therapy (CBT), interpersonal psychotherapy (IPT), mindfulness- based cognitive therapy, problem solving therapy and long term psychodynamic psychotherapy. However, only CBT and IPT have good quality evidence in the treatment of depression either as monotherapy or in combination with antidepressants (Sagar et al., 2009).

Cognitive- behavioural therapy has become a standard treatment for mild and moderate depressive disorders. It may be particularly useful for patients who experience relapse in spite of continuous anti-depressant treatment or for patients with partial response. CBT combines elements from both cognitive theory and behaviour theory of depression. According to cognitive theory maladaptive thinking with regard to self, future and environment (cognitive triad) causes depression. These "core beliefs" become active when people face certain life situations and lead to depressed mood mediated by negative automatic thoughts associated with them. CBT helps patients to understand the links between the thoughts, the emotions and the consequent behaviours and then equip them with alternative thinking styles to cope with day to day problems.

CBT has good efficacy in both achieving remission and reducing the risk of recurrence of depression (Vittengl et al., 2009; Hollon et al., 2005). Combination of CBT and antidepressant is more effective than CBT alone (Cuijpers et al., 2009). Therefore current treatment guidelines recommend combing CBT with antidepressant in partial remissions or treatment resistant patients. CBT can also be implemented in different ways such as internet based CBT, self-help guidebooks or even telephone CBT which can be helpful in primary care (Kessler et al., 2009; Simon et al., 2009).

Interpersonal psychotherapy is another effective psychological intervention used in the treatment of depression. IPT incorporates elements from psychodynamic psychotherapy and CBT. Similar to CBT, it is time-limited and includes structured sessions and homework tasks (Weissman et al., 2007). The therapy focuses on current interpersonal relations and their influence in the development of depression. It frequently focuses on role changes (e.g. job loss, becoming a new mother) and role disputes (e.g. relationship problems, work difficulties). It is equally as effective as CBT in mild and moderate depression. However, CBT has a better response rate in severely depressed patients (Luty et al., 2007). The response rate for combination of interpersonal psychotherapy and medication is higher than IPT or medication alone (Schramm et al., 2007) and the benefits are sustained even after remission (Frank et al., 2007).

14.2. Physical treatments

Physical treatments for depression have been increasingly acknowledged in recent years. They include electro- convulsive therapy (ECT), transcranial magnetic stimulation (TMS), deep brain stimulation, magneto-convulsive therapy and vagus nerve stimulation.

Electro-convulsive therapy has been a well recognised treatment for depression even before the discovery of psychotropic drugs. However over the years its usage has declined and now it is indicated mainly for severe depression with a high risk of suicide, depressive stupor, treatment resistant depression and patients in danger to their physical health secondary to poor dietary intake. At the same time, ECT has become a more sophisticated procedure with advances in the field of anaesthesia and improved technology of ECT machines. ECT is a rapid and effective treatment for major depression. A recent meta-analysis showed ECT has significant superiority to antidepressants in both severe and treatment resistant depression (Pagnin et al., 2008). The most common side-effects reported are headaches and short term confusion following the treatment. In some patients, there is an increased risk of long-term memory loss but the evidence base for this side-effect remains controversial.

Transcranial magnetic stimulation (TMS) has now been approved in United States for the treatment of major depression, particularly for patients who have not responded to antidepressant medications (Kim et al., 2009). TMS produces a magnetic field around brain and the main target areas are dorsolateral prefrontal cortex in both sides of the brain. Two meta-analyses (Kim et al., 2009; Slotema et al., 2010) showed that repetitive-TMS has higher efficacy than placebo and comparable efficacy to antidepressants. However it was less effective than ECT. Patients reported headaches following the treatments and seizures can be a rare side-effect.

Deep brain stimulation, magneto-convulsive therapy and vagus nerve stimulation appear to be promising in the treatment of depression but they are all still in the experimental stages.

In deep brain stimulation, electrodes are implanted in the brain and controlled by the internal pulse generator. The stimulation modulates the neurotransmission in the cortico –striatal – thalamic- cortical circuit. It is a reversible procedure and the stimulation can be adjusted according to the patient's needs (Giacobbe et al., 2006).

Magneto-convulsive therapy is another experimental treatment where seizures are induced by repetitive-TMS in a controlled way targeting the brain structures essential for treatment response, particularly the temporal lobes.

In vagus nerve stimulation, bipolar electrodes are attached to the left cervical vagus nerve and stimulation periods are controlled. The side-effects include hoarseness of voice, pain, cough and dysphagia.

15. The future of pharmacotherapy of depression

Despite the advances in the treatment of depression, the efficacy of currently available antidepressants is still relatively modest and there are patients who do not respond to them. The limitations of the monoamine based antidepressants include slow onset of action, poor impact on certain symptoms such as disturbed sleep and fatigue and they cause multiple side-effects. Numerous innovative approaches have been studied looking at new and different mechanisms for the treatment of depression. Some of these promising approaches are discussed below.

15.1. Selective versus multi–transmitter antidepressants

It has always been a debate whether selective neurotransmission is better than multiple neurotransmission. This issue of selectivity versus efficacy has re-emerged as the newer antidepressants are less selective than SSRIs but relatively more selective than the TCAs.

Burke (2004) reviewed the topic comparing SSRIs against TCAs and somewhat more selective venlafaxine. The review concluded that SSRIs' success is presumably not because of their efficacy, but rather to ease of use, minimal need for titration, better tolerability and improved safety in overdose. The difference in tolerability is due to the fact that TCAs act on multiple receptors causing more adverse effects. In comparing SSRIs with venlafaxine, Thase et al., 2001 found that venlafaxine had higher remission rates and they attributed this to its "dual action". However venlafaxine does not have substantial effects on noradrenaline until the dose is increased above 150mgs/day and therefore technically it cannot be considered as a dual acting agent at lower doses.

Perhaps a better way to increase the efficacy is to target the specific receptor rather than increasing overall neurotransmission. If a drug acts only at the specific receptor and alleviates the depressive symptoms then its unnecessary action at other receptors can be avoided. Therefore more receptor specific drugs have to be designed rather than those aiming at greater than previous neurotransmission.

One approach is developing new formulations with existing antidepressants. Some of these are more acceptable to patients (fluoxetine once weekly, paroxetine CR), some have faster onset of actions (mirtazapine soluble tablets & intravenous preparations) and others such as venlafaxine XL have clear pharmacokinetic benefits (Norman & Oliver 2004).

15.2. Other agents in development

The other approach to address the issue of efficacy is developing new agents. The agents in development include multimodal serotonergic agents, triple uptake inhibitors, neurokinin (NK1) antagonists, glutamate antagonists, dopamine agonists and antiglucocorticoid agents.

Multimodal serotonergic agents are simply an extension of SSRIs and SNRIs. They have both serotonin reuptake inhibition and either blocks 5HT2a receptor and/or act as partial agonist at 5HT1a receptor. **Vilazodone**, the first agent of this group,is already available in clinical practice and there are few other drugs in development.

Triple uptake inhibitors combine the inhibition of serotonin, noradrenaline and dopamine transporters. Their development is based on the assumption that targeting dopamine neurotransmission would enhance overall efficacy and diminish certain symptoms such as anhedonia, apathy, sleepiness and fatigue as well as counteract sexual side-effects induced by SSRI (Fava et al., 2007). **Sibutramine** is the only available drug with triple uptake inhibition and it is currently used in weight loss therapy. One of the limitations associated with this mechanism might be the risk of abuse linked with increased dopamine neurotransmission.

Neurokinin receptors (NK1 and NK2) and their endogenous ligand **Substance P** are found in brain areas known to be involved in the regulation of mood, stress and anxiety responses (Bergstrom et al., 2004). However NK1 antagonist **aprepitant** failed to show greater efficacy to placebo (Keller et al., 2006). Currently studies focusing on NK2 antagonists are underway.

Glutamate modulating agents such as **ketamine (**NMDA antagonist) generated significant interest in the field when rapid and sustained antidepressant effects were seen after injections of ketamine (Berman et al., 1999). Another NMDA antagonist and dopaminergic drug **amantadine** showed efficacy in depressed imipramine non-responders (Rogoz et al., 2007). It may be useful in depressed patients with prominent cognitive dysfunction. The main limiting factor in using these agents is the risk of inducing psychotic symptoms due to their hallucinogenic properties (Smith 2008).

Dopamine agonists, similar to DNRI bupropion, seem to be promising in the treatment of depression. A review showed that dopamine agonists had anxiolytic, antidepressive and antianhedonic effects which were related to its action on dopamine D2 and D3 receptors (Lenke 2007). Two agents, **ropinirole and pramipexole** proved efficacy as additional treatment to mood stabiliser in bipolar depression but further research is required to prove their efficacy and usefulness as antidepressants.

Biological studies of depression have shown that the secretion of hypothalamic neuropeptides such as corticotrophin releasing hormone (CRH) and vasopressin is elevated in depressed patients. CRH acting through CRH1 receptor may cause symptoms of depression. Depressed patients also have increased cortisol levels which might be responsible for psychotic symptoms of depression. A review of the hypothesis that **CRH1 receptor antagonists and antiglucocorticoid agents** may be useful in the treatment of depression supports this direction in the development of future antidepressants (Nemeroff 2002).

16. Conclusions

Major depressive disorder is a complex psychiatric condition, with multiple aetiological factors. The pathophysiology of depression is still evolving with ongoing molecular, genetic and neuroimaging studies. Evidence from neurobiological studies indicates that monoamine hypothesis of depression cannot fully explain the causation of depression. Further research into the aetiology of depression beyond monoamine hypothesis may provide new directions in developing novel agents in the treatment of major depressive disorder.

The initial focus on increasing the synaptic levels of neurotransmitters, especially serotonin and noradrenaline, has already shifted towards dual action and receptor specific antidepressants. Although there have been considerable advances in the treatment of depression since TCAs were discovered in the 1950's, the current treatments are not fully satisfactory for either patients or clinicians. Research evidence on several new pharmacological and non-pharmacological interventions is still preliminary and further studies are needed to prove their actual benefits.

Acknowledgements

We would like to thank Mrs Jean Kenning for her secretarial support in the preparation of the manuscript.

Author details

Ashok Kumar Jainer[1], Rajkumar Kamatchi[1,2], Marek Marzanski[1,2] and Bettahalasoor Somashekar[1]

1 Coventry & Warwickshire Partnership NHS Trust, Coventry, UK

2 Warwick Medical School, Coventry, UK

References

[1] Anderson, I. M., Parry-Billings, M., Newsholme, E. A., et al. Decreased plasma tryptophan concentration in major depression: relationship to melancholia and weight loss. Journal of Affective disorders (1990). , 20, 185-191.

[2] Aguglia, E., Casachia, M., Cassano, G. B., Ferrari, G., Giodano, P., et al. Double-blind study of efficacy and safety of sertraline vs. fluoxetine in major depression. Int Clin Psychopharmacol (1993). , 8, 197-202.

[3] Azorin, J. M., Llorca, Pm., Despiegel, N., & Verpillat, P. Escitalopram is more effective than citalopram for the treatment of severe major depressive disorder. L'Encephale (2004). , 30, 158-166.

[4] Baldwin, Thomas. J. C., & Birtwistle, J. Effect of antidepressant drugs on sexual function. Int J Psych Clin Pract (1997). , 1, 47-58.

[5] Berman, R. M., Cappiello, A., Anand, A., et al. Antidepressant effects of ketamine in depressed patients. Biol Psychiatry (1999). , 47, 351-354.

[6] Berman, R. M., Narasimhan, M., Miller, H. L., et al. Transient depressive relapse induced by catecholamine depletion: potential phenotypic vulnerability maker? Arch Gen Psychiatry (1999). , 56, 395-403.

[7] Bergstrom, M., Hargreaves, R. J., Burns, H. D., et al. Human positron emission tomography studies of brain neurokinin 1 receptor occupancy by aprepitant. Biol Psychiatry (2004)., 55, 1007-1012.

[8] Berzewski, H., Van Moffaert, M., & Gagiano, . Efficacy and tolerability of reboxetine compared with imipramine in a double-blind study in patients suffering from major depressive episodes. European Neuropsychopharmacology (1997)., 7, 37-47.

[9] Brown GL, Linnoila MI. CSF serotonin metabolite (5-HIAA) studies in depression, impulsivity and violence. J Clin Psychiatry 1990; 51(suppl 4): 31-41

[10] Blier, P., Ward, H. E., Tremblay, P., Laberge, L., Hébert, C., & Bergeron, R. Combination of antidepressant medications from treatment initiation for major depressive disorder: a double-blind randomized study. Am J Psychiatry (2010)., 167, 281-288.

[11] Burke WJ. Selective versus multi- transmitter antidepressants: are two mechanisms better than one? J Clin Psychiatry 2004; 65 (suppl 4): 37- 45

[12] Chen, Z., Wang, h., & Jin, W. Selective serotonin reuptake inhibitor is more likely to induce sexual dysfunction than mirtazapine in treating depression. National Journal of Andrology(2008)., 10, 896-899.

[13] Cipriani, A., Furukawa, T. A., Salanti, G., Geddes, J. R., et al. Comparative efficacy and acceptability of 12 new-generation antidepressants: a multiple- treatments meta-analysis. Lancet (2009)., 373, 746-758.

[14] Czeisler CA, Buxton OM, Khalsa SBS.The human circadian timing system and sleep-wake regulation.In Kryger MH, Roth T, Dement WC, eds. Principles and practice of sleep medicine. 4thedn. Philadelphia: WB Saunders, (2005)., 2005, 375-394.

[15] Cuijpers, P., van Straten, A., Warmerdam, L. ., & Andersson, G. Psychotherapy versus the combination of psychotherapy and pharmacotherapy in the treatment of depression: a meta-analysis. Depression and Anxiety (2009)., 26, 279-288.

[16] De Beradis, D., Di Iorio, G., Acciavatti, T., et al. The emerging role of melatonin agonists in the treatment of major depression: focus on agomelatine. CNS Neurol Dis Drug Targets (2011)., 10, 119-132.

[17] de Bodinat C, Guardiola- Lemaitre B, Mocaer E, Renard P & et al.,. Agomelatine, the first melatonergic antidepressant: discovery, characterisation and development. Nat Rev Drug Discov 2010; 9: 628- 642

[18] De Boer, T. H., & Ruigt, G. The selective alpha 2 agonist Org 3770 enhances noradrenergic and serotonin 1a mediated serotonergic neurotransmission. CNS Drugs (1995). suppl1): 29-38

[19] Dubini, A., Bosc, M., & Polin, B. Noradrenaline selective versus serotonin-selective antidepressant therapy; differential effects on social functioning. J Psychopharmacology (1997)., 11, 17-23.

[20] Fava, M., Thase, M., De Battista, C., et al. Modafinil augmentation of selective serotonin reuptake inhibitor therapy in MDD partial responders with persistent fatigue and sleepiness. Ann Clin Psychiatry (2007). , 19, 153-159.

[21] Frank, E., Kupfer, D. J., Bysse, D. J., et al. Randomised trial of weekly, twice-monthly, monthly interpersonal psychotherapy as maintenance treatment for women with recurrent depression. Am J Psychiatry (2007). , 164, 761-767.

[22] Selective serotonin reuptake inhibitors (SSRIs) for depression (Cochrane Review). In: The Cochrane Library, Oxford, England: update software;(3)

[23] Germain A & Kupfer DJ.Circadian rhythm disturbances in depression.Human Psychopharmacology 2008; 23: 571- 585

[24] Giacobbe, P., & Kennedy, S. H. Deep brain stimulation for treatment resistant depression: a psychiatric perspective. Curr Psychiatry Rep (2006). , 8, 437-444.

[25] Guelfi, White. C., Guichoux, J. Y., & Magni, G. Effectiveness of venlafaxine in patients hospitalized for major depression and melancholia.J Clin Psychiatry (1995). , 56, 450-458.

[26] Hale, A., Corral, R. M., Mencacci, C., Ruiz, J. S., et al. Superior antidepressant efficacy results of agomelatine versus fluoxetine in severe MDD patients: a randomised, double-blind study. Int Clin Psychopharmacol (2010). , 25, 305-314.

[27] Harris CR, Gualtieri J & Stark G. Fatal bupropion overdose. J Clin Toxicology 1997; 35: 321- 324

[28] Healy D, Savage M. Reserpine exhumed. Br J Psychiatry 1998; 172: 376-378

[29] Hickie I & Davenport T. A behavioural approach based on reconstructing the sleep-wake cycle. Cogn Behav Pract 1999; 6: 442- 450

[30] Holliday SH, Benfield P. Venlafaxine.A review of its pharmacology and therapeutic potential in depression. Drugs 1995; 49: 280-294

[31] Hollon SD, DeRubeis RJ, Shelton RC & et al.,.Prevention of relapse following cognitive therapy vs. medications in moderate to severe depression.Arch Gen Psychiatry (2005). , 62, 417-422.

[32] Inskip, H. M., Harris, E. C., & Barraclough, B. ". Lifetime risk of suicide for affective disorder, alcoholism and schizophrenia". Br J Psychiatry (1998). , 172, 35-7.

[33] Kasper, S., Hajak, G., Wulff, K., et al. Efficacy of the novel antidepressant agomelatine on the circadian rest- activity cycle and depressive and anxiety symptoms in patients with major depressive disorder: a randomised, double-blind comparison with sertraline. J Clin psychiatry (2010). , 71, 109-120.

[34] Katon WJ.Clinical and health services relationships between major depression, depressive symptoms, and general medical illness. Biol Psychiatry (2003). , 54, 216-226.

[35] Kennedy SH, Rizvi S, Fulton K, Rasmussen J.A double-blind comparison of sexual functioning, antidepressant efficacy and tolerability between agomelatine and venlafaxine XR.J ClinPsychopharmacol 2008; 28: 329- 333

[36] Keller, M., Montgomery, S., Ball, W., et al. Lack of efficacy of the substance antagonist aprepitant in the treatment of major depressive disorder. Biol Psychiatry (2006)., NK1.

[37] Kessler, R. C., Angermeyer, M., Anthony, J. C., et al. Lifetime prevalence and age-of-onset distributions of mental disorders in the World Health Organization's World Health Survey Initiative. World Psychiatry (2007)., 6, 168-76.

[38] Kessler, D., Lewis, G., Kaur, S., et al. Therapist delivered internet psychotherapy for depression in primary care: a randomised controlled trial. Lancet (2009). , 374, 628-634.

[39] Kim DR, Pesiridou A, O'Reardon JP.Transcranial magnetic stimulation in the treatment of psychiatric disorders.Curr psychiatry Rep 2009; 11: 447- 452

[40] Lenke MR.Antidepressant effects of dopamine agonists. Experimental and clinical findings.Der Nervenarzt (2007)., 78, 31-38.

[41] Lopes-Ibor J, Guelfi JD, Platen Y, Tournoux A, Prost JF.Milnacipran and selective serotonin reuptake inhibitors in major depression.IntClinPsychopharmacol 1996; 11(suppl4): 41-46

[42] Lorinquivst, j., Sintonen, H., Syvalati, H., et al. Antidepressant efficacy and quality of life in depression: a double-blind study with moclobemide and fluoxetine. Acta Psychiatr Scand (1994)., 89, 363-369.

[43] Luty SE, Carter JD, McKenzie JM & et al.,.Randomised controlled trial of interpersonal psychotherapy and cognitive- behavioural therapy for depression. Br J Psychiatry (2007)., 190, 496-502.

[44] Mallinchdrodt, C., Prakash, A., Andron, A., Watkin, J. ., & Wohlreich, M. Duloxetine for the treatment of major depressive disorder; a closer look at efficacy and safety data across the approved dose range. Journal of Psychiatric Research (2006). , 40, 337-348.

[45] Montgomery, S. A., Prost, J. F., Solles, A., & Briley, M. Efficacy and tolerability of milnacipran: an overview. Int Clin Psychopharmacol (1994). suppl4): 47-51

[46] Nakagawa, A., Wantanbe, N., Omor, I. M., Barbui, C., et al. Efficacy and tolerability of milnacipran in the treatment of major depression compared with other antidepressants: a systematic review and meta-analysis. CNS drugs (2008)., 22, 587-602.

[47] Nemeroff CB.New directions in the development of antidepressants: the interface of neurobiology and psychiatry. Human Psychopharmacology: Clinical and Experimental (2002). suppl 1): 13-16

[48] Nierenberg AA, Feighner JP, Rudolph.Venlafaxine for treatment resistant depression.J Clin Psychopharmacol (1994). , 14(6), 419-423.

[49] Nierenberg AA, Petersen TJ & Alpert JE.Prevention of relapse and recurrence in depression: the role of long term pharmacotherapy and psychotherapy. J Clin Psychiatry (2003). suppl 15): 13-17

[50] Norman TR & Oliver JS.New formulations of existing antidepressants: advantages in the management of depression. CNS Drugs (2004). , 18, 505-520.

[51] Nutt, D., Demyttenaere, K., Janka, Z., Aarre, T., et al. The other face of depression reduced positive effect: the role of catecholamines in causation and cure. J Psychopharmacol(2007). , 21, 461-471.

[52] Pagnin D, de Queiroz V, Pini S, Cassano GB. Efficacy of ECT in depression: a meta-analytic review. Focus 2008; 6: 155- 162

[53] Palzanis, E., Renoir, T., Lelievre, V., et al. Behavioural and neuroplastic effects of the new- generation antidepressant agomelatine compared to fluoxetine in glucocorticoid receptor-impaired mice. Int J Neuropsychopharmacology (2010). , 13, 759-774.

[54] Papakostas, G., Nutt, D., Hallett, L., Tucker, v., Krishen, A., & Fava, M. Resolution of sleepiness and fatigue in major depressive disorder: A comparison of bupropion and the selective serotonin reuptake inhibitors. Biol Psychiatry (2006). , 60, 1350-1355.

[55] Papakostas G & Fava M.A meta-analysis of clinical trials comparing the serotonin 5HT2 receptor antagonist trazodone and nefazodone with selective serotonin reuptake inhibitors for the treatment of major depressive disorder.European Neuropsychopharmacology 2007; 22: 444-447

[56] Papakostas G, Homberger C & Fava M.A meta-analysis of clinical trials comparing mirtazapine with selective serotonin reuptake inhibitors for the treatment of major depressive disorder.Journal of Psychopharmacology 2008; 22: 843- 848

[57] Price JS, Waller PC, Wood SM, Mackay AP.A comparison of the post-marketing safety of four selective serotonin reuptake inhibitors including investigation of symptoms occurring on withdrawal.Br J ClinPharmacol 1996; 42: 757- 763

[58] Quasim, M., & Kumar, A. J. Recent advances in antidepressant drug therapy. Int J Psychiatry in ClinPract(1999). , 3, 17-22.

[59] Rickels, K., Robinson, Schweizer. E., et al. Nefazodone: aspects of efficacy. J Clin Psychiatry (1995). suppl 6): 43-46

[60] Rocha, F. L., Fuzikawa, C., Riera, R., & Hara, C. Combination of antidepressants in the treatment of major depressive disorder: A systematic review and meta-analysis. J ClinPsychopharmacol (2012). , 32, 278-281.

[61] Rogoz, Z., Skuza, G., Daniel, W. A., et al. Amantadine as an additive treatment in patients suffering from drug- resistant unipolar depression.Pharmacol Rep (2007). , 59, 778-784.

[62] Sagar, P. V., Segal, Z. V., Grigoriadis, S., Ravidran, A. V., et al. Canadian Network for Mood and Anxiety Treatments (CANMAT) clinical guidelines for the management of major depressive disorder in adults. II. Psychotherapy alone or in combination with antidepressant medication. J Aff Disorders (2009). suppl 1): 15-25

[63] Schramm, E., van Calker, D., Dykierek, P., et al. An intensive treatment program of interpersonal psychotherapy plus pharmacotherapy for depressed inpatients: acute and long-term results. Am J Psychiatry (2007). , 164, 768-777.

[64] Shrier, M., Diaz, J. E. ., & Tsarouhas, N. Cardiotoxicity associated with bupropion overdose. Ann Emergency Med (2000).

[65] Simon GE, Ludman EJ, Rutter CM.Incremental benefit and cost of telephone care management and telephone psychotherapy for depression in primary care. Arch Gen Psychiatry (2009). , 66, 1081-1089.

[66] Slotema CW, Blom JD, Hoek HW, Sommer IE.Should we expand the toolbox of psychiatric treatment methods to include repetitive transcranial magnetic stimulation (r-TMS)? A meta-analysis of the efficacy of rTMS in psychiatric disorders.J Clin Psychiatry (2010). , 71, 873-884.

[67] Smith EJ.Amantadine induced psychosis in a young healthy patient. Am J Psychiatry (2008).

[68] Smith KA, Fairburn CG, Cowen PJ.Relapse of depression after rapid depletion of tryptophan. Lancet (1997). , 349, 915-919.

[69] Soares, C., Kornstein, S., Thase, M., Jiang, Q., et al. Assessing the efficacy of desvenlafaxine for improving the functioning and well-being outcome measures in patients with major depressive disorder: a pooled analysis of 9 double-blind, placebo-controlled, 8-week clinical trials. J Clin Psychiatry (2009). , 70, 1365-1371.

[70] Stewart, J. Treating depression with atypical features.J Clin Psychiatry (2007). suppl3): 25-29

[71] Thase, M., Entsuah, R. A., & Rudolph, R. L. Remission rates during treatment with venlafaxine or selective serotonin reuptake inhibitors. Br J Psychiatry (2001). , 178, 234-241.

[72] Thase, M. What role do atypical antipsychotic drugs have in treatment- resistant depression? J Clin Psychiatry (2002). , 63, 95-103.

[73] Thase, M., Haight, B., Richard, N., Rockett, C., Mitton, M., et al. Remission rates following antidepressant therapy with bupropion or selective serotonin reuptake inhibitors: a meta-analysis of original data from 7 randomized controlled trials. J Clin Psychiatry (2005). , 66, 974-981.

[74] Thase, M., Kornstein, S., Germain, J., Jiang, Q., et al. An integrated analysis of the efficacy of desvenlafaxine compared with placebo in patients with major depressive disorder. CNS Spectrums (2009). , 14(3), 144-154.

[75] Thase, M., Nierenberg, A., Vrijland, P., Van Oers, H., et al. Remission with mirtazapine and selective serotonin reuptake inhibitors: a meta-analysis of individual patient data from 15 controlled trials of acute phase treatment of major depression. Int Clin Psychopharmacol (2010). , 25, 189-198.

[76] Van Harten, J. Clinical pharmacokinetics of selective serotonin reuptake inhibitors.Clin Pharmacokinet (1993). , 24, 203-220.

[77] Duloxetine and Venlafaxine-xr in the treatment of major depressive disorder: a meta-analysis of randomised clinical trials. The Annals of Pharmacotherapy: , 39, 1798-1807.

[78] VittenglJR, Clark LA, Jarrett RB. Continuation- phase cognitive therapy's effects on remission and recovery from depression. J Consult ClinPsychol (2009). , 77, 367-371.

[79] Weaver DR.Melatonin and circadian rhythmicity in vertebrates.Physiological roles and pharmacological effects. In: Turek FW, Zee PC, eds. Regulation of sleep and circadian rhythms. New York: Dekker, (1999). , 1999, 197-262.

[80] Weissaman MM, Markowitz JC & Klerman GL.Clinician's quick guide to interpersonal psychotherapy. (2007). New York: Oxford University Press

[81] WHO.Facts and Figures. (http://www.euro.who.int/en/what-we-do/health-topics/noncommunicable-diseases/mental-health/facts-and-figures)- accessed on 1st August 2012

Chapter 13

The Association Between Tinnitus and Mental Illnesses

Adeyi A. Adoga and Taiwo J. Obindo

Additional information is available at the end of the chapter

1. Introduction

Tinnitus is defined as a perception of sound which is unrelated to an external acoustic source (Kompis et al., 2004). Some sufferers usually describe the noise as "ringing" but others describe it with various hyperboles such as grinding, whistling, humming, roaring, chirping, howling, buzzing or clicking. It is a symptom of unknown patho-physiology with few therapeutic measures (Tan et al., 1999). Even as there are many available potential treatment modalities, there has never been a single intervention which has been identified to consistently eliminate this symptom. It has become a source of increasing health concern affecting all strata of the public manifesting with comorbid psychological stresses which necessitate psychiatric treatment (Halford& Anderson, 1991; Schaaf et al., 2003).

It impinges on the quality of life of affected individuals to varying degrees occurring as a minor irritation to some and in extreme cases result in the intentional or ambivalent self destructive act of suicide (Simpson & Davies, 1999). Tinnitus sufferers often give reports of associated co-morbidities. They may complain of impairment in lifestyle, emotional difficulties, sleep deprivation, hindrance with work and social life and a general decrease in health status (Folmer & Griest, 2000; Folmer et al., 1999; Tyler & Baker, 1983). Patients with tinnitus have been known to have an increased risk for depression, anxiety and insomnia although the causative relationships are rare (Folmer & Griest, 2000; Crocetti et al., 2009; Schleuning, 1991).

2. History of tinnitus

Famous people who had suffered tinnitus are often mentioned in its history. These include Joan of Arc (1412-31), Ludwig van Beethoven (1770-1827), Bedrich Smetana, a great music composer of his time who described his tinnitus as a "high E". Others were Charles Darwin (1809-82) who recorded the amplitude and frequency of his tinnitus daily. Michelangelo and his fellow Italian rival Leonardo da Vinci were other famous people who suffered tinnitus.

The work on tinnitus was of modest scope in the past, not until the development of modern electroacoustic equipments. In the past, the description of tinnitus was highly dependent on cultural factors. For example in ancient oriental mysticism, tinnitus was regarded as sensitivity to the divine. Old Egyptians believed that tinnitus occurred from a bewitched ear and instilled oils or herbs into the external auditory canal as a form of treatment. This practice continued through the middle Ages. In the 400 century BC, Hippocrates and Aristotle introduced the masking of tinnitus suggesting the probability of a greater sound driving out the lesser sound of tinnitus.

In the Babylonian Talmud, tinnitus was referred to as the "curse of Titus". It was described as a buzzing sound in the brain which responded to sound therapy and habituation. In recent times, sound therapy is commonly used in treating tinnitus. It was first administered in high levels to mask tinnitus (Feldmann, 1971; Vernon, 1977) and subsequently replaced by low-dose white band noise generators (Jastreboff & Hazel, 1993).

As far back as during the Roman times, tinnitus was regarded as being associated with depression and seizure disorders. These three disorders were thought to have a common pathophysiology. However, these days the pathways are explained in a completely different way (Holgers et al., 2005).

Due to the heterogeneity of tinnitus patients from the stand point of symptoms and etiological factors, understanding of tinnitus requires a multivariate approach that were not available in the past until the advent of modern methods for assessment and treatment. The overall goal is to develop better methods for treatment and prevention.

3. Epidemiology

Tinnitus is a widespread distressing symptom affecting 30-40% of the adult population with 0.5-2.5% of affected individuals experiencing significant distress from it, interfering with their quality of life (Krog et al., 2010; Nondahl et al., 2011; Shargorodsky et al., 2010a; Sindhusaki et al., 2003). An estimated 16 (50 million) percent of Americans experience tinnitus with about 16 million of these seeking medical help and 2 million unable to lead normal enjoyable lives because of distressing tinnitus (American Tinnitus Association, 2012). The prevalence reported from Nigeria is 15.1% (Adoga et al., 2008). It is estimated that at least one third of the population experience tinnitus once in their lifetime and about 1-5% experience serious psychosocial complications (Martinez et al., 2010). The overall prevalence of depression and anxiety in a population based study in Nigeria reveals 17.4% and 22.8% respectively (Adoga et al., 2008). Twenty percent of individuals are said to endure the distress they experience (Robinson et al., 2003). The prevalence is higher in men (Hoffman & Reed, 2004). Tinnitus frequency is lower in women but its characteristics are more complex in men who are reported to present at a younger age and have a greater hearing loss.Adults and children experience tinnitus but its development is said to increase with age and with exposure to loud sounds (Hoffman & Reed, 2004) especially in young adults (Bulbul et al., 2009) presumed to be from exposure to high volume music from portable or mini devices (Shargorodsky et al., 2010b). However the rate in children has been reported to be as high as 13%.

4. Pathophysiology and risk factors

It is important to note that tinnitus is a symptom and not a disease therefore reflecting one or more underlying abnormalities. These abnormalities range from impaction of wax in the external auditory canal to acoustic tumours which will require medical or surgical attention.

A number of risk factors have been associated with tinnitus and they include increasing age, hearing loss and exposure to loud noise (Axelsson & Ringdahl, 1989; Nondahl et al., 2002). Exposure to noise is the largest attributed aetiological factor in tinnitus (American Tinnitus Association, 2011). People can develop hearing loss and tinnitus when exposed to loud military, industrial and recreational noise. Military personnel are commonly exposed to high levels of sound. Tinnitus is the most common military service related disability amongst veterans of the United States of America returning from Iraq and Afghanistan (American Tinnitus Association, 2012). These events can be classed under Post Traumatic Stress Disorders (PTSD) in which tinnitus in these individuals may serve as a constant reminder of a traumatic event such as exposure to a blast.

Environmental sound is of importance for the awareness of tinnitus with 94 percent of individuals experiencing transient tinnitus in completely silent surroundings (Heller & Bergman, 1953). Tinnitus has been suggested to be an early symptom of hearing loss particularly noise induced hearing loss (Griest & Bishop, 1998) but then there are studies to dispute this statement (Rubak et al., 2008). However, tinnitus is not always secondary to hearing loss. There are individuals with normal hearing who experience tinnitus.

Tinnitus shares similar risk factors with hearing loss. In addition to those mentioned above, these risk factors are exposure to toxins and otologic diseases such as cerumen auris, ear infections, acoustic neuromas, Meniere's disease. Others are dizziness, head injury, poor socioeconomic and general health status of individuals and ototoxic drugs e.g. aspirin, quinine, aminoglycosides and cancer chemotherapeutics especially cisplatin. The effects of these drugs may be temporary or permanent. The relationship between tinnitus and these risk factors are however unclear but there may be a bidirectional relationship between them (Guitton,2006).

The patho-physiology of tinnitus is unknown; however, central nervous system mechanisms are believed to play a role in its patho-physiology (Saunders, 2007). Therefore, risk factors related to homeostatic neural plasticity may be of importance. Neural plasticity is an ongoing dynamic process and it describes the ability of the brain to adapt its nerve cell, synapses or even the whole brain and its organisation to modified biological requirements. There are two types of neural plasticity;

1. *Cortical plasticity* describes the activity dependent changes in size, connectivity or the activation patterns in the cortical networks of the brain.

2. *Synaptic plasticity* describes the activity dependent changes in the strength of transmission of impulses across the synapse which can affect both the morphology and physiology of the synapse. From the standpoint of molecular biology, this type of neural plasticity is said to be important for the development and persistence of tinnitus. Stimulation of afferent nerve fibres causes long term changes in synaptic transmission, a process called long-term potentiation or long-term depression. An imbalance between these two processes which results from damage to the hair cells and vestibulocochlear nerve leads to changes in gene expression and involves changes in neurotransmission, in the expression of receptors, ion channels, regulatory enzymes and direct changes on the synapses. These events increase the level of cellular activity leading to hyperactivity in the dorsal cochlear nucleus, inferior colliculus and in the auditory cortex causing changes in cortical plasticity leading to tinnitus (Mazureck et al., 2010).

It has also been suggested that tinnitus results from an abnormally synchronised action potential pattern of the spontaneous activity within the central auditory pathways due to inner ear damage (Lenarz et al., 1993). This hypothesis however neither explains why some patients with sensorineural deafness due to damage to hair cells perceive tinnitus while others do not, nor does it explain the suffering experienced from tinnitus. Not all individuals who have tinnitus complain of comorbid debilitating conditions.

Whether tinnitus results from the amplification of contrasts between neighboured frequencies with differences in the input has been a subject of debate for many years. Findings from animal models however clearly suggest that it is the homeostatic mechanisms which are responsible for tinnitus generation. This is an important step forward in the understanding of tinnitus especially since the molecular mechanisms that are involved have been identified (Mazureck et al., 2010; Knipper et al., 2012). This generally believed mechanism of the generation of tinnitus also conforms to the clinical observation that in most cases the tinnitus frequency is in the same frequency area like the hearing loss. For example a patient with noise induced hearing loss around 4 kHz also perceives the tinnitus at 4 kHz. However tinnitus is not a disease of the auditory system alone.

It is postulated that the difficulty to ignore tinnitus, the annoyance patients experience from tinnitus, the anxiety that tinnitus becomes worse, the experience of irritability and concentration difficulties are related to functional changes in non-auditory brain systems (Jastreboff, 1990). Neuro-imaging studies such as electroencephalography (EEG), functional magnetic resonance imaging (fMRI) and positron emission tomography (PET) in tinnitus patients have helped to identify the structures in the central nervous system believed to be responsible for the patho-physiology of tinnitus (De Ridder et al., 2011; Schecklmann et al., 2011; Van de Heyning et al., 2008) demonstrating in the auditory cortex of patients suffering from tinnitus a reduction of alpha wave activity and an increase in the delta and gamma wave activities. Therefore, altered activity in the central auditory pathways is not sufficient for the perception of tinnitus. This explains that many patients with hearing loss (and consequent increased activity in the central auditory pathways) do not perceive tinnitus. It is only when the auditory activity is connected to activity in the "attentional network" that the tinnitus is consciously perceived (De Ridder et al., 2011).

The complex nature of changes associated with tinnitus in the central nervous system may very well explain its treatment difficulty.

5. Classification and aetiology

The noise of tinnitus can present in different forms but it is classified into two major types and these are;

1. *Objective tinnitus*- also described as pulsatile is a type of tinnitus that is perceptible to the patient and other people. It is rare, affecting 3percent of patients. It is mostly caused by myoclonic contractions of the tensor tympani muscle or blood vessels, eustachian tube dysfunction and tumours of the middle ear. Its presence signifies a serious underlying disease such as hypertension, vascular aneurysms, otitis media, brain tumours and glomusjugulare tumours. Diagnosis and appropriate treatment of these conditions makes the tinnitus to cease.

2. *Subjective tinnitus*- also described as idiopathic is a type of tinnitus that is perceptible only to the patient. It is the most common type and causes the most nuisances to patients. The causes of subjective tinnitus are prolonged exposure to loud sounds, ototoxicity, otosclerosis, head injuries, meningitis and brain tumours. It is the type mostly associated with psychosocial comorbidities.

As a result of the rarity of objective tinnitus, it is argued that all tinnitus is subjective and should be classified based on origin either as somatic or neurophysiologic. By this classification, somatic tinnitus (somatosounds) is described as tinnitus that has an underlying medical condition which creates internal acoustic mechanical sounds i.e. this type is of a vascular, muscular, respiratory and temporomandibular joint origin (Henry et al., 2010). The sounds produced in this type of tinnitus is commonly described as pulsatile and can be heard when an examiner uses a stethoscope or a microphone. The treatment therefore for this type of tinnitus is finding the underlying cause and treating it. Neurophysiologic (subjective idiopathic) tinnitus is the commonest type, non-pulsatile, mostly bilateral and difficult to evaluate. Matching the loudness and pitch of this type of tinnitus to external sounds with known acoustical parameters is helpful in the management of patients.

The causes of tinnitus are shown in Table 1.

TYPE OF TINNITUS	CAUSES
Subjective tinnitus	
Otologic	Noise-induced hearing loss, presbycusis, otosclerosis, otitis, impacted cerumen sudden deafness, Meniere's disease, and other causes of hearing loss
Neurologic	Head injury, whiplash injury, multiple sclerosis, vestibular schwannoma (acoustic neuromas) or other cerebellopontine-angle tumours
Infectious	Otitis media and sequelae of Lame disease, meningitis, syphilis, and other infectious or inflammatory processes that affect hearing
Drug-related	Common side effect of many drugs, such as salicylates, nonsteroidal anti-inflammatory drugs, aminoglycosides antibiotics. Loop diuretics and cancer chemotherapeutics (e.g. , cisplatin and vincristine)
Others	Temporomandibular-joint dysfunction and other dental disorders
Objective tinnitus	
Pulsatile	Carotid stenosis, arteriovenous malformations, other vascular anomalies, vascular tumours (e.g., the glomusjugulare), valvular heart disease (usually aortic stenosis), states of high cardiac output (anaemia and drug-induced high output) , and other conditions causing turbulent blood flow
Muscular or anatomical	Palatal myoclonus, spasm (of stapedius or tensor tympani muscle, patulousEustachian tube
Spontaneous	Spontaneous otoacoustic emissions

Table 1. Causes of subjective and objective tinnitus (Adapted with the permission of Matthews RJ).

6. Comorbidities and severity

Several studies have demonstrated the close association between tinnitus and comorbid psychological disorders (Adoga et al, 2008; Harter et al., 2004; Reynolds et al., 2004; Londero et al., 2006) showing that tinnitus causes distresses leading to deterioration in psychological well being and hampering the daily life enjoyment of affected individuals. There could also be a reversal in this relationship with increase in tinnitus severity during periods of poor psychological well being (Rauschecker et al., 2010). Therefore this association can be said to be dual. A population study has reported that emotional exhaustion is a strong predictor of tinnitus severity which indicates the degree to which an affected individual is worried, bothered or angry about the tinnitus (Hebert et al., 2012) with the severity of tinnitus depending on these comorbid psychological disorders.

Some researchers group tinnitus severity into the following; help-seekers, non-help-seekers; complainers and non-complainers (Attias et al., 1995; Hallberg et al., 1993). Others classify tinnitus severity into three subgroups based on the predictive factors for incapacitating tinnitus and these are: audiological tinnitus, somatic tinnitus and depression and anxiety related tinnitus with the latter group being the largest subgroup (Holgers et al., 2000).

The neurophysiologic model explains the severity of tinnitus to be a conditioned response focusing on the network of neural activity in the auditory system, the sympathetic and para-sympathetic autonomic nervous systems and the limbic system (Jastreboff & Hazel, 1993).

Some of the psychological disorders associated with tinnitus are anxiety, depressive disorders, hysteria, insomnia, anger, fear and despair. Researchers have found associations between tinnitus and anxiety disorders (Shargorodsky et al., 2010) and depression (Krog et al., 2010). However, patients with tinnitus and depression may not meet the clinical criteria for the diagnosis of major depressive disorder (Shargorodsky et al., 2010). Patients with tinnitus and comorbid anxiety and depressive disorder often present with exaggerated symptoms or non-tolerance of tinnitus. The clinical manifestations which may be seen in these patients are highlighted in Table 2 and 3.

Type of symptom	Manifestations
Increased arousal	Restlessness, increased startle response, disturbance with sleep
Mood	Fearfulness, apprehension, worries, irritability
Thoughts	Unrealistic appraisal of danger, belief in inability to cope, fear of impending death or a sinister background illness for the tinnitus
Behaviour	Constriction of purposeful activities, avoidance
Overactivity of autonomic nervous system	Tachycardia, hot and cold flushes, dry mouth, diarrhoea, urinary frequency, sweating
Somatization	Sense of retrosternal constriction, hyperventilation, faintness, muscular tension, fatigue, pain, tremor

Table 2. Manifestations of anxiety disorder

Type of symptom	Manifestations
Loss of interest	Inescapable sadness, loss of capacity for enjoyment or interest in previously pleasurable activities
Loss of energy	Staying indoors and avoidance of social interactions, inactivity with degeneration in physique, strength and physical well being
Biologic symptoms	Change in appetite and weight, disturbance of sleep and loss of libido
Disorders of thought content	Feeling of guilt, worthlessness, hopelessness
Psychomotor agitation	Incoherent conversation, expansive gesturing, pacing and hair twirling
Psychomotor retardation	Slow speech, coordination and impaired articulation
Others	delusions, depersonalization, derealization, obsessive-compulsive phenomena

Table 3. Manifestations of depressive disorders

Researchers have also found out a strong association between hearing loss (which is a strong predictor of tinnitus) and mental illnesses (Hebert et al., 2012; Dalton et al., 2003). Hearing loss reduces an individual's ability to communicate with people and this can worsen a mental health disorder like anxiety and depression. Tinnitus severity ratings also strongly correlate with levels of psychological distress indicating that tinnitus may worsen mental illnesses (Fagelson, 2007; Henry et al., 2007; Mrena et al., 2002). Anxiety and depression often increase in patients with tinnitus suggesting that tinnitus and these mental illnesses may affect similar neuronal mechanisms in the central nervous system which affect attention, emotions and perception (Fagelson, 2007; Henry et al., 2007).

7. Clinical assessment

One of the most criticized points in the clinical studies of tinnitus is the lack of consensus about the methods available for assessment of patients (Figueiredo et al., 2010). The aim of clinical assessment is to determine the underlying etiological factor that had led to tinnitus. As a result of the large number of differential diagnoses of tinnitus this assessment is difficult. However, the diagnosis is largely dependent on a thorough clinical history, physical examination and indicated laboratory investigations. All of these require attention to detail in picking the exact risk and etiological factors responsible for the symptoms and the absence or presence of comorbid psychological distresses for the effective treatment of patients. Many patients with associated psychological distresses will require various psychological evaluation techniques to assist in their management.

The time taken to listen to patients in obtaining a history is not a wasted venture although many details may be obscured by the number of factors that have taken place since the onset of the tinnitus. Since tinnitus is mostly subjective in type, a systematic approach to the history and physical examination should be geared towards differentiating subjective from objective tinnitus (Figure 1), identifying those conditions that are treatable, protect the patient's hearing and treat comorbid psychological distresses. Questions to patients should largely attempt to determine the presence, development, time course and the severity of any hearing loss as most cases of tinnitus are associated with hearing loss.

It is vital to get a description of the type of sound the patient hears and this can be ascertained by asking if the sound is constant or episodic; unilateral or bilateral; sudden or gradual in onset; the circumstances of onset; the duration of the tinnitus; the pitch and loudness of the sound- audiological protocols can be used to match the loudness and pitch of tinnitus experienced by patients to external sounds with known acoustical parameters (Holgers, 2003). Subjective tinnitus can be measured using numeric rating scales which provide a high measurement resolution and are easy to score (Stouffer & Tyler, 1990; Meikle et al., 2008).

Other questions to be asked are the presence of vertigo, otalgia, otorrhea or temporomandibular joint disorder; exposure to loud sounds, history of head injuries, otologic surgeries or the ingestion of ototoxic drugs. It is also important to elicit the presence of psychiatric illnesses by assessing the mental status- ask how the tinnitus affects the patient's daily life and the ability to function. These related distresses are measured using various psychometrically validated questionnaires (Robinson et al., 2003).Questionnaires can be used for diagnosis, treatment and for follow up of patients to measure the level of progress.

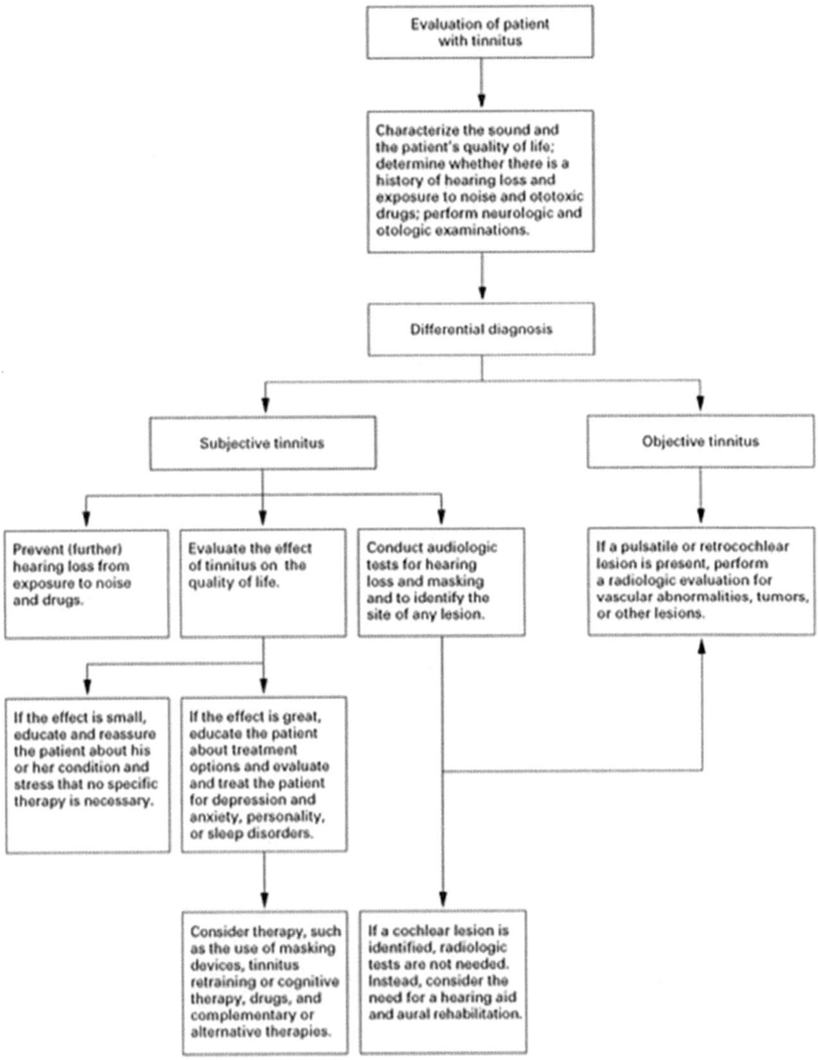

Figure 1. Algorithm for evaluation of tinnitus patients (Adapted with the permission of Matthews RJ).

Physical examination of patients should focus on the ears and the entire head and neck region.

The ears should be examined for cerumen impaction, otitis media with effusion or the presence of suppuration in the external auditory canal indicating otologic infection. Otomicroscopy may reveal a bluish tint on the tympanic membrane indicating an uncovered jugular vein, a bluish red mass in the tympanum which blanches on positive pressure with pneumatic otoscopy indicating the presence of a glomusjugulare tumour or a red hue suggesting otosclerosis. Auscultation of the periauricular region to listen for tinnitus is also helpful. The stethoscope can also be used to listen to the carotid vessels in the neck for bruits and venous hums, the cranium to check for arteriovenous malformations as well as listening to the heart.

Understanding that tinnitus is as much a medical condition as it is psychological gives room for a thorough psychological assessment of patients with a view to instituting appropriate treatment, the aim of which is to reduce the impact of tinnitus on the quality of life of patients. Psychological assessment is achieved via interviews of patients, use of questionnaires, tinnitus severity ratings etc. Dairies may have to be employed to document the characteristics of the tinnitus experienced.

In psychological assessment of patients, perceptual, emotional, attentional and behavioural parameters are considered. In doing this the following are sought; the characteristics of the tinnitus i.e. loudness, localization and the pitch, onset, duration, intensity, aggravating and relieving factors of the tinnitus. The visual analogue scale can be used for this analysis indicating a position along a continuous line between two endpoints (Figueiredo et al., 2009). Tinnitus questionnaires contain a series of questions from which patients select a response from the given choices which is usually recorded as a graded scale. In this way the severity of the tinnitus is graded. However, some questionnaires were not designed to measure the effectiveness also called responsiveness of tinnitus interventions (Kamalski et al., 2010). This effectiveness emphasizes effect sizes, content validity and response scaling which enables the detection of changes in condition of the patients during treatment (Kazdin, 2003; Lipsey, 1990). The Tinnitus Functional Index (TFI) is a new self-report type of questionnaire developed to scale the severity and negative impact of tinnitus and used for measuring changes during treatment (Meikle et al., 2012).

Cognitive evaluation of these patients is also vital finding out if they feel anger, sadness, helpless or have suicidal tendencies as a result of the tinnitus. Evaluate for psychological or mental comorbid disorders such as anxiety depression and sleep disorders which may have an impact on the general life quality of the patient. Assessing tinnitus also involves finding out what the patient perceives of his/her condition. Some considerations have to be given to the peculiar characteristics of an affected individual and not just the features of the tinnitus related psychological distress because individuals vary in the manner they can cope to these tinnitus related distresses. This will categorise individuals who simply experience tinnitus from those who have incapacitating psychological or mental disorders from tinnitus and therefore require psychological treatment (Sweetow, 1986).

Following history and physical examination of patients, some investigations are vital in helping to arrive at a diagnosis;

A complete audiogram with speech discrimination score and tympanometry is mandatory for all patients with tinnitus. An audiogram is done even though the patient does not make a complaint of hearing loss. The audiologist in this process can complete the subjective tinnitus matching evaluation to have a better understanding of the patient's condition. The pitch and loudness matching should be assessed remembering that 90 percent of tinnitus patients match their tinnitus at 20dB or less and 84 percent match theirs at 9dB or less. Other important audiological evaluations are the minimum tinnitus masking level and residual inhibition. The minimum masking level measures the degree to which tinnitus can be masked by external acoustic sources. This test employs a band of noise extending from 2000Hz to 12000Hz as the masking sound which is applied to the affected ear using earphones. The masking sound is gradually increased until it is detected by the patient. The pitch of the sound is increased until the patient no longer hears the tinnitus. In most people the minimum masking level is 8dB or less. Residual inhibition records the time the tinnitus is reduced or eliminated following a masking period. This is achieved by masking the tinnitus at a minimum level plus 10dB for 60 seconds and the length of time it takes the tinnitus to improve is determined.

Poor speech test performance indicates pathology in the central nervous system (Brechtelsbauer, 1990). Tympanometry identifies a previously undetected middle ear effusion, tympanic membrane stiffness from a patulous eustachian tube or stapedial and palatal muscle myoclonus (Meyerhoff & Cooper, 1991).

If suggested by the presence of a medical comorbidity, a full blood count, thyroid function tests, autoimmune tests e.g. rheumatoid factor, lipid profile may be done.

A computed tomography (CT) scan of the temporal bone can delineate a sigmoid sinus or a bony defect over the jugular bulb. Magnetic resonance imaging (MRI) with or without magnetic resonance angiography can pick up a glomusjugulare tumour, an arteriovenous and other vascular malformations.

8. Treatment

The development of therapeutic measures for tinnitus has been made difficult as a result of the complex relationship between tinnitus and its comorbid mental illnesses. However, a range of treatment modalities are available with varying degrees of statistical reliability. These comorbidities may modulate the experience of tinnitus and treatment of these conditions will alleviate patients' conditions. It is argued that psychological treatment should be employed before the consideration of drugs of which there is no single agent or groups of agents specifically recommended for this treatment.

There are no clear cut clinical standards or practice guidelines for the management of tinnitus, however, an evidence based review and tinnitus triage guide (Henry et al., 2010) has been developed to help family physicians who may be the first contact point for these patients (Table 4).

If patient	Refer to	Status/Considerations
Has neural deficits such as facialweakness, head trauma, orother urgent medical condition	Otolaryngology *or* ED	Emergency
Has unexplained suddenhearing loss	Audiology *and* otolaryngology	Emergency; must seeaudiologist prior tootolaryngologist on same day
Expresses suicidal ideation *or*manifests obvious mental illness	Mental health *or* ED	May be emergency;report suicide ideation; provideescort, if necessary
Has *any* of the following: • symptoms suggestive ofsomatic origin of tinnitus(eg, tinnitus that pulses withheartbeat) • persistent otalgia or otorrhea • vestibular symptoms (eg,dizziness/vertigo)	Otolaryngology *and* audiology	Urgent; scheduleotolaryngology exam as soonas possible
Has symptoms that suggesta neurophysiologic origin oftinnitus*without*: • ear pain, drainage, ormalodor • vestibular symptoms • sudden hearing loss • facial weakness or paralysis	Audiology *and* otolaryngology	Nonurgent; schedule audiologyexam before patient seesotolaryngologist

Table 4. Tinnitus Triage Guide (Henry et al., 2010)

Treatment depends on the cause and in a host of patients; the cause is inner ear damage. In these patients, reassurance of the benign nature of their condition usually suffices.

The treatment for tinnitus is classified into medical, otopsychiatric, sound modulation and surgical.

Medical treatment- Is further subdivided into pharmacological treatment, electrical stimulation, psychological counselling and homeopathic therapy.

Pharmacological treatment: There is no single pharmacological agent approved for the treatment of tinnitus. Most medications available are used in the modulation of tinnitus related comorbidities especially psychological conditions hence the use of anxiolytics, antidepressants, vasodilators and even intravenous anaesthetic agents like lidocaine have been used (Noble, 2008; Johnson et al., 1993; Agrawal & Pothier, 2009; Kalcioglu et al., 2005). Newer medications are being investigated with promising results which attempt to modulate the central auditory pathways and reducing tinnitus. Examples are Pramipexole and Acamprosate (Sziklai et al., 2011; Azevedo & Figueiredo, 2005; Sharma et al., 2012).

Drugs presently in use are tricyclic antidepressants (Amytryptiline 50 to 100mg daily at bedtime; Nortryptiline 50mg given at bedtime). Beneficial effects are noticed in about three to four weeks of treatment. Selective serotonin reuptake inhibitors have also been used such as Sertraline (50mg daily) and Paroxetine (10mg at bedtime). Alprazolam has been found to improve the visual analogue scales in patients who did not have anxiety or depression (Jalali et al., 2009). Others are Gabapectin, prostaglandin E1 and botulinium toxin A.

Electrical stimulation: The mechanism by which this works is still largely unknown but stimulation of the auditory system has been found to relieve tinnitus. There are many types of electrical stimulation which have been attempted, cutaneous, transcranial, promontory etc. Reports suggest relieve of tinnitus in 80 percent of patients but the effects are only transient.

Psychological counselling: Many patients consider tinnitus to be a very severe condition, afraid that it will worsen with deafness setting in over time. Therefore, patients need to be thought about tinnitus especially the relationship between selective attention on tinnitus and its cognitive emotional and behavioural effects. Educating the patients that they are able to cope with their tinnitus usually suffices.

Homeopathic therapy: The use of alternative medical therapies for tinnitus has been on the increase over the years. This is because for some patients modern medical therapies may not provide relief from this symptom. Though there seem to be a strong suggestion of a placebo effect with some of these therapies indicating that the belief of the patient and the provider of the therapy are strong factors in treatment success. The therapies used include gingko biloba extracts, niacin, acupuncture and hyperbaric oxygen. Others which are largely available to individuals especially as information on the internet are diet modification e.g. avoidance of caffeine, nicotine, refined sugar, chocolate, saturated and unsaturated fats e.t.c. and a combination of vitamins and supplements.

The extract of the gingko biloba tree is an antioxidant which increases blood flow to the brain and small blood vessels, inhibits platelet activating factor, alter neuron metabolism and prevent free radicals from damaging cell membranes. Bleeding time should be checked if treatment is to last longer than 4 weeks since it inhibits platelet aggregation.

About half the patients on niacin express successful treatment reporting that it reduces the severity and intensity of the tinnitus. Niacin provides smooth muscle relaxation especially of tiny blood vessels hence increasing blood flow to the inner ear. Skin blushes are the drawback of its use.

Acupuncture as treatment for tinnitus originated in Asia with the belief that the discomfort from tinnitus is reduced when needles are applied to the hand and face on the affected side (Park et al., 2000). However, there are doubts in this form of therapy as controlled studies indicate a strong component of faith by the patients in the physician or the treatment.

Hyperbaric oxygen which is used for the treatment of certain medical conditions such as carbon monoxide poisoning, necrotising fasciitis, gas gangrene etc has been reported to relieve tinnitus associated with sensorineural hearing loss by increasing the blood hence oxygen supply to the inner ear (Bennett et al., 2005).

Otopsychiatric treatment- Psychological comorbidities are often times neglected with the physician giving medications for tinnitus alone and when improvement is not noticeable by the patients they tend to go doctor shopping and the eventual result will be disappointment and frustration. Seeking the help of a psychologist and psychotherapist early is quite vital. The other spectrum is the referral of these patients to the psychologist and/ or psychotherapist without full medical and audiological assessment. Therefore, the close collaboration of the physician, audiologist, psychologist and psychotherapist is important in the effective management of these patients.

The ultimate objective of otopsychiatric treatment is to help patients direct their attention away from the tinnitus and putting negative cognitive processes under control.

Cognitive behavioural therapy: Psychological assessment/treatment should be an integral part of the tinnitus management protocol and not just based on the presence of a mental illness. Referral to the psychologist and psychotherapist which has to be carefully planned is essential to assessing associated comorbid mental disorders because tinnitus patients may be psychologically vulnerable (Langguth et al., 2001). This type of therapy will help improve patients' quality of life by restructuring thought patterns and habituating these patterns when the patient reacts to tinnitus (Martinez et al., 2010). Habituation or adaptation takes place when an originally new stimulus becomes well known and has no relevance for the patient taking any actions. It fails when it leads to the development of comorbid psychological distresses and impairment in the quality of life. It is explained that tinnitus occurs when habituation fails. Research has shown that tinnitus can be equated to any other auditory stimulus to which a patient may or may not attend and the normal response is adaptation to this stimulus (Hallam, 1987). Three variables or factors are influential in the process of habituation and are;

1. *Sensory factors*- The characteristics i.e. intensity and quality of the stimulus. It is assumed that noises which are more irregular in pattern are more require a longer period of adaptation or habituation.

2. *Perceptual factors*- Environmental conditions such as the intensity of other stimuli and the competing demands on attention. Natural sounds will mask tinnitus in some patients. Different daily activities and various competing sensory perceptions should help distract a patient's attention from tinnitus.

3. *Psychological factors*- The more meaningful or threatening a stimulus is the more a patient pays attention to it creating a positive feedback loop i.e. the more attention is paid to tinnitus the more the patient develops negative cognitive emotional processing resulting in various comorbidities.

Biofeedback, Education and relaxation therapies: First described for the successful treatment of pain and other stress related disorders, biofeedback in combination with educating patients about their tinnitus and relaxation therapies aim to teach the patients to focus on adapting to the tinnitus and subsequent comorbid psychological stresses (Dobie, 1999). This method of treatment does not eliminate tinnitus but helps improve the patient's quality of life. It involves listening to audio signal produced electromyography (EMG) of the frontalis muscle. This helps to reduce the tinnitus and muscle tension.

8.1. Sound modulation therapy

Hearing aids: Especially useful for patients with associated hearing loss. For such patients hearing aids with sound generators are used (Henry et al., 2008). Hearing aids can increase the level of ambient sound delivered to the patient which achieves all the objectives targeted for sound therapy.Studies have shown a benefit of hearing aids in patients enrolled in comprehensive tinnitus management programs (Foliner & Carroll, 2006). However, a success rate of 50 percent is recorded.

Cochlear implants: These work by masking tinnitus or by electric stimulation of the auditory nerve as mentioned above but are only beneficial in patients who have bilateral profound sensorineural hearing loss.

Tinnitus maskers: Create and deliver constant low level wideband sounds to the patient's ear. This helps to give relieve from tinnitus and its attendant psychological stresses. Bedside clocks or radios can be used for those experiencing tinnitus at bedtime. These fill the ambient silence with low level noise which masks the tinnitus.

Neuromonics: This is a combination of acoustic stimulation with a structured program of counselling and support given by a clinician trained specifically in tinnitus rehabilitation (Davis et al., 2008).

Tinnitus feedback retraining: This method of therapy involves generation of a background sound to make the tinnitus less noticeable. It is based on the neurophysiologic model (Jastreboff & Hazel, 1993) helping patients to understand that tinnitus sounds are actually meaningless. This should also lead to habituation. Another important component of this type of treatment is counselling of patients.

When treatment is finished, the audiologist must assess to determine if the patient needs further psychological counselling. If further counselling is required, the audiologist should consider if there are patient conditions beyond his/her scope of management and refer appropriately. The treatment options may include any combination of biofeedback, imagery training and muscle relaxation. If counselling is unnecessary, the audiologist should measure outcomes and recommend an appropriate patient follow up schedule (Steiger & Hamill, 2004).

Surgical treatment- Tinnitus which results from surgical lesions in and around the ears is treated surgically. These lesions as mentioned earlier include acoustic tumours which when excised relieves tinnitus in 50 percent of cases; Meniere's syndrome for which auditory nerve section, endolymphatic shunt, labyrinthectomy and ototoxic antibiotic injections gives relief in 40 to 80 percent of patients themechanism of which is unknown; temporomandibular joint diseases for which dental orthotics suffice.

Others are glomusjugulare tumours, sigmoid sinus diverticulum and arteriovenous malformation.

9. Prevention

A large number of the aetiological factors implicated in tinnitus are unpreventable. However, some precautions can help to prevent tinnitus. These are avoidance of over exposure to noise at social events or gatherings, at work or at home. Turning down the volume of musical appliances will be of help and at work when exposed to loud machinery, using ear protectors or ear muffs are helpful.

Other helpful measures are regular exercises and eating right to prevent cardiovascular diseases that cause tinnitus.

10. Conclusion

The treatment of tinnitus is as multifaceted as its aetiology.

Its close association with comorbid psychological distresses requires thorough clinical assessment by an audiologist, psychologist/psychotherapist and neuro-otologist to establish the presence of these comorbidities in order to institute adequate treatment.

Author details

Adeyi A. Adoga* and Taiwo J. Obindo

*Address all correspondence to: adeyiadoga@gmail.com

Departments of Otorhinolaryngology, Head and Neck Surgery and Psychiatry, University of Jos & Jos University Teaching Hospital, Jos, Plateau State, Nigeria

References

[1] Adoga AA, Adoga AS, Obindo JT. Tinnitus and the prevalence of comorbid psychological stress. Nig J Med. 2008; 17(1): 95-97.

[2] American Tinnitus Association.ATA's top 10 most frequently asked questions. Available at: http://www.ata.org/for-patients/faqs. Assessed July 2nd, 2012.

[3] American Tinnitus Association. Press Release: August 24th, 2011. Available at: http://www.ata.org/about-ata/news-pubs/press-release#DoDGrant.

[4] Agarwal L, Pothier DD. Vasodilators and vasoactive substances for idiopathic sudden sensorineural hearing loss. Cochrane Database Syst Rev. 2009; 7(4): CD003422.

[5]. Attias J, Shemech Z, Bleich A, Solomon Z, Bar-oR G et al. Psychological profile of help-seeking and non-help-seeking tinnitus patients. ScandAudiol. 1995; 24: 13-18.

[6] Azevedo AA, Figueiredo RR. Tinnitus treatment with Acamprosate: double blind study. Braz J Otorhinolaryngol. 2005; 71(5): 618-23.

[7] Axelsson A, Ringdahl A. Tinnitus- a study of its prevalence and characteristics. Br J Audiol.1989; 23: 53-62.

[8] Bennett M, Kertesz T, Young P. Hyperbaric oxygen therapy for idiopathic sudden sensorineural hearing loss and tinnitus: a systematic review of randomized controlled trials. J Laryngol Otol. 2005; 119(10): 791-8.

[9] Brechtelsbauer DA. Adult hearing loss.Prim Care.1990; 17: 249-65.

[10] Bulbul SF, Muluk NB, Cakir EP, Tufan E. Subjective tinnitus and hearing problems in adolescents. Int J PedOtorhinolaryngol. 2009; 73: 1124-1131.

[11] Crocetti A, Forti S, Ambrosetti U, Bo LD. Questionnaires to evaluate anxiety and depressive levels in tinnitus patients. Otolaryngol Head Neck Surg. 2009; 140: 403-405.

[12] Dalton DS, Cruickshanks KJ, Klein BE, Klein R, Wiley TL et al. The impact of hearing loss on quality of life in older patients.Gerontologist. 2003;43(5): 661-68.

[13] Davis PB, Wilde RA, Steele LG, Hanley PJ. Treatment of tinnitus with a customized acoustic neural stimulus: a controlled clinical study. Ear Nose Throat J. 2008; 87(6): 330-9.

[14] De Ridder D, Elgoyhen AB, Romo R, Langguth B. Phantom percepts: Tinnitus and pain as persisting aversive memory networks. ProcNatlAcadSci U.S.A. 2011; 20: 8075-8080.

[15] Dobie RA. A review of randomized clinical trials in tinnitus.Laryngoscope. 1999; 109(8): 1202-11.

[16] Fagelson MA. The association between tinnitus and post-traumatic stress disorder.Am J Audiol. 2007; 16(2): 107-17.

[17] Feldmann H. Homolateral and contralateral masking of tinnitus by noise-bands and by pure tones.Audiology. 1971; 10(3): 138-44.

[18] Figueiredo RR, Azevedo AA, Oliveira PM. Correlation analysis of the visual-analogue scale and the Tinnitus Handicap Inventory in tinnitus patients. RevistaBrasileira de Otorrinolaryngologia. 2009; 75(1): 76-9.

[19] Figueiredo RR, Rates MA, Azevedo AA, Oliveira PM, Navano PB. Correlation analysis of hearing thresholds validated questionnaires and psychoacoustic measurements in tinnitus patients. Braz J Otorhinolaryngol. 2010; 76(4): 522-6.

[20] Folmer RL, Carroll JR. Long term effectiveness of ear-level devices for tinnitus. Otolaryngol Head Neck Surg. 2006; 134(1): 132-137.

[21] Folmer RL, Griest SE. Tinnitus and insomnia. Am J Otolaryngol.2000; 21: 287-293.

[22] Folmer RL, Griest Se, Meikle MB, Martin WH. Tinnitus severity , loudness and depression. Otolaryngol Head Neck Surg. 1999; 121: 48-51.

[23] Griest SE, Bishop PM. Tinnitus as an early indicator of permanent hearing loss: A 15 year longitudinal study of noise exposed workers. AAOHN J. 1998; 46:325-9.

[24] Guitton MJ. Tinnitus and anxiety: more than meets the ear. Curr Psychiatry Rev. 2006; 2: 333-8.

[25] Halford JB, Anderson SD. Anxiety and depression in tinnitus sufferers. J Psychosom Res. 1991; 35(4-5): 383- 90.

[26] Hallam RS. Psychological approaches to the evaluation and management of tinnitus distress. Tinnitus. J. Hazell (Ed). Edinburgh, Churchill Livingstone; 1987: 156-175.

[27] Hallberg L, Erlandsson SI. Tinnitus characteristics in tinnitus complainers and non-complainers.Br J Audiol.1993; 27: 19-27.

[28] Harter M, Maurischat C, Weske G, Laszig R, Berger M. Psychological stress and impaired quality of life in patients with tinnitus.HNO. 2004; 29(6): 628-634.

[29] Hebert S, Canlon B, Hasson D. Emotional exhaustion as a predictor of tinnitus. PsychotherPsychosom. 2012; 81(5): 324-326.

[30] Heller MF, Bergman M. Tinnitus in normally hearing persons.Ann Otol. 1953; 62: 73-93.

[31] Henry JA, Schechter MA, Zaugg TL, Myers PJ. Progressive audiologic tinnitus management.ASHA leader. 2008; 13(8): 14-7.

[32] Henry JA, Trune DA, Robb MJ, Jastreboff PJ. Tinnitus retraining therapy: clinical guidelines. San Diego (CA): Plural Publishing, Inc; 2007.

[33] Henry JA, Zaugg TL, Myers PJ, Kendall CJ, Michaelides EM. A triage for tinnitus. J FamPract. 2010; 59(7): 389-93.

[34] Hoffman HJ, Reed GW. Epidemiology of tinnitus. In: Snow JB.ed. Tinnitus: Theory and management. Leviston, NY: BC Decker Inc; 2004: 16-41.

[35] Holgers KM. Mechanisms and classification of tinnitus: a discussion paper. Audiol Med. 2003; 1(4): 238-41.

[36] Holgers KM, Erlandsson SI, Barrenas ML. Predictive factors for auditory somatic and depression/anxiety related tinnitus.Audiol.2000; 39: 284-291.

[37] Holgers KM, Zoger S, Svedlund K. Predictive factors for development of severe tinnitus suffering- further characterization. Int J Audiol. 2005; 44(10): 584-92.

[38] Jalali MM, Krusha A, Naghavi SE, Suleiman R, Banan R. The effects of Alprazolam n tinnitus: a cross-over-randomized clinical trial. Med SciMonit. 2009; 15(11): 155-60.

[39] Jastreboff PJ. Phantom auditory perception (tinnitus): mechanism of generation and perception. Neurosci Res. 1990; 8: 221- 254.

[40] Jastreboff PJ, Hazell JWP. A neurophysiological approach to tinnitus: clinical implications. British J Audiol.1993; 27: 7-17.

[41] Johnson RM, Brummett R, Schleuning A. Use of Alprazolam for relief of tinnitus: A double blind study. Arch Otolaryngol Head Neck Surg. 1993; 119(8): 842-5.

[42] Kalcioglu MT, bayindir T, Erdem T, Ozturan O. Objective evaluation of the effects of lidocaine on tinnitus. Hear Res. 2005; 199(1-2): 81-8.

[43] Kamalski DM, Hockstra CE, van Zanten BG, Grolman W, Rovers MM. Measuring disease specific health related quality of life to evaluate treatment outcomes in tinnitus patients: a systematic review. Otolarygol Head Neck Surg. 2010; 143(2): 181-5.

[44] Kazdin AE. Research design in clinical psychology. 2003. 4th ed. Needham heights, MA: Allyn& Bacon.

[45] Knipper M, Muller M, Zimmerman U. Molecular mechanisms of tinnitus.Springer handbook of Auditory Research.2012; 44: 59-82.

[46] Kompis M, Neuner NT, Hemmeler W, Hausler R. Tinnitus.TherUmsch. 2004; 61(1): 15-20.

[47] Krog NH, Engdahl B, Tambs K. The association between tinnitus and mental health in a general population sample: results from the HUNT study. J Psychosom Res. 2010; 69: 289-298.

[48] Langguth B, Kleinjung T, Landgrebe M. Tinnitus: the complexity of standardization. Eval Health Prof. 2001; 34(4): 429-33.

[49] Lenarz T, Schreiner C, Snyder RL, Ernst A. Neural mechanisms of tinnitus. Eur Arch Otorhinolaryngol. 1993; 249(8): 441-446.

[50] Lipsey MW. Design sensitivity: Statistical power for experimental research. 1990. Newbury Park, CA: Sage Publications, Inc.

[51] Londero A, Peignard P, Malinvaud D, Avan P, Bonfils P. Tinnitus and cognitive behavioural therapy: results after 1 year. PresseMedicale. 2006; 35(9): 1213-1221.

[52] Martines F, Bentivegna D, Martines E, Sciacca V, Martinciglio G. Assessing audiological, patthophysiological and psychological variables in tinnitus patients with or without hearing loss. Eur Arch otorhinolaryngol.2010; 267: 1685-1693.

[53] Martinez-Devesa P, Perera R, Theodoulou M, Waddell A. Cognitive behavioural therapy for tinnitus. Cochrane Database Syst Rev. 2010; 8(9): CD005233.

[54] Mazureck B, Olze H, Haupt H, Klapp BF, Adili M et al. Molecular biological aspects of neuroplasticity: approaches for treating tinnitus and hearing disorders. HNO. 2010; 58(10): 973-82.

[55] Meikle MB, Henry JA, Griest SE, Stewart BJ, Abrams HB et al. The Tinnitus Functional Index: development of a new clinical measure for chronic intrusive tinnitus. Ear Hear. 2012; 33(2): 153-76.

[56] Meikle MB, Stewart BJ, Griest SE, Henry JA.Tinnitus outcomes assessment.Trends Amplif.2008; 12: 223-235.

[57] Meyerhoff WL, Cooper JC. Tinnitus. In: Paparella MM, ed. Otolaryngology. 3d ed. Philadelphia: Saunders. 1991:1169-75.

[58] Mrena R, Svolainen S, Kuokkanen J, Ylikoski J. Characteristics of tinnitus induced by acute acoustic trauma: a long term follow up. AudiolNeurootol. 2002; 7(2): 122-30.

[59] Noble W. Treatments for tinnitus. Trends Amplif. 2008; 12(3): 236-41.

[60] Nondahl DM, Cruickshanks KJ, Huang GH, Klein BE, Klein R et al. Tinnitus and its risk factors in the Beaver Dam offspring study.Int I Audiol.2011; 50: 313-20.

[61] Nondahl DM, Cruichshanks KJ, Wiley TL, Klein R, Klein BE et al. Prevalence ad 5 year incidence ot tinnitus among older patients: the epidemiology of hearing loss study. J Am AcadAudiol. 2002; 13: 323-331.

[62] Park J, White AR, Ernst E. Efficacy of acupuncture as a treatment for tinnitus: a systematic review. Arch Otolaryngol Head Neck Surg. 2000; 126(4): 489-92.

[63] Rauschecker JP, Leaver AM, Muhlau M. Tuning out the noise: limbic-auditory interactions in tinnitus. Neuron.2010; 66: 819-826.

[64] Reynolds P, Gardner D, Lee R. Tinnitus and psychological morbidity: a cross-sectional study to investigate psychological morbidity in tinnitus patients and its relationship with severity of symptoms and illness perceptions. ClinOtolaryngol Allied Sci. 2004; 29(6): 628-634.

[65] Robinson SK, McQuaid JR, Viirre ES, Betzig LL, Miller DL et al.The relationship of tinnitus questionnaires to depressive symptoms, quality of well-being and internal focus.Int tinnitus J. 2003; 9(2): 97-103.

[66] Rubak T, Kock S, Koefoed-Nielsen B, Lund SP, Bonde JP et al.The risk of tinnitus following occupational noise exposure in workers with hearing loss or normal hearing.Int J Audiol. 2008; 47: 109-14.

[67] Saunders JC. The role central nervous system plasticity in tinnitus.J CommunDisord. 2007; 40: 313-34.

[68] Schaaf H, Dolberg D, Seling B, Martner M. Comorbidity of tinnitus and psychiatric disorders. Nervenarzt. 2003; 74(1): 72-5.

[69] Schecklmann M, Landgrebe M, Poeppl TB, Kreuzer P, Manner P et al. Neural correlates of tinnitus duration and distress: A positron emission tomography study. Human Brain Mapp. 2011; 22: doi 10.1002/hbm.21426.

[70] Schleuning AJ 2nd. Management of the patient with tinnitus.Med Clin North Am. 1991; 75: 1225-1237.

[71] Shargorodsky J, Curhan SG, Curhan GC, Earvey R. Change in prevalence of hearing loss in US adolescents. JAMA.2010; 304: 772-778.

[72] Shargorodsky J, Curhan GC, Farwell WR. Prevalence and characteristics of tinnitus among US adults.Am J Med. 2010; 123: 711-718.

[73] Sharma DK, Kaur S, Singh J, Kaur I. Role of Acamprosate in sensorineural tinnitus.Indian J Pharmacol. 2012; 44(1): 93-6.

[74] Simpson JJ, Davies WE. Recent advances in the pharmacological treatment of tinnitus. Trends Pharmacol Sci. 1999; 20(1): 12-8.

[75] Sindhusake D, Golding M, Newall P, Rubin G, Jakobsen K et al. Risk factors for tinnitus in a population of older adults: the blue mountains hearing study. Ear Hear. 2003; 24: 501-507.

[76] Steiger JR, Hamill TA. A proposed clinical pathway for tinnitus evaluation and management. Hear J. 2004; 57(7): 26-28.

[77] Stouffer JL, Tyler RS.Characterization of tinnitus by tinnitus patients. J Speech Hear Disord.1990; 55(3): 439-453.

[78] Sweetow RW. Cognitive aspects of tinnitus- patient management. Ear Hear. 1986; 7: 390-396.

[79] Sziklai I, Szilvassy J, Szilvassy Z. Tinnitus control by dopamine agonist pramipexole in presbycusis patients: a randomized, placebo-controlled double-blind study. Laryngoscope. 2011; 121(4): 888-93.

[80] Tan J, Tange RA, Dreschler WA, vdKleij A, Tromp EC. Long-term effect of hyperbaric oxygenation treatment in chronic distressing tinnitus.ScandAudiol. 1999; 28(2): 91-6.

[81] Tyler RS, Baker LJ. Difficulties experienced by tinnitus sufferers. J Speech Hear Disord. 1983; 48: 150-154.

[82] Van de Heyning P, Vermeire K, Diebl M, Nopp P, Anderson I et al. Incapacitating unilateral tinnitus in single sided deafness treated by cochlear implantation. Am OtolRhinolLaryngol. 2008; 17(9): 645-652.

[83] Vernon J. Attempts to relieve tinnitus, j Am Audiol Soc. 1977; 2(4): 124- 31.

Chapter 14

The Characteristics of Nicotine Addiction Among Patients with Schizophrenia

Ewa Wojtyna and Agnieszka Wiszniewicz

Additional information is available at the end of the chapter

1. Introduction

Premature death connected mainly with somatic disorders is observed among patients with schizophrenia. The major reason for this phenomenon are metabolic disorders caused on the one hand by side effects of pharmacological treatment [1], on the other by genetically determined differences in metabolism. Finally, the importance of behavioral factor, which is the lifestyle of patients with schizophrenia, must not be ignored here. Obesity, physical inactivity, poor diet, and smoking are the major factors contributing to the development and intensification of cardiovascular diseases. These factors are so important because they can be modified, as opposed to the genetic factors or necessary pharmacological treatment.

This article addresses the issue of nicotine addiction among patients with schizophrenia.

1.1. Schizophrenia and nicotine addiction

1.1.1. Scope of phenomenon

The phenomenon of tobacco dependence involves 60-90% of patients with schizophrenia, and it is a much higher rate than among the general population, where the percentage of smokers varies between 25-47% [2-6].

A study by de Leon et al. [7] and Gurpegui et al. [8] has shown that in adults (over twenty years old) who are in the group of increased susceptibility to schizophrenia, or are already suffering from the disease there is a significantly higher risk of taking up smoking than among the general population [9]. No wonder then that the problem of nicotine addiction and its consequences is becoming more and more urgent in clinical psychiatry.

Schizophrenics are most often among the so-called heavy smokers, which means, first of all, smoking at least 20 cigarettes a day, and often a shorter interpuff interval, and smoking cigarettes with a higher nicotine content [3, 10].

In this group of patients a higher risk of dependence on nicotine is observed [11], as well as a more severe abstinence syndrome when trying to quit smoking [12]. This last phenomenon probably results from the fact that in schizophrenics there are, independent of metabolism, higher levels of nicotine and cotinine than in the blood of non-schizophrenics smoking the same amounts of cigarettes [13]. This fact can be explained by a greater number of puffs per cigarette and shorter interpuff intervals [10]. It is not surprising, therefore, that schizophrenics stop smoking more rarely than non-psychotic people [14], and the treatment of nicotine addiction - behavioral and pharmacological - in this group is much less effective [15-18].

1.1.2. Health consequences of smoking in schizophrenics

Research shows that patients suffering from schizophrenia live roughly 20% shorter than healthy people, while cigarette smoking is here one of the main risk factors for premature death [19]. It was also shown that due to smoking these patients die on average 10 years earlier than the general population [20, 21].

This increased mortality is largely the result of cancer, cerebrovascular disease, respiratory diseases, and coronary heart disease. It is estimated that approximately 33% of psychotic patients suffer from this illness and in this group it accounts for more premature deaths than suicide [22].

This phenomenon is particularly relevant in the light of reports which indicate that in schizophrenics who smoke regularly there is a higher risk of coronary heart disease and stroke than in the general population [23]. It is estimated that, in the group with schizophrenia, the risk of death from cardiovascular problems is about 2.2 times higher than among the general population [24].

Also, in schizophrenia patients, respiratory diseases [25, 26] such as chronic obstructive pulmonary disorder (COPD) and pneumonia are frequently observed. Although lung cancer occurs less frequently in patients with schizophrenia than among the general population, the effects of cigarette smoking are clearly seen here [27]. In the case of COPD and lung cancer, cigarette smoking is undoubtedly a significant etiologic factor [28]. Smoking can also increase susceptibility to pneumonia [29]. As shown in the Copeland et al. [26] study, COPD and pneumonia are the diseases more frequently occurring in the last year of life in schizophrenics than in those mentally healthy. In this group of patients the risk of dying from respiratory diseases is estimated to be approximately 3.2 times higher than among the general population [30].

1.1.3. Biological determinants of smoking

1.1.3.1. Genetic background

The empirical data available suggest the existence of common risk factors for schizophrenia (and other mental illnesses) and smoking. The possibility of a genetic risk factor, particularly associated with the regulation of cholinergic neurotransmission is emphasized here [31-35].

1.1.3.2. Self-medication hypothesis

Self-medication hypothesis is based on the assumption that the use of psychoactive substances helps patients compensate for neurobiological deficits underlying a variety of ailments [36, 37]. Accordingly, intuitive reaching for cigarettes by schizophrenics would facilitate both dealing with the symptoms of the disease – positive and negative or with cognitive impairment, as well as with the side effects of treatment.

However, the importance of smoking in coping with the disease symptoms is not clear [38]. Some studies show an improvement within the range of negative symptoms by increasing the dopamine release in the prefrontal cortex [39-42]. These results, however, are subject to a number of constraints - sample size and methodological limitations. It is also worth remembering that research on animal models indicated that while occasional acute administration of nicotine did increase the dopamine release in the brain, chronic administration of nicotine resulted in a decrease in dopamine level, but these effects varied in different areas of the brain [41-43].

There is more data on the relief of drug-induced symptoms and on the cognitive deficits.

1.1.3.2.1. Neuroleptics

Referring the self-medication hypothesis to the problem of antipsychotic treatment [38], it should be assumed that smoking helps to reduce the adverse symptoms of antipsychotic treatment. The mechanism that may explain the reduced severity of extrapyramidal symptoms associated with high-dose neuroleptic treatment, may be the nicotine-induced acceleration of drug metabolism by cytochrome P450 (CYP1A2, CYP2D6 polymorphisms) [4, 44]. Thus alleviation of drug induced effects of the CYP1A2 metabolized neuroleptics can be expected but there should be no such effects in case of drugs metabolized in a different way. The empirical data do not provide conclusive evidence that heavy smoking has a really important role in alleviating the side effects of antipsychotic treatment, especially such as tardive dyskinesis or akathisia [38].

Antipsychotic drugs with anticholinergic properties influence the expression of nicotine acetylcholine receptors (nAChRs) [45]. This translates into a deterioration of neurotransmission in the cholinergic system in patients with schizophrenia.

1.1.3.2.2. Cognitive factors – The role of the cholinergic system

The cholinergic neurotransmission is one of the key phenomena important for cognitive functioning. This applies in particular to such areas of the brain as the prefrontal cortex and hippocampus, whose functions are regulated by cholinergic projections from other parts of the brain [46]. Cholinergic system dysfunction is manifested, among others, in impaired cognitive functions such as memory and attention disorders. On the other hand stimulation of this system results in memory improvement.

Research shows that administration of nicotine to schizophrenics, both smokers and non-smokers, activating the cholinergic system, reduces the cognitive deficits connected with e.g. working memory, attention, and spatial organization [47-49].

It was also observed that in schizophrenics cognitive deficits worsen with the increase of withdrawal symptoms, and restarting smoking alleviates these unwanted changes in cognitive functioning [49]. This suggests that the treatment of cognitive deficits connected with schizophrenia could contribute to increasing the chance of successful smoking cessation, and indirectly to improving the patient's overall health.

1.1.4. Psychological determinants of smoking

As shown above, in a group of schizophrenics there are a number of biological factors, specific to a lesser or greater extent to schizophrenia which explain the increased incidence of nicotine dependence in this group of patients. However, these factors are not the only ones that are relevant here. The psychosocial factors should not be ignored, especially that these factors are largely modifiable, and thus possible to be included in a therapeutic process.

Many reasons for smoking, mentioned by patients suffering from schizophrenia, are similar to those mentioned by healthy people. Some of the common arguments are: pleasure, addiction, weight control, the need for relaxation, or a desire to calm down.

Schmitz et al. [50] presume the possibility of an increased susceptibility to nicotine addiction in people who have difficulty coping with stress, tension, anxiety, or depression. Anxiety and depressive disorders have been repeatedly identified as a risk factor for taking up and continuing smoking [51]. In psychotic patients, the coexistence of these various disorders can further increase the tendency to smoking.

Patients with schizophrenia often emphasize that cigarettes are for them a product of first necessity, just like food, and help them endure life with the illness and prevent schizophrenia relapses [52]. Not without reason, therefore, schizophrenics often mention the sedative effect of nicotine as the main reason for smoking [38]. This temporary way of dealing with unpleasant symptoms, however, puts in motion a vicious circle, because the inability to cease smoking is also the cause of stress and can lead to a greater anxiety than in the beginning. After lighting a cigarette waiting for the calming effect is also important. However, in many cases of agitation, such an effect does not appear, which results in smoking more and more cigarettes in the hope that a higher dose of nicotine will eventually help [38].

Schizophrenics often emphasize that smoking is the fulfillment of a strong need related to addiction, it is also an opportunity to escape and helps to control emotions. In Solway et al. clinical studies [53] the psychotic patients singled out three main roles that smoking plays in their daily functioning. Smoking is a tool used to control stress, helps to make interpersonal contacts and meet the need for peace and comfort. Facilitating interpersonal relations occurs here by entering a group of smokers, which helps to cope with the sense of exclusion and of being different (tobacco use is thus understood as supporting the development of social networks and a source of social support). Solway et al. [53], however, draw attention to the fact that the respondents are increasingly aware of the fact that smoking - contrary to expectations - does not accomplish its purpose in terms of interpersonal contacts. Although many of the schizophrenics examined began to smoke in order to reduce discomfort in social situations, there is currently a trend towards unfavorable attitudes to smokers, which, in individuals suffering from mental illnesses, may create an additional barrier in the process of socializing.

People suffering from schizophrenia find it more difficult to quit smoking partly because of the withdrawal symptoms, including irritability, poor concentration, impatience and anxiety [6], and partly because they do not have enough support and motivation to do it successfully. The balance of gains and losses related to smoking cessation is in favor of the benefits of tobacco use [53]. The decision to maintain the addiction is often connected with the opinions functioning in society (especially among relatives), suggesting many obstacles and losses resulting from the process of smoking cessation.

According to de Leon et al. [54] the socio-economic status and poor education about the negative effects of smoking have a major impact on the initiation of smoking in people with severe mental illnesses. De Leon et al. [54] also suggest that in some countries where tobacco use by women is prohibited, the relationship between smoking and schizophrenia cannot be proven. This points to the fact that the number of cigarettes smoked by people with schizophrenia depends on their availability [54]. In Poland, the price of cigarettes is relatively high compared to the income of the mentally ill. However, patients cope with these economic constraints by selecting the cheapest cigarettes, usually without a filter, from illegal sources, or they roll the cheap tobacco cigarettes. Also, the surrounding people often provide the patient with cigarettes. In the Solway's research [53] some smokers suffering from severe mental illnesses stated that the reason for their initiation of smoking was the addiction of one of their family members or friends.

In the Solway's research [53], some respondents answered that they do not feel the need for smoking when cigarettes are not in sight, but at the time of distress, anxiety, or in a situation where there is a person smoking nearby, they feel a strong desire to smoke a cigarette. Meanwhile, in Poland, the functioning of patients is often based on life in communities which are dominated by smokers. Many smokers define the sole physical act of holding a cigarette as a highly satisfactory form of relaxation.

In conclusion, a number of biological and psychosocial phenomena are observed in patients with schizophrenia that exacerbate the problem of nicotine addiction and hinder the process of smoking cessation. A better understanding of the mechanisms associated with cigarette smoking in this group of patients may help to improve their quality of life, their general health, but also reduce the economic effects associated with the treatment and the consequences of tobacco-related diseases in schizophrenics.

1.1.5. Aim of the research

The research was designed to characterize nicotine dependence in schizophrenics compared to smokers not having mental health problems. Indirectly, the research was also to determine whether the affective psychological factors such as anxiety or depression and the level of distress are important predictors of smoking in a group of psychotic patients.

2. Material and methods

2.1. Participants

204 smokers participated in the research, including 104 people with paranoid schizophrenia and 100 healthy persons. The schizophrenic smokers recruited for the research were in remission of psychotic symptoms or had residual symptoms and their condition was stable. These people have been treated for schizophrenia for at least 1 year. The control group were smokers who have not been diagnosed with a serious mental or somatic illness. At the time of the research, all the participants were in the active phase of nicotine dependence.

2.2 Design of research

The research was cross-sectional and was carried out in Mental Health Outpatient Clinics and Psychiatric Day Hospitals. The control group, consisting of mentally healthy people, was recruited in the Occupational Medicine Outpatient Clinics, where they came for periodic employee medical examinations. The research participants underwent a structured interview concerning smoking, and then the respondents were asked to complete five self-report questionnaires.

2.3. Tools

2.3.1. Interview

The interview with the respondents concerned their smoking history and included questions about the time of smoking initiation, the addiction process over time, the daily rituals related to smoking, number of attempts to stop smoking, length of periods of abstinence, the average number of puffs per cigarette, and the type of cigarettes smoked. Also, in the interview information was obtained about basic socio-demographic data, such as economic status, family, place of residence. In the case of patients with schizophrenia the interview contained additional questions about the course of the disease and its treatment.

2.3.2. Fagerström test for nicotine dependence

The study used the Fagerström Test for Nicotine Dependence (FTND) in order to estimate the severity of nicotine dependence [55]. This tool consists of 8 questions concerning factors associated with smoking. The result obtained is in the range of 0-11 points. The 0-4 points result corresponds to a low degree of dependence, 5-7 points – to a high degree, and the result of more than 7 points corresponds to a very high dependence. Although Steinberg et al. [56] demonstrated that, in the schizophrenic group, this tool carries the risk of underestimating the size of the problem, yet, in this study, the introduction of a detailed interview is an attempt to compensate for these deficiencies.

2.3.3. The test of motivation for smoking cessation

The test of motivation for smoking cessation consists of 12 items containing statements about the smoker dependent factors that contribute to smoking cessation (e.g., *Do you decide to quit smoking for yourself?, Do you know why you smoke?, Do you know how to cope in crisis situations?*). The respondent gave his own answers to these items by indicating whether the statement referred to him or not. The Cronbach's α coefficient for this scale is 0.91. Predominance of positive responses (> = 6 points) corresponds to a relatively strong motivation to smoking cessation.

2.3.4. The test of readiness to change

This tool has been designed on the basis of the Transtheoretical Model of Behavioral Change (TTM) [57] assumptions. According to this model, the current smokers are at the stage of precontemplation, contemplation or preparation. The precontemplation stage is defined as the lack of need for changes in behavior. At the stage of contemplation an intention to change behavior within the next 6 months emerges (here: to stop smoking) (but making this change is not planned within the next 30 days). And finally, the preparation stage is referred to as planning changes within the next month and attempts to stop smoking (lasting a minimum of 24 hours) can be indicated in the past year [58].

The Test of Readiness to Change used in this research consists of 8 questions, making it possible to identify persons at the stage of precontemplation, contemplation, preparation, and action (i.e. the act of smoking cessation).

2.3.5. Hospital Anxiety and Depression Scale (HADS)

The Hospital Anxiety and Depression Scale (HADS) is a widely used, short, 14 item tool for studying anxiety and depression [59]. Each of the tool subscales consists of seven statements to which the tested person responds on a four point scale, where 0 corresponds to no intensity or to the weakest intensity of a given symptom, and 3 indicates the presence of a severe symptom.

This questionnaire was initially recommended as an ambulatory screening tool, but is now also commonly used to assess symptoms of depression and anxiety in different groups of patients [60]. The sensitivity and specificity of this tool is satisfactory and is about 0.8 [61]. In our study, the scale reliability (Cronbach's α coefficient) was 0.86 for the depression subscale and 0.87 for the anxiety scale, which is consistent with the results obtained by other researchers [62, 63].

2.3.6. Distress thermometer

The Distress Thermometer is a single item screening tool that allows a subjective assessment of the severity of distress in the recent time. The respondent marks, on a scale of 0 to 10, how high was the level of stress he or she experienced during the last week. The validation studies of the Polish version of the tool have shown that the 4 point or more result indicates a high risk of comorbid depression and / or anxiety [64].

3. Results

The demographic characteristics of the respondents are shown in Table 1. The schizophrenics were more often single people, less educated, unemployed, and of worse financial situation than those in the control group.

Table 2 presents the comparison of the schizophrenics and the control group in terms of smoking.

The psychotic patients smoked more, took a greater number of puffs, showed a higher level of dependence and were less motivated to give up smoking than the mentally healthy persons.

It was also observed that the schizophrenics taking atypical medications (n = 58), smoked less and took puffs less frequently than those treated with conventional drugs (n = 46). There were no differences between the groups with respect to the age of smoking initiation (first cigarette), while the schizophrenics started smoking on a daily basis earlier than the healthy individuals. Those in the control group made attempts to quit smoking more often, and their abstinence periods were longer. It was also observed that as the period of being ill with schizophrenia gets longer, the number of cigarettes smoked grows ($r = 0.16$, $p < 0.05$) and the level of dependence increases ($r = 0.31$, $p < 0.01$).

Most schizophrenics had no intention to quit smoking, while people in the control group were more often at the contemplation or preparation stage for smoking cessation (Table 3).

Other motives for smoking cessation were also shown. In the mentally healthy individuals the major motive was their relatives' pressure, the desire to save money and, to a lesser extent, the beginning of health problems. The dominant motive in the schizophrenics, however, was the appearance of tobacco-related disease, manifested mainly by shortness of breath. The rarest motive turned out to be the pressure of relatives.

Smokers (N=204)	Schizophrenics (N=104)	Non-psychiatric (N=100)
Gender [*n(%)*]		
Male	61 (58.7)	54 (54.0)
Female	43 (41.3)	46 (46.0)
Age [years]		
Mean (SD)	44.31 (13.94)	44.02 (11.40)
Range	20 – 67	20 – 65
Marital status [*n(%)*]		
Single	32 (30.8)	25 (25.0)
Married	39 (37.5)	48 (48.0)
Widowed	13 (12.5)	15 (15.0)
Divorced	20 (19.2)	12 (12.0)
Level of education [*n(%)*]		
Primary	29 (27.9)	5 (5.0)
Vocational	54 (51.9)	35 (35.0)
Secondary	20 (19.2)	42 (42.0)
Higher	1 (1.0)	18 (18.0)
Residence[*n(%)*]		
With family	54 (52.0)	59 (59.0)
Alone	15 (14.4)	41 (41.0)
In a nursing home	35 (33.6)	-
Financial Situation [*n(%)*]		
Poor	60 (57.7)	18 (18.0)
Average	31 (29.8)	56 (56.0)
Good	13 (12.5)	26 (26.0)
Employment status [*n(%)*]		
Employed	18 (17.3)	69 (69.0)
Unemployed	23 (22.1)	16 (16.0)
Disability Pension	50 (48.1)	9 (9.0)
Retirement	13 (12.5)	6 (6.0)

Table 1. Socio-demographic characteristics of the smokers with schizophrenia and non-psychiatric controls.

Smoking	Schizophrenics (N=104)	Non-psychiatric (N=100)	Comparisons *t*
Cigarettes			
Cigarettes smoked per day [*M*(*SD*)]	25.98 (13.40)	20.09 (8.58)	3.72***
Range [*n* (%)]			
1-10	14 (13.5)	20 (20.0)	
11-20	42 (40.4)	46 (46.0)	
21-30	28 (26.9)	30 (30.0)	
"/>30	20 (19.2)	4 (4.0)	
Nicotine yield of cigarettes [*M*(*SD*)]	1.03 (0.22)	0.85 (0.22)	5.97***
Puffs per cigarette [*M*(*SD*)]	12.12 (3.57)	8.64 (2.39)	8.14***
Min to first cigarette of the day [*M*(*SD*)]	7.23 (4.58)	7.54 (3.97)	0.36
Nicotine dependence			
FTND [*M*(*SD*)]	7.63 (2.62)	6.30 (1.95)	4.12***
Years of daily smoking [*M*(*SD*)]	23.87 (14.26)	24.35 (12.02)	-0.26
Age of first smoking [*M*(*SD*)]	17.00 (4.49)	17.31 (5.59)	0.43
Age of daily smoking [*M*(*SD*)]	19.67 (3.84)	20.44 (8.53)	0.83
Smoking cessation			
Motivation to quit [*M*(*SD*)]	5.47 (3.54)	8.39 (2.24)	-7.07***
Past quit attempts [*M*(*SD*)]	2.05 (1.78)	3.92 (3.04)	-5.34***
Longest abstinence period [months] [*M*(*SD*)]	3.39 (4.55)	5.52 (6.18)	-2.80**

Notes: ** $p<0.01$; *** $p<0.001$

FTND – Fagerström Test for Nicotine Dependence

Table 2. Smoking characteristic of schizophrenic patients and healthy participants.

Stage of change	Schizophrenics (*N* =104) *n* (%)	Non-psychiatric (*N* =100) *n* (%)
Precontemplation	61 (58.6)	29 (29.0)
Contemplation	35 (33.7)	46 (46.0)
Preparation	8 (7.7)	25 (25.0)

Table 3. Readiness to smoking cessation

In the schizophrenics a higher level of distress and anxiety was observed than in the control group. Depression of the psychotic patients was also higher than in the healthy persons, but the difference did not reach statistical significance (table 4).

Factors	Schizophrenics (N=104)		Non-psychiatric (N=100)	Comparisons t
	subgroups	*M (SD)*		
Anxiety	all	9.20 (4.43)	6.28 (3.44)	5.28***
	typical treat.	9.49 (4.27)[a]		5.70***
	atypical treat.	7.50 (5.97)[a]		2.68
Depression	all	7.48 (3.65)	6.56 (3.10)	1.94
	typical treat.	7.53 (3.72)		2.01
	atypical treat.	6.87 (3.10)		0.68
Distress	all	5.42 (2.64)	4.20 (2.37)	3.47**
	typical treat.	5.67 (2.67)[b]		3.64***
	atypical treat.	5.31 (1.92)[b]		2.79*

Notes: * $p<0.05$; ** $p<0.01$; *** $p<0.001$

typical treat. – typical neuroleptics (n=46)

atypical treat. – atypical neuroleptics (n=58)

[a] comparison between typical and atypical treatment subgroups: $t=4.32$ ($p<0.001$)

[b] comparison between typical and atypical treatment subgroups: $t=2.15$ ($p<0.05$)

Table 4. Level of anxiety, depression and distress among participants

In the subgroup of schizophrenics, in the patients treated with atypical neuroleptics, a lower level of distress appeared (but still significantly higher than in the control group) and anxiety.

The analysis of the correlation between the affective factors and distress and the parameters characterizing smoking, indicated that in both groups – in the schizophrenics and in the control group - higher levels of anxiety, depression and distress are associated with a greater number of cigarettes smoked (table 5).

To determine the predictive power of the affective factors and distress for the number of cigarettes smoked multivariate linear regression analysis was carried out (table 6).

Affective factors and distress explain a greater percentage of variance of the number of cigarettes in the group of mentally healthy persons ($adj.R^2 = 0.56$) than in the group of schizophrenics ($adj.R^2 = 0.34$).

Smoking	Anxiety	Depression	Distress
Schizophrenic patients			
Cigarettes smoked per day	0.57***	0.64***	0.67***
Puffs per cigarette	-0.07	-0.03	-0,04
Nicotine dependence (FTND)	0.53***	0.49***	0.55***
Motivation to quit	-0.02	0.04	0.13
Non-psychiatric participants			
Cigarettes smoked per day	0.56***	0.21*	0.62***
Puffs per cigarette	0.12	-0.01	0.07
Nicotine dependence (FTND)	0.55***	0.17	0.53***
Motivation to quit	-0.14	-0.02	-0.06

Notes: * *p<0.05; *** p<0.001*

FTND – Fagerström Test for Nicotine Dependence

Table 5. Correlation between the affective factors and distress and the parameters characterizing smoking.

Factors	Schizophrenic patients (*N*=104)		Non-psychiatric smokers (*N*=100)	
	adj.R²=0.34		*adj.R²*=0.56	
	β	***ΔR²***	***β***	***ΔR²***
Anxiety	0.14	0.04	0.48***	0.24
Depression	0.36**	0.11	0.18	0.05
Distress	0.47***	0.19	0.55***	0.27

Notes: ** *p<0.01; *** p<0.001*

Table 6. Predictors of numbers of cigarettes smoked per day (multivariate linear regression model).

In both groups, the strongest predictor of smoking was distress and the predictive power of anxiety and depression was distributed differently in the group of schizophrenics and the control group. In the mentally ill patients depression was more strongly correlated with smoking, and in the control group, a stronger correlation with the number of cigarettes smoked was observed for anxiety.

4. Discussion

The study confirmed the observations of other researchers that schizophrenics smoke more than the mentally healthy and take a greater number of puffs per cigarette [10,

65]. In the group of mentally ill patients, similarly as in the Tidey et al. [10] studies, a variation in the number of cigarettes smoked and the number of puffs taken was observed depending on the type of treatment applied. The fact that patients taking atypicals smoked less than the patients receiving typical medication, may result from the different effect of taking these drugs. Several studies have shown that atypical drugs such as clozapine and olanzapine, are conducive to reducing smoking, reduce the desire to smoke and, finally, relieve the withdrawal symptoms [10, 66, 67]. Also, in patients taking atypicals, a lower level of distress is observed [68]. In this study, distress turned out to be a significant predictor of smoking, therefore it is possible that this mechanism is important in explaining the observed difference. In the presented work, however, neither the timing nor the doses of the administered medication were controlled, so these dependencies are worth researching more closely in the future.

The analysis of the factors motivating schizophrenics to stop smoking indicates a very serious problem. Only a significant deterioration of health, to be precise, shortness of breath making smoking impossible, inclined patients to consider reducing or giving up smoking. Lack of finances and bans on smoking in public places and in the place of residence were not a sufficient bareer for people with schizophrenia. Lack of pressure from the close environment to reduce smoking should also be noted. This may result from the fact that the closest people here are often smokers themselves (often these are other patients). Interviews with the patients showed that most often it was the family who supplied the patients with cigarettes, and thus contributed to continuing this addiction in schizophrenics.

The results of the study show the important role of affective factors and a feeling of distress in nicotine dependence. This importance is greater in the group of healthy persons than in schizophrenics, but the results obtained in this study (26% of the explained variance of the number of cigarettes smoked) suggest introducing psychological (and/or pharmacological) interactions, aimed at improving coping with stress and reducing the negative affect. These results also confirm the fact that cigarette smoking in schizophrenics is probably, to a much greater extent than in the mentally healthy, determined by factors other than affective [31-37].

The study also confirmed a significant relationship between distress and the number of cigarettes smoked. These results are consistent with other studies. It should be noted, that distress may have different sources and may be understood differently by the respondents. It is therefore a very general construct, and in this study should be understood as the so called aggregate variable [69].

5. Conclusion

The relationship between distress, affective factors, and cigarette smoking has important clinical implications. First of all - apart from the typical pharmacological treatment and nicotine replacement therapy – psychological treatment should be implemented into programs for nicotine dependence to improve the functioning of schizophrenics in terms of coping with stress and maintaining good mood.

Secondly, it seems interesting to study the causes of the perceived distress. Knowing the sources of stress and the strategies of coping with it can help to build more effective programs supporting the treatment of nicotine addiction.

Weak pressure of the environment on the mentally ill to quit smoking, and even strengthening the addiction by the closest ones, points to a need for actions targeted at the schizophrenics' environment. Such interventions should be aimed at increasing the knowledge about smoking and its consequences, including families in the process of motivating to quit smoking and improving support given to patients.

Author details

Ewa Wojtyna and Agnieszka Wiszniewicz

*Address all correspondence to: ewa.wojtyna@us.edu.pl

Institute of Psychology, University of Silesia, Katowice, Poland

References

[1] Stahl SM. Podstawy psychofarmakologii [Essentiale psychopharmacology]. Gdańsk: ViaMedica; 2009.

[2] Chapman S, Ragg M, McGeechan K. Citation bias in reported smoking prevalence in people with schizophrenia. The Australian And New Zealand Journal Of Psychiatry 2009; 43(3) 277-282.

[3] de Leon J, Diaz F. A meta-analysis of worldwide studies demonstrates an association between schizophrenia and tobacco smoking behaviors. Schizophrenia Research 2005; 76; 135-157.

[4] Dervaux A, Laqueille X. Tabac et schizophrénie: aspects épidémiologiques et cliniquess. L'encéphale 2008; 34(3) 299–305.

[5] Goff DC, Cather C, Evins, AE, Henderson DC, Freudenreich O, Copeland PM, Bierer M, Duckworth K, Sacks FM. Medical morbidity and mortality in schizophrenia: Guidelines for psychiatrists. Journal of Clinical Psychiatry 2005; 66(2) 183-194.

[6] Wang CY, Xiang YT, Weng YZ, Bo QJ, Chiu HF, Chan SS, Lee EH, Ungvari GS. Cigarette smoking in patients with schizophrenia in China: prospective, multicentre study. The Australian And New Zealand Journal Of Psychiatry 2010; 44(5) 456-462.

[7] de Leon J, Diaz FJ, Rogers T, Browne D, Dinsmore L. Initiation of daily smoking and nicotine dependence in schizophrenia and mood disorders. Schizophrenia Research 2002; 56; 47-54.

[8] Gurpegui M, Martínez-Ortega JM, Aguilar MC, Diaz FJ, Quintana HM, de Leon J. Smoking initiation and schizophrenia: A replication study in a Spanish sample. Schizophrenia Research 2005; 76; 113-118.

[9] Dome P, Lazary J, Kalapos MP, Rihmer Z. Smoking, nicotine and neuropsychiatric disorders. Neuroscience and Biobehavioral Reviews 2010; 34(3) 295-342.

[10] Tidey JW, Rohsenow DJ, Kaplan GB, Swift RM. Cigarette smoking topography in smokers with schizophrenia and matched non-psychiatric controls. Drug and Alcohol Dependence 2005; 80; 259–265.

[11] Spring B, Pingitore R, McChargue DE. Reward value of cigarette smoking for comparably heavy smoking schizophrenic, depressed, and nonpatient smokers. American Journal of Psychiatry 2003; 160; 316-322.

[12] Weinberger AH, Sacco KA, Creeden CI, Vessicchio JC, Jatlow PI, George TP. Effects of acute abstinence, reinstatement, and mecamylamine on biochemical and behavioral measures of cigarette smoking in schizophrenia. Schizophrenia Research 2007; 91; 217-225.

[13] Williams JM, Ziedonis DM, Abanyie F, Steinberg ML, Foulds J, Benowitz NL. Increased nicotine and cotinine levels in smokers with schizophrenia and schizoaffective disorder is not a metabolic effect. Schizophrenia Research 2005; 79(2-3) 323-35.

[14] Lasser K, Boyd JW, Woolhandler S, Himmelstein DU, McCormick D, Bor DH. Smoking and mental illness: A population-based prevalence study. JAMA 2000; 284; 2606-2610.

[15] Addington J, el-Guebaly N, Campbell W, Hodgins DC, Addington D. Smoking cessation treatment for patients with schizophrenia. American Journal of Psychiatry 1998; 155; 974-976.

[16] George TP, Ziedonis DM, Feingold A, Pepper WT, Satterburg CA, Winkel J, Rounsaville BJ, Kosten TR. Nicotine transdermal patch and atypical antipsychotic medications for smoking cessation in schizophrenia. American Journal of Psychiatry 2000; 157; 1835-1842.

[17] George TP, Vessicchio JC, Termine A, Bregartnera TA, Feingold A, Rounsaville BJ, Kosten TR. A placebo controlled trial of bupropion for smoking cessation in schizophrenia. Biological Psychiatry 2002; 52(1) 53–61.

[18] Richmond R, Zwar N. Therapeutic review of bupropion slow release. Drug and Alcohol Review 2003;22; 203–220.

[19] Hennekens CH, Hennekens AR, Hollar D, Casey DE. Schizophrenia and increased risks of cardiovascular disease. American Heart Journal 2005; 150;1115–1121.

[20] Hannerz H, Borga P, Borritz M. Life expectancies for individuals with psychiatric diagnoses. Public Health 2001; 115; 328–337.

[21] Culhane MA, Schoenfeld DA, Barr RS, Cather C, Deckersbach T, Freudenreich O, Goff DC, Rigotti NA, Evins AE. Predictors of early abstinence in smokers with schizophrenia. Journal of Clinical Psychiatry 2008; 69(11) 1743–1750.

[22] Baker A, Lubman DI, Hides L. Smoking and schizophrenia: Treatment approaches within primary care. Primary Psychiatry 2010; 17(1) 49-54.

[23] Takeuchi T, Nakao M, Shinozaki Y, Yano E. Validity of self-reported smoking in schizophrenia patients. Psychiatry and Clinical Neurosciences 2010; 64: 274–278.

[24] Curkendall SM, Mo J, Glasser DB, Rose Stang M, Jones JK. Cardiovascular disease in patients with schizophrenia in Saskatchewan, Canada. Journal of Clinical Psychiatry 2004; 65(5) 715-720.

[25] Chafetz L, White M, Collins-Bride G, Nickens J. The poor general health of the severely mentally ill: Impact of schizophrenic diagnosis. Community Mental Health Journal 2005; 41(2) 169-184.

[26] Copeland LA, Mortensen EM, Zeber JE, Pugh MJ, Restrepo MI, Dalack GW. Pulmonary disease among inpatient decedents: Impact of schizophrenia. Progress in Neuro-Psychopharmacology and Biological Psychiatry 2007; 31(3) 720-726.

[27] Bushe CJ, Hodgson R. Schizophrenia and cancer: in 2010 do we understand the connection? Canadian Journal of Psychiatry 2010; 55(12) 761-767.

[28] Shapiro SD, Ingenito EP. The pathogenesis of chronic obstructive pulmonary disease: advances in the past 100 years. American Journal of Respiratory Cell and Molecular Biology 2005; 32(5) 367-372.

[29] Sherman CB. The health consequence of cigarette smoking. Pulmonary diseases. Medical Clinics of North America 1992; 76(2) 355–371.

[30] Joukamaa M, Heliövaara M, Knekt P, Aromaa A, Raitasalo R, Lehtinen V. Mental disorders and cause specific mortality. British Journal of Psychiatry 2001; 179(6) 498–502.

[31] Chambers RA, Krystal JH, Self DW. A neurobiological basis for substance abuse comorbidity in schizophrenia. Biological Psychiatry 2001; 50; 71-83.

[32] de Leon J. Smoking and vulnerability for schizophrenia. Schizophrenia Bulletin 1996; 22; 405–409.

[33] D'Souza MS, Markou A. Schizophrenia ad tobacco smoking comorbidity: nAChR agonists in the treatment of schizophrenia-associated cognitive deficits. Neuropharmacology 2012; 62; 1564-1573.

[34] Leonard S, Gault J, Adams C, Breese CR, Rollins Y, Adler LE, Olincy A, Freedman R. Nicotinic receptors, smoking and schizophrenia. Restorative Neurology and Neuroscience 1998; 12(2-3) 195-201.

[35] Leonard S, Gault J, Hopkins J, Logel J, Vianzon R, Short M, Drebing C, Berger R, Venn D, Sirota P, Zerbe GO, Olincy A, Ross RG, Adler LE, Freedman R. Association of promoter variants in the alpha-7-nicotinic acetylocholine receptor subunit gene with an inhibitory deficit found in schizophrenia. Archive of General Psychiatry 2002; 59; 1085-1096.

[36] Khantzian EJ. The self-medication hypothesis of addictive disorders: Focus on heroin and cocaine dependence. American Journal of Psychiatry 1985; 142; 1259-1264.

[37] Markou A, Kosten TR, Kobb GF. Neurobiological similarities in depression and drug dependence: a self-medication hypothesis. Neuropsychopharmacology 1998; 18; 135-174.

[38] de Leon J, Diaz FJ, Aguilar MC, Jurado D, Gurpegui M. Does smoking reduce akathisia? Testing a narrow version of the self-medication hypothesis. Schizophrenia Research 2006; 86(1-3), 256-268.

[39] Domino EF, Mirzoyan D, Tsukada H. N-methyl-D-aspartate antagonists as drug models of schizophrenia: a surprising link to tobacco smoking. Progress in Neuro-Psychopharmacology and Biological Psychiatry 2004; 28(5) 801-811.

[40] Glassman AH, Covey LS, Dalack GW, Stetner F, Rivelli SK, Fleiss J, Cooper TB. Smoking cessation, clonidine, and vulnerability to nicotine among dependent smokers. Clinical Pharmacology and Therapeutics 1993; 54(6) 670–679.

[41] Lohr JB, Flynn K. Smoking and schizophrenia. Schizophrenia Research 1992; 8; 93–102.

[42] Lyon E. A Review of the effects of nicotine on schizophrenia and antipsychotic medications. Psychiatric Services 1999; 50; 1346-1350.

[43] Brody AL, Mandelkern MA, Jarvik ME, Lee GS, Smith EC, Huang JC, Bota RG, Bartzokis G, London ED. Differences between smokers and nonsmokers in regional gray matter volumes and densities. Biological Psychiatry 2004; 55(1) 77-84.

[44] Carrillo JA, Herraiz AG, Ramos SI, Gervasin G, Vizcaino S, Benitez J. Role of the smoking-induced cytochrome P450 (CYP)1A2 and polymorphic CYP2D6 in steady-state concentration of olanzapine. Journal of Clinical Psychopharmacology 2003; 23(2) 119–127.

[45] Grinevich VP, Papke RL, Lippiello PM, Bencherif M. Atypical antipsychotics as non-competitive inhibitors of alpha4beta2 and alpha7 neuronal nicotinic receptors. Neuropharmacology 2009; 57(2) 183–191.

[46] Hasselmo ME, Sarter M. Modes and models of forebrain cholinergic neuromodulation of cognition. Neuropharmacology 2011; 36; 52-73.

[47] Barr RS, Culhane MA, Jubelt LE, Mufti RS, Dyer MA, Weiss AP, Deckersbach T, Kelly JF, Freudenreich O, Goff DC, Evins AE. The effects of transdermal nicotine on cognition in nonsmokers with schizophrenia and nonpsychiatric controls. Neuropsychopharmacology 2008; 33(3) 480-490.

[48] Harris B, Kongs S, Allensworth D, Martin L, Tregellas J, Sullivan B, Zerbe G, Freedman R. Effects of nicotine on cognitive deficits in schizophrenia. Neuropsychopharmacology 2004; 29; 1378-1385.

[49] Sacco K, Termine A, Seyal A, Dudas M, Vessicchio J, Krishnan-Sarin S, Jatlow PI, Wexler BE, George TP. Effects of cigarette smoking on spatial working memory and attentional deficits in schizophrenia: Involvement of nicotinic receptor mechanisms. Archives of General Psychiatry 2005; 62; 649-659.

[50] Schmitz N, Kruse J, Kugler J. Disabilities, quality of life, and mental disorders associated with smoking and nicotine dependence. American Journal of Psychiatry 2003; 160; 1670-1676.

[51] Ziedonis D, Hitsman B, Beckham JC, Zvolensky M, Adler LE, Audrain-McGovern J, Breslau N, Brown RA, George TP, Williams J, Calhoun PS, Riley WT. Tobacco use and cessation in psychiatric disorders: National Institute of Mental Health report. Nicotine and Tobacco Research 2008; 10(12) 1691-1715.

[52] Forchuk C, Norman R, Malla A, Martin ML, McLean T, Cheng S, Diaz K, McIntosh E, Rickwood A, Vos S, Gibney C. Schizophrenia and the motivation for smoking, Perspectives in Psychiatric Care 2002; 38(2) 41–49.

[53] Solway ES. The lived experiences of tobacco use, dependence, and cessation: Insights and perspectives of people with mental illness. Health and Social Work 2011; 36(1) 19-32.

[54] de Leon J, Gurpegui M, Diaz FJ. Epidemiology of comorbid tobacco use and schizophrenia: Thinking about risks and protective factors. Journal of Dual Diagnosis 2007; 3(3/4) 9-25.

[55] Heatherton TF, Kozlowski LT, Frecker RC, Fagerström KO. The Fagerström Test for Nicotine Dependence: A revision of the Fagerström Tolerance Questionnaire. British Journal of Addiction 1991; 86(9) 1119–1127.

[56] Steinberg ML, Williams JM, Steinberg HR, Krejci JA, Ziedonis DM. Applicability of the Fagerström Test for Nicotine Dependence in smokers with schizophrenia. Addictive Behaviors 2005; 30(1) 49-59.

[57] Prochaska JO, DiClemente CC, Norcross JC. In search of how people change. Applications to addictive behaviors. American Psychologist 1992; 47(9) 1102–1114.

[58] DiClemente CC, Prochaska JO, Fairhurst SK, Velicer WF, Velasqquez MM, Rossi JS. The process of smoking cessation: An analysis of precontemplation, contemplation, and preparation stages of change. Journal of Consulting and Clinical Psychology 1991; 59; 295-304.

[59] Zigmond A, Snaith R. The Hospital Anxiety and Depression Scale. Acta Psychiatrica Scandinavica 1983; 67(6) 361-370.

[60] McCue P, Buchanan T, Martin CR. Screening for psychological distress using internet administration of the Hospital Anxiety and Depression Scale (HADS) in individuals with chronic fatigue syndrome. British Journal of Clinical Psychology 2006; 45(4) 483–498.

[61] Bjelland I, Dahl A, Haug T, Neckelmann D. The validity of the Hospital Anxiety and Depression Scale: An updated literature review. Journal of Psychosomatic Research 2002; 52; 69-77.

[62] McPherson A, Martin CR. Is the Hospital Anxiety and Depression Scale (HADS) an appropriate screening tool for use in an alcohol-dependent population? Journal of Clinical Nursing 2011; 20; 1507–1517.

[63] Olsson I, Mykletun A, Dahl A. The Hospital Anxiety and Depression Rating Scale: a cross-sectional study of psychometrics and case finding abilities in general practice. BMC Psychiatry 2005, 5; 46.

[64] Wojtyna E. Termometr Dystresu jako narzędzie przesiewowe u osób chorych psychicznie. (in press).

[65] Olincy A, Young DA, Freedman R. Increased levels of the nicotine metabolite cotinine in schizophrenic smokers compared to other smokers. Biological Psychiatry 1997; 42; 1-5.

[66] McEvoy J, Freudenreich O, McGee M, VanderZwaag C, Levin E, Rose J. Clozapine decreases smoking in patients with chronic schizophrenia. Biologic Psychiatry 1995; 37; 550-552.

[67] Hutchison KE, Rutter MC, Niaura R, Swift RM, Pickworth WB, Sobik L. Olanzapine attenuates cue-elicited craving for tobacco. Psychopharmacology 2004; 175; 407-413.

[68] Ritsner M, Perelroyzen G, Ilan H, Gibel A. Subjective response to antipsychotics od schizophrenia patients treated in routine clinical practice: A naturalistic comparative study. Journal of Clinical Psychopharmacology 2004; 24(3) 245-254.

[69] Spendel Z. O pewnych niebezpieczeństwach nadużywania etykiet zastępczych. Niespecyficzne Zmienne Zagregowane (NZZ) w badaniach psychologicznych. In: Popiołek K, Bańka A (eds.) Kryzysy, katastrofy, kataklizmy w kontekście narastania zagrożeń. Poznań: Stowarzyszenie Psychologia i Architektura; 2007. p335-356.

Chapter 15

Post Traumatic Eco-Stress Disorder (PTESD): A Qualitative Study from Sundarban Delta, India

Arabinda N. Chowdhury, Ranajit Mondal,
Mrinal K Biswas and Arabinda Brahma

Additional information is available at the end of the chapter

1. Introduction

International Classification of Diseases, ICD– 10, [78] defined PTSD (code F43.1) as: "Arises as a delayed or protracted response to a stressful event or situation (of either brief or long duration) of an exceptionally threatening or catastrophic nature, which is likely to cause pervasive distress in almost anyone.... Typical features include episodes of repeated reliving of the trauma in intrusive memories ("flashbacks"), dreams or nightmares, occurring against the persisting background of a sense of "numbness" and emotional blunting, detachment from other people, unresponsiveness to surroundings, anhedonia, and avoidance of activities and situations reminiscent of the trauma. There is usually a state of autonomic hyperarousal with hypervigilance, an enhanced startle reaction, and insomnia. Anxiety and depression are commonly associated with the above symptoms and signs, and suicidal ideation is not infrequent. The onset follows the trauma with a latency period that may range from a few weeks to months. The course is fluctuating but recovery can be expected in the majority of cases. In a small proportion of cases the condition may follow a chronic course over many years, with eventual transition to an enduring personality change." *PTSD was first recognized as a clinical entity in the third edition of the* the Diagnostic and Statistical Manual of Mental Disorders in 1980.

In the last 30 years considerable research has accumulated which has provided deep insight not only into the epidemiology but also the conceptual framework of different categories of trauma and its differential impacts and coping psychodynamics. The classification of causes of trauma based on available research findings may be categorized as follows:

1. Eco-Stress traumas resulting from natural disasters like cyclone, earthquake, flood, hurricane, tsunami, bushfire, tornado, drought and wild animal attacks.

2. Technological traumas like plane crash, industrial accidents, domestic accidents, nuclear reactor explosion and oil spills etc.

3. Human induced (direct) trauma like sexual assault and rape, violence, terrorist attack, vehicle accident, combat and military trauma, illness, death and hostage taking etc.

The nature and extent of ecological traumas [2] are usually more pervasive and collective [58] and entail a strong sense of powerlessness and destiny/spiritual dimension among the victims [44]. PTSD is quite common after eco-disasters and it is estimated that the prevalence rate of PTSD related to natural disasters is currently between 8.6% and 57.3% depending on assessment methodologies, instruments and timing [75].

The present work based on the case studies from Sundarban, India, attempting to highlight the development of post-traumatic symptomatology after wild animal attacks, viz., Tiger, Shark and Crocodile, in the context of a unique ecological landscape of the delta region. All natural disasters and incidents are ecological events and their impact on humans (in terms of psychological, physical, economic and social) can be seen as an extraordinary eco-stress that is operative behind the development of post-traumatic stress disorder and hence the defining terms PTESD (to separate it from Technological and Human related traumas).

2. The Study Area: Sundarban

Sundarban is the largest estuarine mangrove forest in the world; stretching over an area of about 10,200 Km^2 (42% is in India and 58% in Bangladesh). It comprises outer deltas of the Ganges, Brahmaputra and Meghna rivers at the confluence of Bay of Bengal. The Indian portion is located about 130 km southeast of Kolkata (West Bengal State), between 21°31′ to 22°53′N and 88°37 to 89°09′E coordinates, at an altitude of 7 m from the sea level.

The Indian Sundarban (Fig.1) extends over some 102 islands (54 are habitable) and mudflats intersected by major distributory rivers and innumerable intricate network of tidal estuaries, creeks, and canals that support the world's largest tidal halophytic mangrove forest (4266 Km^2). UNESCO declared Sundarban National Park as World Heritage site in 1987 and in 1989 it was designated as a Biosphere Reserve under the UNESCO 'Man and Biosphere Programme'. Sundarban Biosphere Reserve covers the delta south to Dampier-Hodges line (an imaginary line that indicates the northern-most limits of estuarine zone affected by tidal fluctuations) and includes Sundarban Reserve Forest (SRF), Tiger Reserve and human settlements. The Sundarban Tiger Reserve (STR) was established in 1973 and Sajnakhali Wildlife Sanctuary in 1976. The name Sundarban comes from mangrove names: the *Sundari* (beautiful) tree (*Heritiera fomes)* and ban from *Bani* (*Avicennia officinalis).* The other meaning of *ban* is forest as well [40].

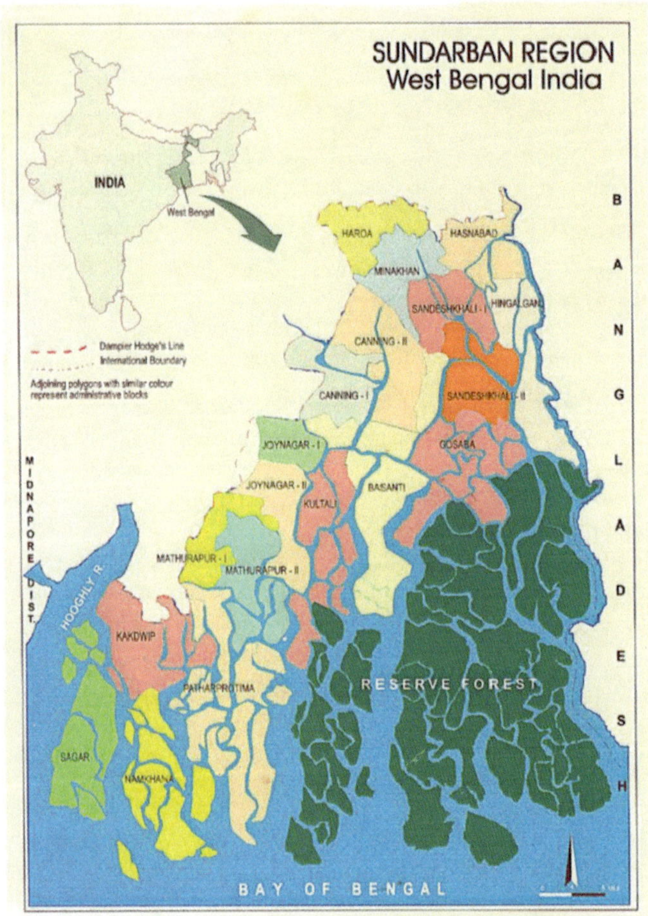

Figure 1. Sundarban Region

The Sundarban ecosystem carries a great regional ecological significance. Sundarban has extremely rich and unique biodiversity of aquatic and terrestrial flora and fauna, which supports 334 species of plants, 44 species of fish, 8 species of amphi-bians, 53 species of reptiles, 161 species of birds and 49 species of mammals [66]. It support one of the sub-continent's largest tiger populations, the Royal Bengal Tiger (*Panthera tigris tigris*), who are well-known for their swimming, man-eating and eco-adaptive behaviours. Census of 2004 (pugmark method) estimated the tiger population at 274 [8]. Its high density relative to the availability of prey, and recurrent encounters with local people in the Tiger Reserve are probably the reasons for its habit of man-eating [13].

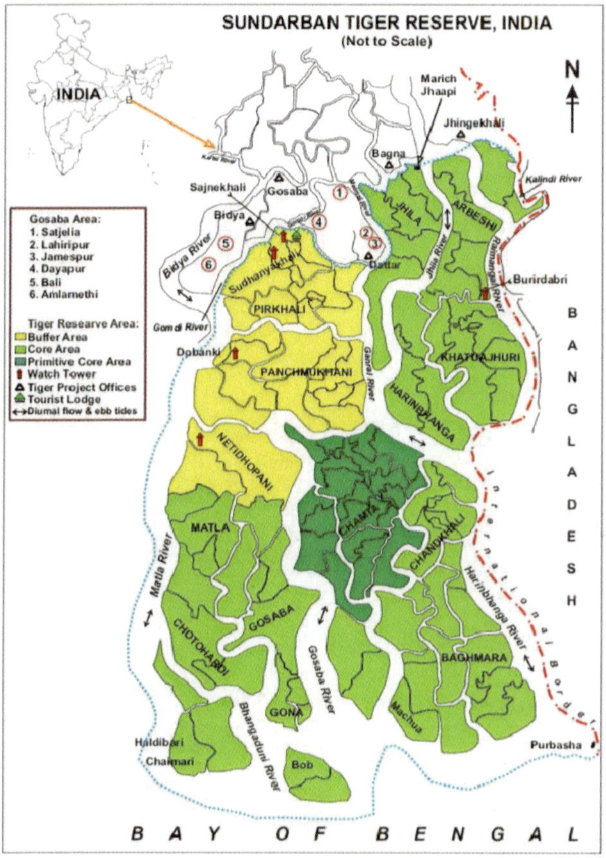

Figure 2. Gosaba and Sundarban Tiger Reserve

STR (Fig.2) is bounded in the East by international boundary with Bangladesh and in the North-West it is surrounded by numerous villages, thus making the reserve vulnerable to ever increasing biotic interference in the form of livelihood forest explorations, illegal fishing, timber smuggling and poaching. STR extends over 2,585 Km^2 (1,600 Km^2 land component, and 985 Km^2 water components) with three designated zones: *Core* or *Wilderness zone*: 1,330 Km^2; Primitive *zone (inside* core): 124.40 Km^2; *Subsidiary wilderness zone*: 241.07 Km^2 and *Buffer zone*: rest of the area, where activities are regulated. Around 0.22 million people are living in 66 villages within 2 Km of the buffer zone of STR. Between 1975 to 1982, an average of 45 people was annually killed by tigers. This casualty rate has fallen (Fig.3) since the introduction of various preventive measures like use of deterrents in the form of electrified human dummies and face masks worn on the back of the head during forest activities.

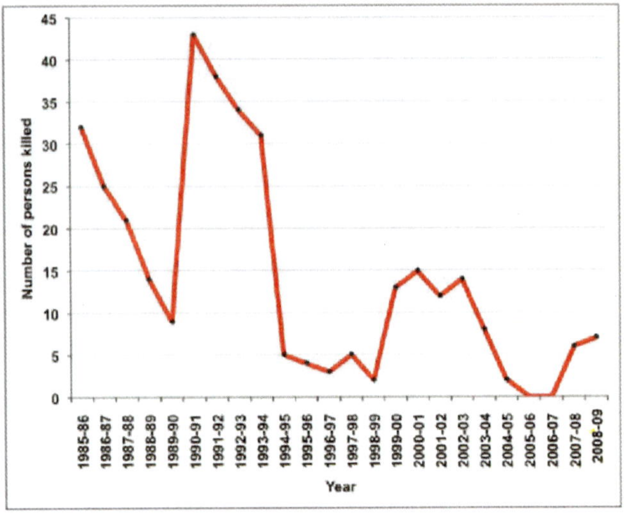

Figure 3. Humans killed by Tigers in STR from 1985 to 2009 (adopted from [50].

SRF and Livelihood measures: The Indian Sundarban comprises thirteen community development blocks in the South 24 Parganas District and six blocks in the North 24 Parganas District of West Bengal State and has a total population of 4.1 million [12]. 85% live on agriculture, of which 90% are landless agricultural labourers and marginal farmers. Around 3.5 million people live around Sundarban, 32% of whom depend on the resources of Sundarban mangrove forest directly or indirectly. Some 35,330 people work in the forest annually, of whom 4,580 collect timber and firewood, 24,900 are fishermen, 1,350 collect honey and 4,500 are involved in other activities. On average some 4,000 fishermen are active each day, and the mean annual fish catch is 2,500 tones (14).

Dependence of fringe population on Sundarban's eco-reserve (resources) is high, and the main groups are:

a. Fisherfolk - catching fish in creeks, rivers and sea.

b. Wood Cutters and fuel wood (Golpatta- *Nypa fruticans* and Hental bush- *Phoenix paludosa* – also used for thatching) collectors: The yearly average timber collection from SRF is about 1, 20,000 quintals. Usually a team of 5-8 wood cutters are led by a *Boulay* inside the SRF. *Boulay* is a man with traditional expertise, who knows the magic of keeping the team out of danger in the forest and they are supposed to have supernatural power to make the work area protected so that tiger cannot enter into the 'chanted' territory.

c. Honey and wax collectors: from wild bee (*Apis indica)* hive - is a seasonal activity (during months of April-May) and 4-5 member group is lead by a *Moulay*. They are traditional experts and especially skilled persons who can locate the beehives in the deep forest by observing the flying directions of bees and they also possess supernatural power to sense forest dangers and prevent tiger attacks by their ritual and chants. On an average 20,000 Kg of honey and 1000 Kg wax is collected yearly.

d. Crab collectors: Estuarine mud crab *Scylla serrata* (locally called *bada kanckara* – mangrove crab) is an edible species found in the mudflat of Sundarban forests and has a good market demand, both locally and overseas. There are many crab fisheries in Sundarban region that are running this lucrative trade [57]. There are different techniques of crab collection from the water or mud flat or burrows like using bamboo trap, bait, hook or hand picking [55], which is a very time-consuming and skilled technique. Many a time crab collectors are taken by the tiger, when they are concentrating on their catch [71].

e. Tiger Prawn (*Penaeus monodon*) Seed (TPS) Collectors (locally called *'meen dhara'*): is a lucrative on the spot earning of about Rs. 50–100 (USD $ 1 - 2) per day per person. Shrimp exports constitute 75% of total marine products to foreign markets from West Bengal. Tiger prawns live in the sea but enter the Sundarban rivers and creeks to lay their eggs. The spawns make their way back to the sea and that is when they are trapped by nets. There is large demand for prawn seeds from the neighbouring shrimp aquaculture industry and also from Bangladesh, resulting in substantial illegal cross border trade.

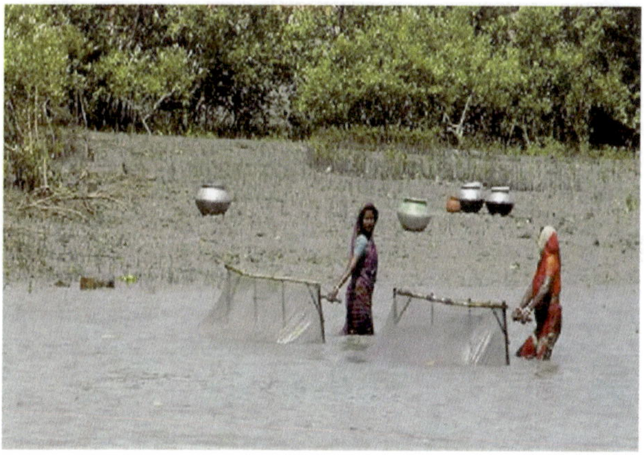

Figure 4. TPS collection by using *Tana jal* in Sundarban river [45].

A significant proportion of the women population of Sundarban is engaged in this non-farm livelihood activity (Fig. 4). The collection of juvenile shrimp has become a major income source with estimates of up to 40,000 collectors involved within the Sundarban. On an average 1,500 to 3,000 million seeds are collected per annum [32]. Two types of fishing gear are used: Hand operated net, locally called *Tana-jal or meen berajal* (Drag net) and Dip net- locally called *Naukar-jal* (boat's net), a triangular net with three bamboo arms. As they are always working in the waist-deep river water, they are prone to shark (Indian Dog Shark - *Scoliodon laticaudus*, locally called *Kamote*) and Crocodile (*Crocodylus porosus*) attack and usually develop some waterborne diseases, skin infections, reproductive tract disease (in female) and musculoskeletal disorders [37]. TPS collection inside the SRF always carries a high risk from tiger attack.

STR issues Boat License Certificate and seasonal Pass to each individual for entering into the forest for permitted activity (fishing, wood cutting or honey collection) in designated area. Fishing violations are legal offence and are registered under Compounded Offence Report (COR). It is reported that COR are increasing: from 361 in 2000-01 to 2,806 in 2007-08 [15]. Illegal trip inside the forest is locally called trip in '*Black*' (like urban use of black money or black market) and in case of any fatality they avoid reporting to the government health facility for the fear of police case and fine. In legal exploration if a death occurs from tiger attack, the victim's family is supposed to get some compensation.

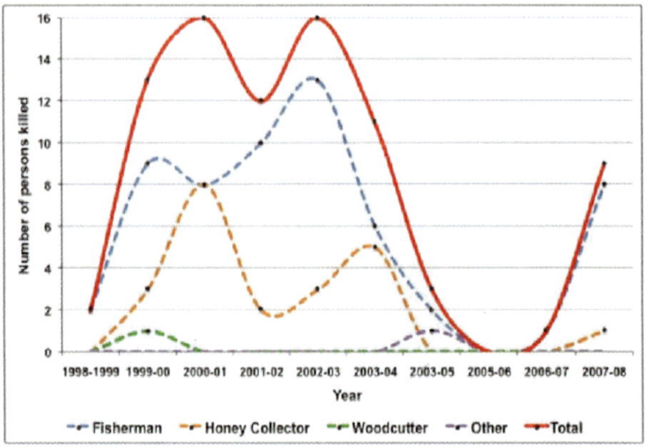

Figure 5. Categories of persons killed by Tigers in STR from 1998 to 2008 (adopted from [50]).

There are some agencies who offer life insurance policy on deposit of some regular money. No compensation is paid for crocodile, shark attacks and snake bites. The whole procedure is very complicated and in most instances the claim remains unmet because they are cheated for their illiteracy, ignorance and unfamiliarity with official rules. All these livelihood measures are highly dangerous and potential for death, mainly from tiger attacks (Fig. 5). Sundarban people mention all animal attacks as 'accident', as a parallel to 'auto accident' in urban locality.

People of Sundarban, both Hindus and Muslims, have a strong faith on mythical cult of *Bonobibi* (Queen of the forest), as protector inside the forest and *Dakshin Ray*, the God of Tiger. Invocation of Tiger God is a mandatory ritual for safe passage throughout the Sundarban forest territory. Inside the forest they never say the word 'Tiger' but to show reverence, they refer to the tigers as *Bara Miah* (Big Uncle). Before entering the forest, it is obligatory to offer *puja* and pray to the Deity for support and safety. In each Sundarban village there is a Bonobibi shrine (*Than*) and at different entrance points to the SRF, there are idols of Bonobibi (Fig.6). Bonobibi Puja is a big social festival in Sundarban, celebrated once a year. Manasa is a cult of Hindu folk Goddess of snakes and protector from snake bite. Almost in every home in Sundarban, there is a sacred alter with a *Manasha shrub* (a Sij plant of a cactus family *Euphorbia genus*). People of Sundarban have deep faith in these mythical cults as their protector and fate-regulator which is being reflected in their day to day socio-cultural discourses [26].

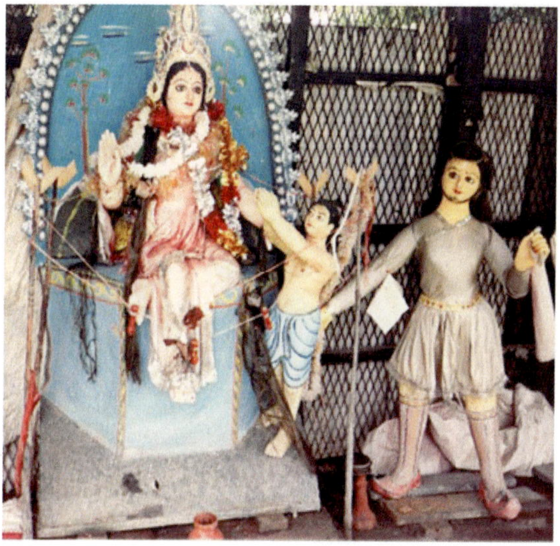

Figure 6. Bonobibi idol at the Sajnekhali forest.

Health care in Sundarban region is pluralistic in nature. Each block has one main government Block Primary Health Centre (BPHC) with indoor beds and 3-5 Primary Health Centres (PHC) and 6-10 Subsidiary Health Centres (SHC). PHC and SHC offer only outpatient services. Distance, inappropriate infra-structure and shortage of health staff hinder the desired services to the people. In addition, many private medical practitioners provide health care to the people. There is an intricate network of Health Care Providers (HCP) mainly of non-registered practitioners, locally known as "Quack" and virtually they are the first line of contact for the vast majority of Sundarban people [23]. There is an extensive network of indigenous magico-religious healers like *Sarpa Baidya* (snake-bite healers), *Gunin, Ojha* and *Fakir* who by supernatural means and rituals (Jhar-Phuk, Chants, herbal roots and enchanted water, amulets or talisman) treat varieties of ailments, ranging from ghost-possession to veterinary problems.

Gosaba block (Fig.7) is at the extreme Eastern side of Sundarban region close to international border with Bangladesh. It is the last inhabited island before the Sundarban forest start. It is located at 22.16°N 88.80°E and has an average elevation of 13 feet from the sea level. It has 14 Gram Panchayats (democratically elected local self-government unit) of which Bali I and II, Gosaba, Rangabelia, Lahiripur and Satjelia are facing the STR buffer zone (and partly Core area), separated by Gomdi, Gomor, Sajna, and Melmel rivers respectively. Gosaba is the most poor and underdeveloped block in Sundarban and a significant proportion of population is thriving on forest resources.

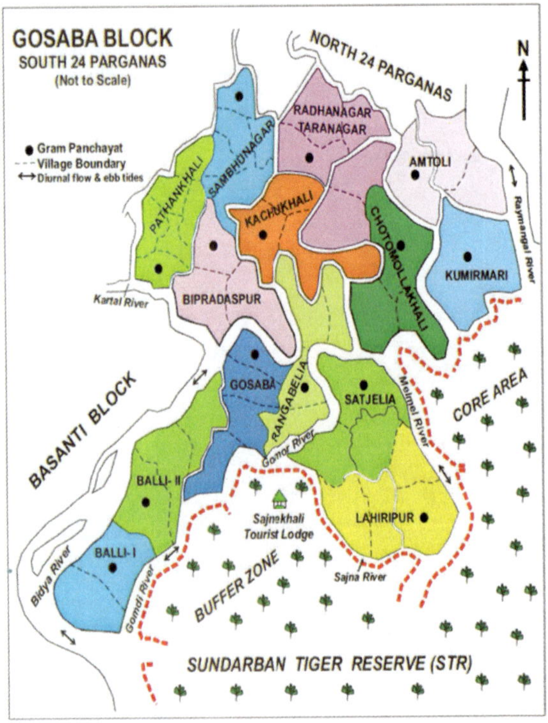

Figure 7. Gosaba Block and Sundarban Tiger Reserve.

Sundarban is one of the underdeveloped, poorest and most densely populated regions of South Asia, with an estimated 8 million people (India and Bangladesh combined) directly dependent on its fragile ecosystem. The level of literacy and per capita income is far below the state average and most of the people fall below the poverty line. The communication and transport network is very poor and most of the areas are inaccessible. Agriculture is hard and difficult and there is no industrial infrastructure. Provision of health care is extremely poor and electricity is almost non-existent. Frequent climatic insult is a regular feature—cyclonic storm; inrush of tidal waves and flooding is the cause of recurrent damage of life, crops and property every year. Sundarban is an extremely backward region with a very poor quality of life of its inhabitants [16, 20].

3. Method

In the context of a rural mental health programme in the Sundarban Delta [17], a community study had previously identified deliberate self-harm by pesticide poisoning and human-animal conflicts as a locally recognized priority problem. This research was thus undertaken with reference to a framework that examined the problem of human-animal conflicts in relation to occupational nature, socio-economic factors and its impact on mental health and environment. The details of this study were reported elsewhere [24]. The present case studies were conducted in two villages of Gosaba block, namely Satjelia and Lahiripur during August 2005 to January 2006. A total of 111 (male 83, female 28) cases of human-animal conflicts were identified from those two villages among which 12 males (14.4%) and 17 (60.7%) females survived.

The present study group comprises a total of 13 cases (7 female and 6 male). 3 males and 4 females were from the survivor group. The other 2 males and 3 females were seen at the community mental health clinic conducted in Gosaba during this period. One case (7) was seen immediately after the accident with a follow up. Among the 13 cases, one was a post-humous study. 10 cases developed PTESD symptoms after tiger attack, 2 after shark attack and 1 after crocodile attack. An ethnographic history including the details of situation analysis of the encounter and physical injuries sustained and subsequent help seeking were elicited. In some cases detailed clinical examination including Mental State Examination was also done. Depending on the clinical presentation and history, an attempt was made to arrive at a provisional diagnosis and treatment was offered to those who agreed. In the clinical description all the animals are referred as 'it' because the sex of the animals was not known. All the in-depth interviews conducted separately and all of them have given written consent/ thumb impression for tape recording of the interview which was transcript later. They also gave written consent to publish their case studies in academic journals or meeting and use their photographs in academic papers. All the names used were changed or abbreviated.

4. Results: Case Studies

4.1. Case 1:

Mrs. Mondal, a 39 years old married woman, was in a fishing (tiger prawn) trip in the middle of February, opposite to Bali I block near Sajnakhali jungle in the SRF, 11 years ago. During the netting exercise, four people were on the *dingi* (country boat) and five were on the bank of the *khari* (narrow canal). She was on the bank on the right, behind the other four. A big aluminum pot, to collect juvenile prawns, was to her left while with her right hand, she was pulling the *mean-bera jal* in the river. It was about 3 am and as it was cold, she covered her head with a wrapper. Suddenly the tiger jumped from the slope of the *khari* onto her from behind. Having not landed on her precisely, the tiger's left paw hit the metal bowl and right paw hit her head. The wrapper therefore slid off, she became unbalanced and fell into the river along with the tiger. Immediately the tiger rushed towards her in an attempt to grab her head but that she escaped by going under the tiger's belly. The tiger then started throwing violent paw thrusts. She sustained severe injuries to her right upper arm, beneath the neck and bled profusely. The surrounding water became bright red ('like red chili') and as a last resort she swam deeper into the water, away from the tiger in an attempt to reach middle of the *khari* to get closer to the boat. By this time, people on the boat were shouting and thrusting their long bamboos on the water to ward off the tiger. The tiger left the prey and having reached the bank stared at the people briefly and disappeared into the jungle. She was immediately helped into the boat; she was crying out of terror and pain. It took three hours to reach Gosaba BPHC where she was treated with '56 stitches'. In the hospital she was drowsy and frequently shouted, "the tiger is coming…am I in the jungle?...standing there- run away- run away". She showed extreme fear and apprehension particularly at night. She said to one staff member, "I will not be spared, it will catch me again. Tigers always search for their missed preys."

After being discharged from hospital in a month, she remained very frightened. At night she repeatedly checked doors and windows and developed a conviction that tiger will attack her at home. She was not amenable to any logic. Her thatched cottage was just on the Melmel river bank and every night she put a kerosene lamp by the side of her bed. Any trivial sound outside would wake her from sleep. She took a *katari* (machete) and stood up in an attention stance as if the tiger is entering the room and she will hit with this weapon. In the midst of sleep she shouted "see the tiger is coming… beat it with *baitha* (rowing wooden sticks)" and became extremely emotional and cried profusely. Her religiosity increased many folds; she believed that it was due to kindness of goddess Bonobibi she was saved from the mouth of the tiger and clutches of death. She offered prayer with flowers twice daily at the Bonobibi *than* in the village. She became highly fearful and cried a lot when she heard of any news of a tiger-attack in the locality. She avoided not only any further fishing trip in the SRF but also avoided the jungle where she used to collect fuel wood. Her present living is TPS collection in the river (not inside the forest) and though previously she used to spend the whole day in waist deep water for netting, she was now unable to take a dip in the water to bathe by submerging her head under water. When asked about the reason, she said, "though the possibility of tiger attack no longer present, I feel frightened to take a deep bath. I feel anxious when I am not able to see my surrounding." Though she is doing all household tasks and maintaining regular TPS collection in the river, she still has fear of a tiger. She avoids going outside of her home after sundown and feels quite upset with any news of tiger attack in the jungle. She says, "The memory of the attack haunts my mind like a scary cinema show". She has developed multiple bodily pains, especially in the neck and both shoulders. Health and work ability-wise she said that she is now 40% capable and functional.

Clinical Impression: Chronic PTESD with psychotic symptoms and somatization.

4.2. Case 2:

Mrs. Mistry, 34 yrs old married lady had a *Kamote* attack in Melmel river near Marich Jhappi jungle in May at around 2.30 pm, seven years ago. She was in a fishing trip with three others in this TPS collection. She and another man was immersed waist deep in the water and were pulling the net through the water. It was a low-tide time and there was high force of the water gushing downwards (towards the sea). With some added rain, the water level raised and she was immersed up to her chest. She then felt something heavy under the water and before realizing she was pulled down into the water. She struggled to reach above the water for air but was forcefully pulled down under the water twice. She felt a sharp pain over her left buttock as if someone is cutting it with a sharp saw or "a big leech" is adhering to her body and within a second she realized that it was a *kamote* bite. She noticed the water around her turning bright red. She was repeatedly pulled into the water by the shark. Her right arm below the elbow was also bitten off. "With the salty water the burning sensation increased" and she became unconscious. She was rescued by others immediately and taken to Gosaba BPHC. A big portion of muscle mass from her left buttock and the whole lower right arm was missing. She was treated with multiple stitches. First few days in the hospital she was semiconscious and intermittently shouted "the kamote is coming.. kamote is pulling my legs - save me, save me,.. so much blood, wipe it" Her right arm was amputated below the elbow. After a month she was discharged.

Though physically she was recovering gradually, her fear about a *kamote* attack persisted over almost 4 years. She was always fearful and apprehensive, avoided going to the river, feeling terrified after seeing any floating log of wood or rubbish and misidentified those as *kamote*. Sleep was broken many times at night, having memories of the attack and quite often she jumped off from the bed onto the floor as if she is being attacked by something - she checked and rechecked her legs and muttered to herself "is it alright, is it alright?" She repeatedly and sometimes unnecessarily warned the fellow neighbours not to going fishing. If any animal attack news came to the community, she rushed into her room and cried loudly and profusely. She had fearful dreams of *kamote* attack and disturbed sleep for over two years. Her left leg shrunk and caused pain on pressure leading to difficulties in walking. With the amputed right hand she could not do household work properly. She felt extremely low with high anxiety, intensified by her inability to run the family chores due to the deformity. This brought a constant tussle with the family members. She narrated that: "I am a forest lady, forest is my mother but I cannot dream even to enter the forest or river again. I stopped fishing activities completely. I fear and tremble if I go up to waist-deep water in the river. ... It is my misfortune or rather results of my sin. Many news paper people, forest department people and once a doctor like you came to see me. It is a great disgrace and shame that I have to show my injury by lifting my *shaere* up to the buttock...it is extremely insulting for a woman- I am so unfortunate. Probably it would have been better if it (*kamote*) killed me there, (profuse crying) but I am thankful to Goddess Bonobibi and Ma-Manasa that my life was saved. I don't know when I will get rid of the fear and bad dreams of this accident." She said since this incident she never regained her full strength and always felt morose and low. She always felt fearful without any apparent cause, lacked in energy, had poor appetite and extreme sleep difficulties. She received no governmental financial help. She is now working as a support worker in a local Child Development Centre.

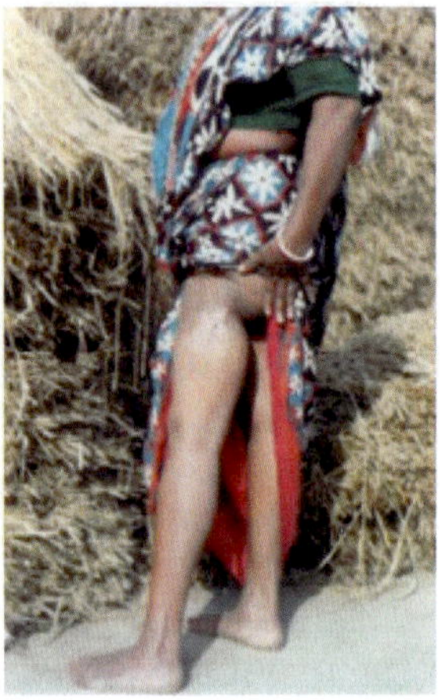

Clinical Impression: Clinical depression with anxiety in addition to her chronic PTESD symptoms. She agreed to take a course of antidepressant and anti-anxiety medication and at follow up after four months she showed significant improvement in her symptoms.

4.3. Case 3:

Mr. Halder, 42 years, was in a crab collection trip for 8 days with other three partners, a year ago. This incident took place on the fourth day of the trip, at about 8 am, in the Dhutra *Khal* (narrow creek) near Netai Jungle of SRF. The men were placing *done* (bamboo made triangular trap) in the river, when the tiger leapt from his back from the *Hental* bush up on the riverbank. He immediately jumped onto the other side of the boat. The tiger attempted to reach him by leaning across the boat. He caught the tiger's fore legs with his two hands and pushed the boat with his chest towards the tiger to injure it. The tiger then lost it's balance and fell into the river. The tiger attacked him again and slashed his right chin and scalp with sharp claws but despite trying was not successful in biting his head. One of the fellow collector lost consciousness and fell on the bank and the other two shouted loudly and took the rowing sticks and thrashed the tiger with all their might. The tiger backed off and disappeared into the forest. He had profuse bleeding and was very restless in pain and fear and constantly shouted saying "save me please, I am dying". He was taken to Gosaba BPHC after 6 hours of rowing. He was much disoriented for the first two weeks, could not detect family members or neighbours, always looked frightened, and tended to cover his head with a blanket. He repeatedly sought reassurance from the doctor if he was alright. He could not eat, so was fed by a tube in the hospital. There was a deep furrow on the right side of the head and his face was also deformed because of loss of muscle and deep scar. He complained of constant pain on the right side of the face. He was discharged after six weeks and stayed a few days in Gosaba with a relative. He was very frightened of returning home which was on the riverbank opposite SRF. He had a strong belief that he, who is once attacked by a tiger, will definitely be attacked by the (same) tiger again.

He was a very courageous man with a strong muscle build. After this tiger attack he changed completely. He became skinny and weak. He became very fearful, even in the daytime while at home and he thought tiger may come at any time to attack him. In the night, things became even worse. He often awoke from sleep shouting "what is that sound?" He enquired if his wife could smell the tiger. He took an iron rod and rehearsed and demonstrated as to how he would strike the tiger if it entered the room. He became very morose; his appetite reduced remarkably and spent the whole day sitting in the courtyard idly. If the neighbors asked how he is doing, he kept silent and tearful. Sometimes he lamented, "All my faith in Bonobibi has gone. I explored the jungle so many times with her blessings, but this time she turned her face away from me. How can I go to forest again! On whose strength I would depend? I will not offer any worship to her again." Since then he never entered the forest again, though the constant fear of tiger attack has subsided considerably. He still presents as fearful and tremulous if he hears any 'accident' news in the jungle, he avoids going out even in the day time, suffers disturbed sleep often with terrible dreams and has lose much weight. When asked about the reason for fear, he said "the scene of *bera-beri* (fierce struggle for life with the tiger) haunts my mind as if it is occurring now, and my body shakes, heart pounds and the terrible *haker* (roaring of tiger) comes to my ear." He completely abandoned any trip to the jungle since then. They received no governmental financial help. They have no land, his wife and elder son run the family by working as day labourers and collecting TPS from the adjoining river (not inside the SRF).

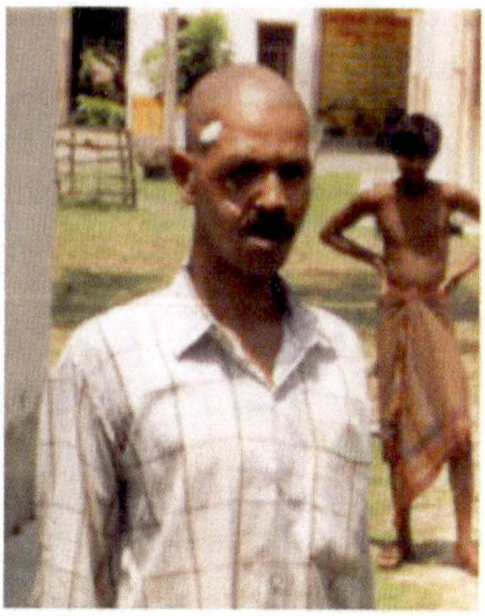

At Gosaba BPHC

Clinical Impression: Acute Stress Disorder followed by PTESD with psychotic symptoms, and with depression. He agreed to take a course of antidepressant and antianxiety medication.

4.4. Case 4:

Mrs. Gayen, 38 yrs married lady, went to a TPS collection with a team of six others, four years ago. They were pulling their net in the high-tide water in a narrow *khari* near Marich Jhappi jungle. It was an April mid day, around 1 pm and they were very active because they had to spread the net properly in the gushing up water from the high-tide. Suddenly one of her fellow fisherman shouted "Alert! Alert! Uncle is coming". She looked back and saw a huge tiger jumping onto her and she immediately jumped into the river but not before sustaining some serious injuries. She narrowly escaped from the full force of the tiger's swing. She kept herself deep inside the river water, but the tiger kept trying to strike her submerged head violently with it's paws. The people started shouting, hitting the boat with sticks and pushing the boat to hit the tiger, which, after several failed attempts to reach its victim, began to recede and eventually disappeared into the forest. People then rescued her. She sustained a deep laceration to the back of her head and upper right shoulder. She bled profusely and became unconscious. They wrapped the wound with a towel and after four hours on the boat, reached a private clinic in Gosaba. The people avoided the government hospital as the incident took place when they were operating in 'Black'. She suffered repeated infections and took more than two months for her wounds to heal.

She developed extreme tiger fear after that. She was always fearful that she may be attacked again by a tiger, even at her home. Her thatched cottage was on a riverbank opposite the SRF. She could not go outside her room, even to use the toilet because of fear of being attacked by the tiger. In the midst of sleep she would wake up and shout "there is a tiger- see… save me, save me" and cried a lot. She was often inconsolable. She cried loudly by holding her head because of constant headache. She developed muscle and bone pain in neck and both shoulders. She left her occupation of TPS collection. Her extreme fear of tiger, even in the day, became a 'talk' in the community. Sometimes kids ridiculed her by saying, "Look there is a tiger" and watch her panic stricken behavior. During these times, she would run back to her cottage and ask her husband to take proper caution to fight away the tiger, as if it is certainly there and coming to attack her. Husband thought she developed some mental problem and thus consulted a *Boulay* and a *Gunin*. Both advised him to offer *puja* to Bonobibi shrine. After being treated (with jhar-fuk and herbal amulets) by the *Gunin*, she became 'somewhat normal' but still remains fearful of the tiger, she cannot go to the market on her own, she never goes out after evening and when she hears any news of such attacks in the forest, she becomes extremely frightened and tremulous.

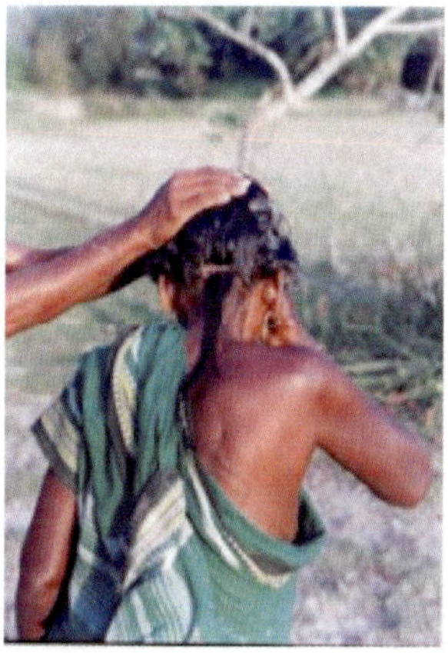

Clinical Impression: Chronic PTESD with psychotic symptoms. She agreed to take a course of anti-anxiety medication.

4.5. Case 5:

Mrs. Mistry, 39 years old, (a tiger widow) accompanied her husband in a boat trip for TPS collection in Garal *khal* near Marich Jhappi jungle, four years ago. They started working at midnight so as to collect the early morning catch from the river and had been working late into the morning. Both husband and wife were busy pulling the drag-net laid in the river. By around 10 am they had collected a good number of juvenile Tiger Prawns. While walking behind her husband in waist deep water, she saw a tiger jump over her and onto her husband. In a split second, his head and part of his neck were inside the tiger's jaws. She described the incident: "I stood there aghast. My husband's head and face were inside the tiger's mouth. The tiger's long pointed teeth plunged into his neck and chest. It's eyes were red and terrifying. Blood was coming out like an open tap-water, he shook violently his both hands and legs in pain and I heard some peculiar sound. I was unsure if it was the tiger's growling or my husband's shrieks of terror and pain. Suddenly I got a supernatural power and courage, as if Bonobibi tranced on me. There was no one nearby. I had to save him. I pulled his legs with all my might to dislodge him from the tiger's jaws. The tiger stepped up on the bank dragging my husband… I was still in the water and kept on pulling his legs towards me but I was no match to the tiger's strength. It snatched my husband's body, my hands slipped and it dragged him into the forest... I could not save him (profuse crying)". By this time another fishing party came and they found her crying loudly and shouting for help. She went along with six others into the forest– all shouted and created sounds with crackers and wooden sticks. After a mile inside, by the side of a dense *Hetal* bush, they found the husband's body in a pool of blood – with the head and left leg missing. She fainted but was attended to. The lacerated body was buried on the river bank. It was not taken back in the village as they went in 'Black'. Because of the risk of police case, if the incident was publicly known, she could not perform the usual mortuary rituals at home, neither did she cry loudly or discuss this extreme misfortune with her neighbours. For the first three months, she could not dress like a widow because forest department may come for enquiry. She said "despite being a widow I had to dress like a married woman. I could not cry loudly or discuss the accident with others to ease my mind. I cried in closed doors, asking Bonobibi to give me strength".

First few weeks after the incident, were extremely sad. She was fearful and suspicious of facing enquiry about the illegal forest trip. Then she developed extreme anxiety, fear about the tiger, cried relentlessly, avoided social mixing and completely stopped TPS collection in the river. She was very suspicious that forest department or police will come to arrest her. She ate very little and confined herself in her cottage. If neighbours visited her she repeatedly asked them about any enquiry from forest department they knew about. At night she repeatedly checked the windows, door and the courtyard as if tiger is hiding there. Throughout the night she had frequent broken sleep and stood up on the bed and shouted "check the room…what is there.. what sound is that outside?.. O God-I could not save him" and cried profusely. A terrible repeated visual image (? dream) occurred often - 'a tiger is extending its paws towards her', which awoke her almost every night. She had insurance but no Pass but got no financial help. She had four kids, all were under 12 and she became overprotective towards them. She didn't allow them to go outside the cottage after evening. Her father came and consulted a doctor who gave some sleeping medicines and a *Gunin*, who by supernatural chant and ritual 'bound her cottage against potential tiger attack'. She was almost dysfunctional for two years and then started a job as a maid servant. She said though the tiger fear has diminished by 50%, she still is fearful and feels bereft of any courage to go out after evening. The recurring images of the 'fight scene' haunt her and she feels terrible with body shakes, uncontrollable tears and feelings of extreme helplessness and hopelessness. She said her mind wandered vacantly, always feeling low without energy in the body, feeling it would be better to die. She felt extreme guilt for not performing the death rituals for her deceased husband. "Whenever I sit alone, the scene of his mutilated body, his cry from the tiger's mouth, the sea of blood, the ferocious look of the tiger shatters me with terrible fear, anxiety and sadness. I only pray to Bonobibi to save my children and me. I can't remember when I had a good night sleep. I have no interest in life, I can't laugh with the neighbours, I have no appetite for food and I am just living for the sake of living". Her life changed completely for the worse, since the incident. Once, she thought about killing herself by hanging but because of the little kids she drove this 'bad thought' out of her mind. Her father took two of her kids to care for them.

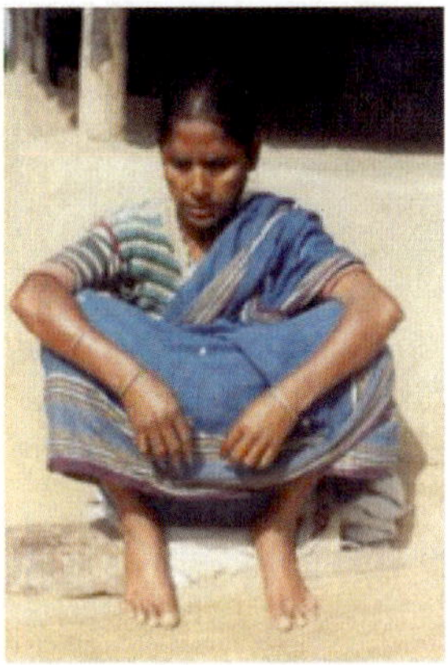

Clinical Impression: Chronic PTESD with depression (with survivor guilt) and expressed her concern about the 'disturbing accident-memory' and agreed to take a course of antidepressant and hypnotic medication.

4.6. Case 6:

Mrs. Mistry, 26 years married lady, when 16 years of age, went to collect TPS along with her mother and five others. They were on a boat trip in Gomar River. It was late March at about 5 pm and they were all pulling the *meenjal* (fishnet) along the bank line. Suddenly she felt a tug and was dragged down deep into the river. Everyone rushed towards her and pulled her with great strength out of the water. It was a *Kamote* that bit her left buttock and the front portion of her thigh. It bled profusely. She fainted after seeing the gush of blood and was taken to the boat. She was treated in the Gosaba BPHC and recovered from the wound after four weeks. But she ended up with an ugly scar extending up to left mid thigh and she had difficulty walking. She later recalled that she felt some slippery big fish-type animal brush against her legs and that she consciously tried to avoid the creature by walking forward into the water. She then suddenly experienced a cutting sensation as if a sharp saw was driven into her thigh. She had excruciating pain and before even shouting for help she had fainted.

First six months was a big trouble for the family as she developed fear of *Kamote*. She avoided the river, abandoned TPS collection and refused to take bath in the river. Mrs. Mistry's mother recalled: "The river is our all time need. When my daughter was taken to the river for bathing, she was very resistive. After going as far as waist deep water, she would shout that there is something in the water underneath her and would rush back to the bank. She cried all the time without any apparent reason and in the night saw Kamote-dream, as if her legs were being pulled into the river. She used to shout in the midst of sleep: "help me, save me,

Kamote is pulling me down". If any neighbour came to their cottage and gave detail about their fishing trip in the jungle, she refused to listen. She confined herself in the room. She was always fearful and asked her parents not to go in the river. She was anxious, fearful and absentminded for about two years after this incident. There was a deep scar mark on her back and the left leg has shrunk. There was a problem in marriage prospects because she had marks of animal scar on her body, which was taken by many as a bad omen. The family somehow managed to find her a match. Though the fear of Kamote has reduced significantly, she remains fearful of water, has abandoned any forest fishing entirely and avoids taking bath in the river, unlike before. When people narrate any such attacks she becomes upset and avoids participation in such discussions. Now she is working as an agricultural labourer. She says "I have no problem now, except my fear of water and that is why I always avoid river".

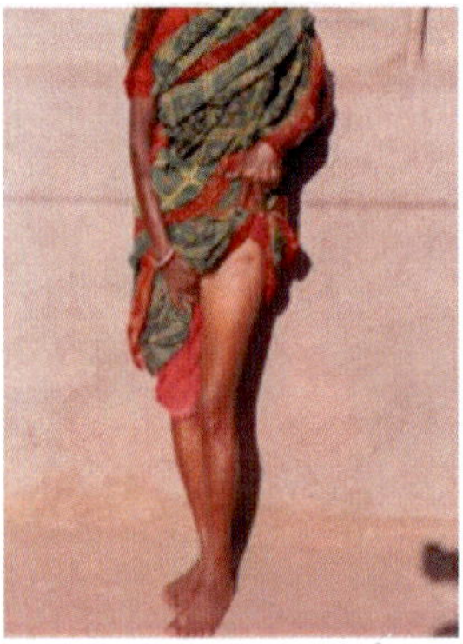

Clinical Impression: Chronic PTESD

4.7. Case 7:

Mr. Jana, a 48 years old man was asleep in his cottage. It was about 8pm in the summer month of May, four years ago. As it was very hot, he was unable to have a good sleep. He heard some sounds of dry hay as if something is moving across the courtyard. He thought of Bonobibi and prayed to save his family. He had heard that a tiger had crossed the river from SRF and thus he was suspicious. As he was tossing and turning in his bed, he heard a sound and got a *'botka'* smell of the tiger. He peeped through the window and saw the shining eyes of the tiger, as if two torch light bulbs were lit. The tiger was standing in the garden adjacent to the courtyard. He closed the door tightly and shouted for help: "tiger is in my house, save me, tiger in the garden". Immediately the neighbours rushed in with machetes, fire on wooden log and bamboo sticks. He, along with others attacked the tiger with sticks and sharp weapons. The tiger jumped on the crowd and knocked him to the ground. As he lay paralysed with fear, he found himself under the tiger's belly while it continually tried to grab him with its paws. Amidst the commotion of screaming, bamboo sticks and clunking metal, the tiger slashed his neck and fled into the forest, while he lay on the ground with excruciating pain and bleeding. He was treated at Gosaba BPHC and developed an extreme fear of the tiger. In the night he cried and shouted repeatedly: "See tiger is there- tiger, kill it-strike it". In the hospital, his constant shouting at night caused inconvenience to other patients and he had to be transferred to a solitary room. After five weeks in hospital, his wound healed properly and one of the authors (ANC) interviewed him at the hospital. He was found in a severe anxiety state, feeling very low and crying. While narrating the incident, he would tremble and stammer, particularly when he described his belief that the tiger would return as it was deprived of its prey. Almost every night he had a fright filled dream- as if the tiger is silently approaching his cottage premises and sat silently with extending fronts paws ready to jump on him. Sleep broke out with intensification of fear and he needed someone to comfort him at that moment. He was also very emotional and concerned about his appearance- his left external ear (pinna) was partly lost with marked deformity on the right forehead and face- the mark of tiger attack for which, he thought, people would ostracize him as a bad sign: "People will avoid to see my face in the morning or before any journey as I would be considered as an "o-*jatra*" (an unholy face to be avoided before any journey).

In a second visit after four months, he still had the tiger-fear, could not go outside his cottage even in daylight, abandoned his kitchen farming, and cleared the area so that tiger could not hide. And with any news of a tiger attack in the jungle he became very upset, trembling and assumed a posture to refuse to hear the story. With time, the frequency of tiger-dream decreased but he continued to have sleep disturbances. He was unable to hear properly and this apparent deafness caused difficulties in communication. He conversed by sign language with hand gestures. For protection and self-confidence, he lit up a kerosene lamp by the side of his bed at night. He felt very insecure and had strong conviction that the tiger will catch him again. He earnestly requested the author (ANC) to find even a minimal-wage menial job in Kolkata, as his life in the village was fraught with fear. He said, "If Bonobibi wishes to save me, she can, otherwise I am doomed". He took a *Manat* (pledge) for a big offering to Bonobibi also. He avoided his forest activities (fishing, wood cutting) entirely and now earns a meager sum of money by TPS collection in the daytime only.

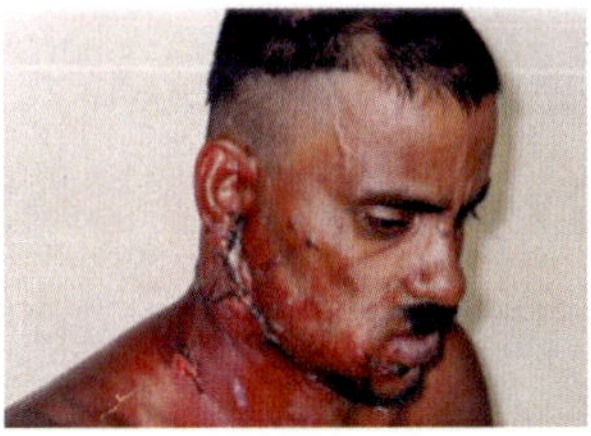

At Gosaba BPHC

Clinical Impression: Acute Stress Disorder followed by PTESD

4.8. Case 8:

Mr. Halder, a 32 years old man, was in a boat trip with six others for Garan wood cutting in Chamta jungle in deep SRF, a year ago. The trip was for three days and was 'Black'. On the second day, at around 8 am, he was cutting the stem of a big tree with his wooden-handle axe. Others were around him in close distance. Suddenly a tiger came like an 'arrow' from the jungle and jumped over his back. As he turned, his axe struck the tiger on the head and it fell on the ground. But it immediately stood up and pounced on him again. His fellow wood-cutters cutters rushed to the scene shouting. They used their wood-axes and wood-logs to injure the tiger. The tiger then fled into the forest. He was severely injured but conscious and requested his fellows to flee away as soon as possible. He was highly apprehensive as he believed that the tiger may come again to collect it's missed prey. He was taken to an Amlamethi private doctor (to avoid government hospital because of police case). The wound was not very deep and the tiger might have been injured sufficiently not to be able to inflict any deeper injury. His wound healed within six weeks but he developed fear of the tiger- as if tiger is coming to attack him again. Particularly at night he could not sleep well- very often shouted and cried loudly "it has come near the door, no more time, it will bite me and eat me in the jungle, coming nearer, leaning on me to take me." He shouted by calling the names of those who were with him in that trip -"save me, hit the tiger, alert-very close by". To stop him, his wife often smacked his face- and he would then look vacantly and sigh "all has gone, gone". His food intake had diminished, as was his sleep. He became very silent and avoided socializing. He always complained of burning sensation and pain over the neck and back. He looked anxious and confined himself within the room the whole day. He asked his wife to check and recheck the cottage and the courtyard repeatedly to ensure that no tiger was there. If there were any noise or shouting in the neighbourhood, he became apprehensive and repeatedly asked what had happened. Sometimes he behaved very oddly, as if he was a different man and nothing has happened to him. His disability was interpreted by neighbours as a 'mental problem'. So an offering was dedicated to Bonobibi and a *Gunin* was consulted, who after detailed ritual gave the verdict that in the jungle there were multiple 'accidental' deaths from tiger attacks and their bodies were buried under the mud without performing any death rituals. So the ghosts of the dead were roaming the forest and one of them has possessed him. He asked him every detail of the incident and then performed a *jhar-fuk* (chanting) with loud voice and burning red dry pepper, dry hay and ginger. He gave him an amulet to wear on his arm. Though he became relatively better, his irrational fear of the tiger prevailed. He cannot go to the local shop on his own or cross the river. He left all forest exploration. He said, "When I venture out, the jungle reminds me of the terrible scene of the accident. I feel shaky and mentally disturbed with anxiety and despair". Now he earns his bread by working as a day-labour.

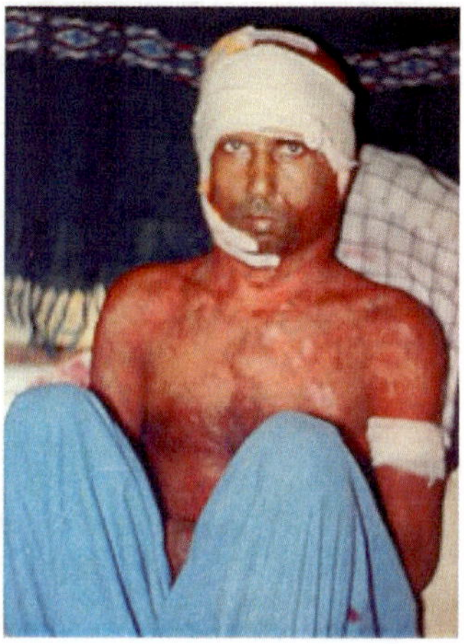

At Gosaba BPHC

Clinical Impression: PTESD

4.9. Case 9:

Mr. Mistry, a 45 years old man, was on a four-day boat trip to Netai jungle for Dhum (Dhundul - *Xylocarpus granatum*) woodcutting illegally, seven years ago. He was with three others. It was around 10 am and everyone was busy identifying which trees to cut. He was engaged in cutting a long tree when a tiger attacked him from behind. He lost balance and fell on the ground. The tiger bit him on the left chest region and the back. He shouted for help and his companions rushed to attack the tiger with their wood-axes. They encircled the tiger from all sides and managed to scare it away. In addition to tiger wounds, Mr. Mistry also sustained head and facial injuries when he fell on the tree and then onto the ground during the tussle. He was disoriented for some time, asking repeatedly whether he is living or dead and he bled profusely from the excruciatingly painful wounds. He was taken to a private doctor (avoided government hospital for legal complication) and was treated for four months. For the first few days he was extremely week, kept absolutely silent, always looked suspiciously and answered questions incoherently. Then he became very frightened of anything related to tiger theme even when he is in the safe confines of his own home. At night he would wake up often and tended to cover his face with a quilt or try to hide under the cot. When asked why he behaved so, he said, "Can you not hear it coming? It will catch me, it is looking at me". He trembled in fear and took long time to become normal again. When there was a storm or loud noise outside, he would hide under the quilt, trembling and would cry out, "few minutes more, it is coming; it will catch me, run away - run away". It was not until six months that he partly recovered, although he continued to avoid the jungle and the river completely. He also avoided social mixing and any discussion relating to tiger attack in the forest. His wife said: "Few days ago a tiger came to the other village and villagers drove it back into the jungle. He was very upset on that day, constantly pacing in and out between the courtyard and the room, looking apprehensively out of the window and muttering to himself. One of his good friends comforted him by staying whole day with him. He is now helping him to go for TPS or crab collection, which he started very slowly again. We are too poor, no land, no boat, if the male of the family sits at home, then we have to starve. We haven't received any help from the forest department."

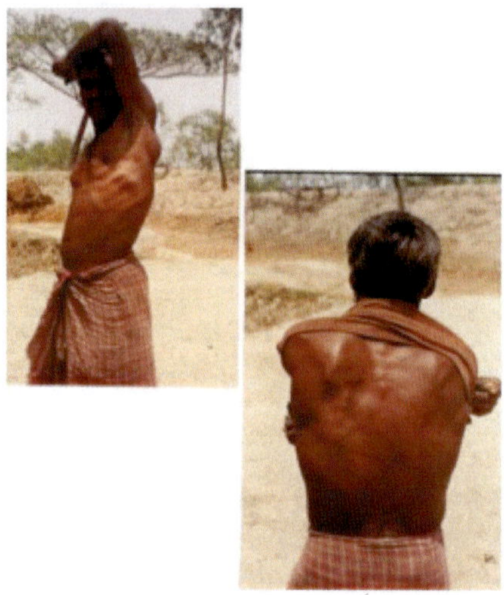

Clinical Impression: Chronic PTESD

4.10. Case 10:

Mrs. Mondal, a 41 years old married lady, was one among a team of five people who left for the jungle to collect TPS, three years ago. As the early morning catch is always good, they started their pursuit at about 4 am, pulling their *meen jal* (drag net) in the Khyal *khal* near Marich Jhappi jungle. The morning light was not very clear and she was wading through knee-deep water along the bank line with her net. The tiger leapt on her from behind and swept its paw on her head and left shoulder. She fell into the river and the tiger followed her into the water but could not bite her head. All others came to her rescue immediately and scared the tiger away with loud noises and creating frenzy with the rowing logs. She was taken to a private doctor in Satjelia and took three months to heal her wounds. First few weeks she was a bit disoriented, stared vacantly, quiet, extremely fright-ridden, with disturbed sleep, diminished appetite, automatic shaking with 'rolling eyes' and was unable to move her head. She then developed fear of the tiger. She thought the tiger might come to the village and detect her. At night she would stand up shouting "tiger is jumping". She had frequent fearful dreams with themes of - a tiger approaching her with a wide-open mouth, tiger sitting inside the room, tiger chasing her etc. Often she heard the *Hakar* (roaring) and dreamt that "the neighbours who were killed by tigers are running with a *Da* (sharp traditional machete) and snatching her from the tiger". She would wake up in fear and often cried holding her husband. She abandoned TPS collection; never entered the forest again and still cannot go outside the cottage in the evening. She has constant neck pain and headache, which increases during the black moon. The scar on the scalp is painful which restricts her from combing her hair. Still she has extreme fear of the tiger and feels upset if any such news is coming in to the village. After this tiger attack she became dysfunctional (multiple bodily pain and headache, weakness, difficulties in turning head, memory problem), cannot do heavy household work, presents as unusually apprehensive and is frequently haunted by terrible memory of the assault.

Clinical Impression: PTESD with somatic symptoms

4.11. Case 11:

Miss. Sarkar, an 18 years old single lady was on a trip to collect TPS with her father and maternal uncle, two years ago. It was end of July at around 10 am when her father was rowing the boat while she and her uncle were pulling the drag net in waist-deep waters of Garal *khal* near Marich Jhappi jungle. Suddenly they heard a terrifying tiger roar and in a blink, a tiger came 'like a kite' and jumped on her back but missed her narrowly. The paws only touched her head and part of right back as the tiger fell in the water. The two men responded instantly shouting to drive the tiger off while the father repeatedly thrashed his rowing log on the tiger's head and injured it enough to bleed and flee. Ms. Sarkar climbed back into the boat from the water. The tiger then went onto the bank, stood there for a second, gave a second glance and walked slowly into the thick jungle. Ms. Sarkar was taken to a private doctor in Tipli-Ghari bazaar and all her injuries healed with time. She is left with a big scar on her head and few scars on the right hand and back. She developed some 'mental' symptoms after the attack like - fear of the tiger, very low mood, suspicions that a tiger is hiding in and around the cottage, inability to go out after evening and feeling too nervous to talk about the incident. Sleep was very poor and dreams were about 'an attacking tiger', 'tiger roaring and thrashing its long tail'. She shouted in the midst of sleep "it is coming, leaping, strike it- strike it" and then cried profusely. She looked very distressed and always apprehensive. Her father gave a big offering to Bonobibi when a few neighbors were invited. She avoided everybody, remained quiet and kept to herself in her room. Few villagers said she is getting '*brain sort*' (mental illness) and advised to consult a *Boulay*. The Boulay from a nearby village presided and listened to the account. He said that his expertise in preventing tiger attacks would be effective only inside the jungle, therefore could not do anything to help in this case and advised to consult a *Gunin*. The *Gunin* then presided and completed a half-day ritual. He then cast a protection circle around the cottage that is meant to prevent the tiger from entering the premises. *Gunin* also gave a chanted Talisman to wear around the waist with red thread. As interesting as these rituals were, they made little difference to Ms. Sarkar's condition. She avoided TPS collection and stopped forest exploration because of the fear. No financial help was received. After a year and half she gradually became relatively better but facing another problem related to her marriage prospects. The groom's family is complaining that she has tiger marks/scars on her body and suspect that in future she may develop a 'mental problem'. Her mother is apprehensive and says, "we have to pay a high cost in dowry for the tiger scar".

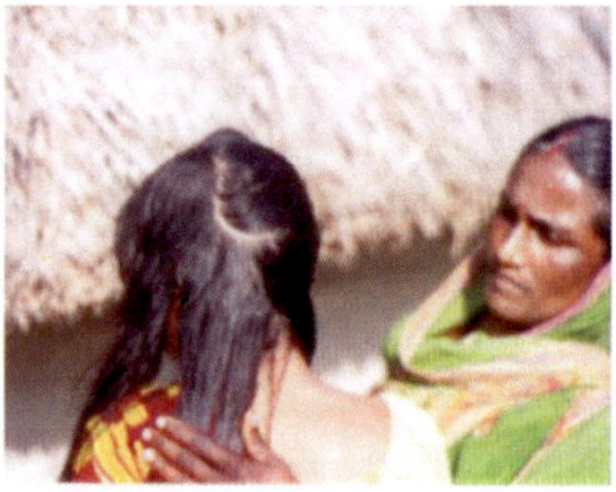

Clinical Impression: PTESD

4.12. Case 12:

Mr. Sardar, a 32 years old man, was invited by his friend for a boat trip for TPS collection on a February morning, nine years ago. He reluctantly accepted the invitation. Both men were pulling the drag-net and collecting the juvenile prawns by washing the net in Ganral river near Pirkhali jungle. He heard a sound but thought that probably the sound was from the bank collapsing into the river. Then he saw a tiger standing about six feet away from him. The tiger leapt on him and he tried to escape by jumping into the water albeit unsuccessfully. The tiger held him by his back and tried to carry him into the forest. Mr. Sardar held onto a lodged log tenaciously and kept his head and body under water. While the tiger tried to strongly pull him away, he could hear his ribs break but he did not give up. The other man came along shouting and thrashing bamboos on water. Being unable to pursue the hunt under water, the tiger jumped back on the riverbank and disappeared. He swam to the boat and to his safety. He had sustained a laceration on his back down to the right arm pit. He was treated in the Gosaba BPHC. He developed lots of problems after this incident. He was profusely distressed by the memories of the 'accident' and was always frightened and had crying spells. In the early morning he would sit up on the bed and ask others to check the room and outside whether any tiger is roaming there, frequently he shouted in the midst of sleep "alert, alert, it is coming, I won't allow" and then sat in the corner of the bed. He stopped going to the jungle, always felt weak with back pain and could not do any work. He often expressed utter hopelessness and helplessness regarding maintaining his health and his family. His elder son added: "We did not receive any financial help from the forest department, though he had a Pass and registry (insurance). He is still having some brain problem- very often he holds his head and his eyes turn red. He cannot work and cannot bear to think of entering the forest to make a living. We experienced some bad signs in the previous night – my mother's vermilion pot fell from her hand. She also broke a *Kalsi* (an earthen pot to collect water). Sometimes he urged us to move from this riverbank to some other village away from forest, but how can we do that? We are too poor, we have no land, and we depend on jungle and the river for livelihood". Mr. Sardar never ventured into the forest or undertook any forest activity after this incident.

Clinical Impression: Chronic PTESD with somatization

4.13. Case 13:

Mr. Mridha, 16 years of age (at the time), accompanied his mother on a crab collection trip in Gomor river, six years ago. At about 9 am he was on the bank and his mother was in waist-deep water. Suddenly his mother shouted, "save me- something is pulling me down". He jumped into water and caught hold of her. He then saw a crocodile's tail splashing on the water and lost his balance and grip on his mother. He then saw his mother being pulled under water. People rushed to the spot and saw the woman's body surfacing and submerging into the river. They chased the crocodile in a boat but it escaped under water along with its prey. Despite these attempts, Mr. Mridha's mother could not be saved. He was terribly upset that he could not save his mother. Since the body was not found, the relatives made a *Nara* (effigy with hay) and burnt it on the riverbank. On the same evening, the body was found floating in the river. Both legs were missing. The relatives left the body in the river (only after they took away the gold ear rings) as the mortuary ritual was already performed. Mr. Mridha struggled for over six months following this terrible incident. He was severely anxious and depressed, stopped going to school, was seen self-absorbed and avoided the river completely. When he saw a banana tree branches or anything floating in the river, he became extremely fearful and pointed to these objects as crocodile and threw bricks at them shouting "kill it, kill it". These 'accidents' are almost a regular event in Jamespur-Lahiripur area and with any such news he became very upset and returned to the cottage and sat quietly in the room. In the night he shouted in the midst of sleep "Mother! Mother! I am here" and woke up with lots of anxiety and crying. He lamented a lot and cursed himself for not being able to rescue his mother. Then a *Gunin* was consulted who performed a ritual and gave some herbal roots and leaves. Mr. Mridha then seemed somewhat settled but continued to remain very low in mood and energy and never went back to school.

He had two brothers and one sister. His father remarried. Family had extreme financial stress and he had to continue fishing trips. Four years from the incident, he was on a fishing trip (with his father) in Sarak Khalir jungle and was killed by a tiger. The above history was collected from his brother.

Clinical Impression: PTESD with depression (with survivor guilt).

5. Discussion

It was a unique opportunity to study people who survived dangerous wild animal attacks during their livelihood measures. Virtually all of them have had near death experience. The detailed situation analysis in each case have shown that how terrible and life-threatening was the experience of these animal attacks. There are some reports of domestic animal like dog attacks to children and PTSD [62, 42] and one report of ASD and PTSD after being mauled by wild bears [35] but no reports available on PTSD following tiger, shark and crocodile attacks in the literature. This is the first comprehensive report of PTSD after wild animal attacks, viz., tiger, crocodile and shark.

All cases here met the criteria of PTSD according to DSM IV [3], viz., all have experienced an actual threat of death and serious bodily injury with a response of intense fear, helplessness, or horror' (Criteria A1, 2)), all of them reexperienced traumatic event either by 'recurrent and intrusive distressing recollections of the event, including images, thoughts, or perceptions' or flashbacks (Criteria B1) or 'recurrent distressing dreams of the event '(B2) or 'acting or feeling as if the traumatic event were recurring' through illusion of tiger perception in the vicinity, hallucinatory hearing of tiger's howling or dissociative flashback episode as if tiger is going to attack them and acted in response (B3), 'intense psychological distress' with related external cues- feeling extremely fearful and anxious while hearing any similar events in the locality (B4). All the cases have 'Persistent avoidance of stimuli associated with the trauma'- by avoiding trauma related conversations (C1), all have avoided activities related to trauma (abandoning their livelihood measures and places where trauma occurred, i.e., Sundarban Reserve forest or rivers) (C2). Most of them have shown 'Persistent symptoms of increased arousal' like difficulty falling or staying asleep (D1), or hypervigilance (D4) or startle response (D5). In all cases the onset of symptoms occurred within a month of the insult and persisted for more than one month (E) and the disturbances caused significant distress and impairment in familial, social and occupational functioning (F). In view of persistence of symptoms more than six months, all cases have had chronic PTESD course. It has to be remembered that there were no therapeutic interventions for their symptoms except some traditional attempts. Some of them had associated symptoms of depression (Case 2, 3, 5, 13), somatic dysfunction (Case 1, 10, 12) and survivor guilt (Case 5, 13). Two cases (3, 7) had an Acute Stress Disorder (DSM IV -TR code 308.3, [4]) immediately after the trauma and three cases (Cases 1, 3, 4) had psychotic symptoms.

In addition to the classical PTSD symptoms (including flashbacks, affective dysregulation and some with dissociative reaction), all the cases here also presented some culture-specific features as well. Some of the interesting features are discussed below. Nightmares are quite common, of the "re-experiencing" symptoms of PTSD, seen in approximately 60% of individuals with PTSD [47]. The cultural interpretation of nightmares influence attitude and help seeking behavior. Some cultures view nightmares as mental health problems, others view them as related to supernatural or spiritual phenomena [38]. In three tiger attack cases (4, 8, 11) and one crocodile attack case (13) here, the nightmares and dream-related behaviours were regarded as mental symptoms and thus traditional healing from *Gunin* was called for. Post-traumatic dream is an important clinical symptom in PTSD. About 50% of post-traumatic dreams comprise replications of the traumatic events [79]. In the present case series all cases, except one (Case 9) had dreams of the animal attacks that disturb their sleep and arouse them with acting-out odd behaviours.

The present PTESD cases shed some interesting light on the situation analysis of trauma in respect to local socio-cultural perspective. It has to be remembered that these are not isolated incidents but rather human-animal conflicts which are ongoing events in SRF [70]. These people are extremely marginal and poor, without any land or wealth for living and all were attacked during their livelihood activities. In that sense these human-animal conflicts may be seen as an occupational hazard due to eco-specificity of SRF area. In fact, among the 13 cases the attack took place while 8 (61.5%) were involved in TPS collection in the river inside SRF; 2 (15.4%) during Crab collection and 2 (15.4%) while wood cutting in the SRF. One was an in-house attack by a straying tiger. Let us discuss the psycho-dynamics of PTESD according to the categories of trauma-causing animals.

Tiger attacks: Tiger and Sundarban Forest are almost synonymous [56]. Fear of tiger attack in the communities around fringe area of SRF and also during forest exploration is a constant threat [17, 60]. Most of the illegal forest intruders are poor and have dual fears during trespassing the forest, i.e., fear of the tiger and fear of the forest guards. Irony of the matter is that after such a life-threatening incident (or death) the whole matter arouses extreme fear of being detected and caught by the forest officials with consequent litigation and penalty. So to keep the attack and related injury secret is another stress to the victims. It not only adds another quantum of anxiety and suspiciousness to their PTESD symptomatology but prevents the inflow of social or community support. This is the reason why most of the cases here took treatment from private medical practitioners and are mostly reluctant to discuss their traumatic episodes publicly. It is also noted that none of the tiger victims here received any financial help, which was so crucial for their treatment and economic support at that point of crisis.

Living on the forest resources is a unique socio-economic dimension of Sundarban region. This enduring life struggle with different adversities including fatal tiger attack raised the status of the tiger to that of God. Counteracting this potential danger, the cult of Bonobibi as a protector, has become deeply ingrained into the belief system of these people. This religiosity is expressed in their day-to-day life pattern like in worshipping Bonobibi before entering the forest or having a strong faith and conviction that Bonobibi will certainly protect them during their in-forest activities. So any such attacks tend to shake their religious devotion and faith because the attack itself is the sign that The Goddess is displeased with the victim and therefore refused to protect them from the tigers. This generates a sense of guilt and sinfulness which impact on their post-trauma psychology immensely. So, some become more devotional to make up their spiritual deficiency by offering *puja* or vows to Bonobibi, while some become frankly disrespectful towards the Goddess. This bidirectional religious trend is also noted among the post-traumatic people after disasters [33, 39].

Post-traumatic grief may be an important psychodynamic contributor to PTSD symptoms [5], which is quite evident in the tiger-widow case (Case 5) here. The trauma scenario she described is horrific, devastating and had a significant impact on her grief and bereavement process. Grief is a healthy process by which an adjustment to loss of loved ones is balanced. Traumatic grief or complicated mourning is a situation where both trauma and grief coincide [67]. Traumatic grief occur when the circumstances of death is sudden and horrific and disrupt the normal mental functioning of the survivor. Grief intensity is related to the suddenness of the trauma and associated feelings of helplessness, powerlessness, threat to one's life, confrontation with shocking deaths and mutilations, and survivor guilt [7, 68]. Prolonged grief among traumatically bereaved relatives after natural disaster (Tsunami) is also reported [43]. The elaborate mortuary rituals act as a supportive social mechanism to channel out the grief reaction. But unfortunately the tiger widows in Sundarban are prohibited from this ritualistic way out (cathartic) process for cultural inhibitions. Most of the bodies of tiger victims are missing and for the recovered dead bodies the usual mortuary rituals are forbidden (as they are unnatural death) thereby hindering productive grieving. Crying, often loudly among solicitous relatives or neighbour is a cultural way of expression of grief in local culture but in case of illegal forest entry, the widows could not cry loudly to avoid the attention of forest guards and risk arrest or fine. For the same reason, the widows have to continue to behave like married women, wearing coloured apparels (widows are supposed to wear white saree) with bangles in both hands. This is a severe form of psychological torture and aggravates the traumatic stress manifold. Moreover, tiger widows are looked down in the community, because they are seen as a bad omen and blamed for their husband's death. They are stigmatized as those that brought misfortune. They are disrespected, and shunned by their in-laws as well as the community. Tiger widows are forced to live in dire poverty, with exclusion from the main stream community as outcasts and always cursed by all. In fact, in some of the forest blocks of Sundarban there are segregated hamlets in each village called *Bidhoba Palli* (Widow Hamlet). The widow has to take the responsibility of running the family with the kids. If the tiger-widow is of younger age group, the misery and hardship is more. In the present case, all these issues were proactively present and intensified her post-traumatic stress with depression. Cultural superstition, stigma and discrimination related to the nature of trauma intensify the stress and thereby cause the clinical course, chronic and more disabling. This is the usual story of other tiger-widows of Indian [6, 10] and Bangladeshi Sundarban [46, 1]. The increasing number of tiger-widows [63] is a serious psycho-social concern in this regard.

Cultural interpretation of trauma is a significant factor in the development of PTSD [64]. The cultural meaning of the trauma experience is crucial to understand PTSD symptoms. One related example may be the trauma of rape, since sexual assault carries elements of social shame and negative social attitude, its burden is more than the burden of a flood or a bomb blast. The myth and social stigma attached with tiger attack (e.g., unholy sign, displeased Bonobibi, cursed family, potential for mental or physical diseases, social isolation etc.) adds further stress to the victims. Two symptoms here, tiger fear and the conviction of reattack need some clarification from eco-specificity and cultural context. Though tiger fear constitutes a core symptom of PTESD here, from ecological perspective this is not unrealistic altogether. Appearance of tiger suddenly within the domestic premises is an ecological reality because very often tigers stray inside the villages (Fig. 8), even into the kitchen or cattle-shed [53, 29, 72, 74, 50]. So this fear is not entirely imaginary but rather has pathological intensification as a part of their PTSD anxiety.

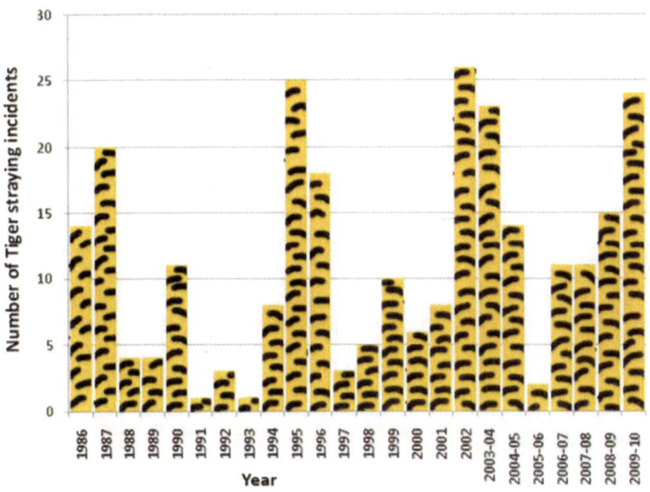

Figure 8. Tiger-straying incidents in Sundarban villages adjacent to SRF (adopted from [50]).

Conviction of reattack has a strong cultural connection with Tiger Cult [59] and folklore myth [41]. It is believed that the tiger always haunts it's missed prey like snakes and elephants and there are many popular anecdotal accounts circulating in the community. The acting out behavior to fight a potential intruding tiger is a symptom which has two components again. Firstly it implies an encroachment on a psychotic domain because inspite of explanation and support by the family member the victim believes that the tiger has come and secondly, it may be a transitory state of heightened anxiety as a part of PTESD flashback. In either component, there is loss of reality testing. Hearing a tiger's roar, hearing tiger's movement or smelling of tiger's odor during flashback – all are indicative of psychotic elements of PTESD. Positive symptoms like delusion and hallucination are not uncommon in PTSD cases [11, 34]. The strong and popular cultural belief that a missed prey will be taken by the tiger again is reported by all the cases here and that this cultural belief triggered lot of anxiety and abnormal behavior to ward off this alleged risk of further attack (by the same tiger). Hence, proper delineation of symptom pattern from the cultural perspective and eco specificity of the local universe [27] is important and will help to understand the PTESD psychopathology and their management.

Cultural experience and interpretation shape various responses to trauma [51], like meaning and implications of the trauma (tiger attack is not just an animal attack but it also reflects a spiritual dimension, i.e., that the Goddess Bonobibi and Tiger God Dakshin Ray, are angry or displeased and further misfortune may ensue), role of belief in 'fate', which increases hopelessness (other family members may fall prey to tiger's rage) and social vulnerability to trauma (stigma and discrimination of tiger attack in the community- hindering marriage prospects because of having a 'tiger mark' or 'Kamote mark' on the body or alleged potential to develop mental health problem after a tiger attack, or people avoid seeing a face with tiger scar etc). Mental symptoms after animal attacks here were considered in terms of supernatural context like possession or displeased God or Goddess in the community and thus called for traditional healing. Non-availability of modern treatment facility in these remote islands coupled with their strong faith on supernatural causation of these 'accidents' prompted them to receive folk treatment from the local HCPs and apparently this has benefitted the victims. So, the understanding of cultural perspective of the local eco-social universe is helpful for the *emic*-insight and may help in planning therapeutic intervention [76].

Crocodile and Shark attacks: Mauling by crocodile and shark are quite frequent in Sundarban rivers and cause significant mortality and morbidity [65, 61]. A survey in 2006 showed that 30 people had been killed by crocodiles in a span of three months in Patharpratima block of Sundarban [73]. Interestingly, one report showed that a crocodile devours a tiger [69]. Crocodiles and Gharials (*Ghavialis gangeticus*- a type of fish-eating crocodile), like tigers, is also straying frequently in the villages and takes shelter in sweet water ponds or inside swampy bushes. Usually the crocodile attacks are severe and since the prey is pulled down under the water, the survival rate is very low, even if rescued immediately. The incidents usually take place in front of many people who are on the river bed and many witness the horrific crocodile-human bloody struggle. Some who are directly involved in attempting to rescue the victim are prone to develop PTESD, as the posthumous case in this study. Some cases survived after losing some body parts, usually the legs. The muddy waters along the river banks are also infested with dog sharks *(Kamots)* and usually they don't kill the victim, but bite off chunks of flesh with their sharp teeth within a second. Often victims don't realise until the water around them turns red and some may bleed to death or lose their body parts (foot or hand or fingers). The author (ANC) has evidenced that after seeing a crocodile, which looks very terrifying and scary in the river of Patharpratima (Fig.9), people become so fearful that they avoid the river for weeks together. The world's largest captive crocodile breeding farm is at Bhagatpur, near Namkhana block of Sundarban. There are more than 300 estuarine crocodiles in the Sundarban National Park. Similar human-crocodile conflicts have been reported from the fringe area of Bhitarakanika wildlife sanctuary, Orissa state, India, where over fifty lives have been lost during the past ten years from saltwater crocodile attacks [54].

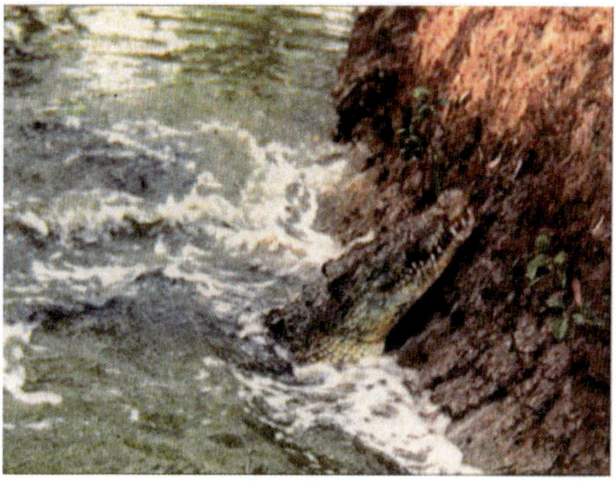

Figure 9. Crocodile in Ramganga river, Patharpratima Block, Sundarban.

The present study, comprising situation analysis of the wild animal attacks during livelihood activities of marginal people and consequent mental health morbidity in the context of Sundarban's unique eco-landscape, offers a new insight into the scope and extent of community mental health programme in the region. The clinical presentation of PTSD in all the cases here manifest a unique cultural component (reattack fear, flashbacks and acting out behaviours) to such an extent that it represent like a culture-bound PTSD syndrome. The therapeutic planning thus goes beyond the usual treatment methods with medications and calls for a multi-level comprehensive psycho-social and eco-cultural approach.

6. Conclusion

Human-animal conflicts are increasing worldwide [31] but there are limited reports regarding their impact on mental health. Ecopsychiatriy tends to unravel ecological influence on mental health. Ecospecificity of the region differs from place to place and thus has different impacts on local people [52]. Ecospecificity of Sundarban region is operative at the background of the morbidities discussed here. Ecological character of the region also influences people's behaviour. One such good example is the alarming rise of Deliberate Self-Harm (DSH), both fatal and nonfatal, by pesticide ingestion [19, 22] in Sundarban region. Eco-stress impacts agriculture in this delta region immensely by frequent storm, cyclone, flood, embankment rupture and tidal inundation of paddy fields, salinity of soil and thus makes agriculture a hard and risk-prone task. To compensate these, poor and illiterate farmers use or overuse pesticides, which are easily available in every grocery shop of each village [25]. This easy availability of pesticides acts as a potential catalyst to enhance the self-harm behaviour among the vulnerable subjects [21]. Similarly, forest-based living is the only available option for the poor and marginal people in the fringe area and during their eco-resource exploration they fall prey to animal attacks. Therefore social and economic development and alternative livelihood opportunities [28] in planning will aid the prevention of these casualties. Direct and indirect ecological influence plays a dynamic role behind human distress. The ecological change, for example climate change and sea-level rise [49] disturb the tiger habitat, thus causing more tiger straying into the villages, thereby increasing the potential for more human-tiger conflicts [9]. Excessive ecoresource, both riverine and forest, exploitation disturbs the food chain web and thus crocodile and sharks are haunting rivers close to human habitat more. The author (ANC) met a group of young students (Class five-six standards) in a Jharkhali village in Basanti block after Cyclone Aila (25 May 2009) who became terrified by at the sight of gathering black clouds in the sky (which reminded them of the devastating Cyclone) and left the school enmass to take secured shelter at home. So understanding of the local ecological landscape is very important eco-clinical task and may help in therapeutic planning and this is the reason that we propose the diagnosis of these cases as Post Traumatic Eco-stress Disorder. Management also needs to address the local cultural and ecological features contributing to the pathology [48, 30]. Cross-cultural research has shown evidently that culture shapes belief systems and thus influences the perception of traumatic events and their meaning, attribution and coping behaviours [76]. Given the importance of cultural context of traumatic experience, the use of DSM-IV Cultural Formulation has been in recent use for diagnostic formulation of patients of PTSD [36].

Conflict of Interest: None

Acknowledgements

The authors thankfully acknowledge the logistic help rendered by Sri Tushur Kanjilal, Tagor Society for Rural Development, Rangabelia, Gosaba, and Dr.Girin Mondal, Block Medical Officer, Gosaba BPHC during this study. World Bank through State Health System Development Project, Department of Health and Family Welfare, Government of West Bengal funded this study. Thanks to Dr. Satyadev Nagari, MRCPsych, Speciality Doctor, Stuart Road Clinic, Corby, Northamptonshire, U.K. for his critical comments on the draft paper.

Author details

Arabinda N. Chowdhury[1*], Ranajit Mondal[2], Mrinal K Biswas[2] and Arabinda Brahma[2]

*Address all correspondence to: arabinda.chowdhury@btinternet.com

1 Northamptonshire Healthcare NHS Foundation Trust, Stuart Road Resource Centre, Corby, Institute of Psychiatry, Kolkata, India

2 U. K. & Research Assistant, Institute of Psychiatry, Kolkata, India

References

[1] ABC News (2012). Tiger widows: Life in the Sundarbans. Available at: http://abcnews.go.com/blogs/headlines/2012/02/tiger-widows-life-in-the-sundarbans/

[2] Aleksareandrovski, I.A. (1991). Ecological disasters and mental health. *Sovetskaia Meditsina*, 12, 3-6.

[3] APA (1994). Diagnostic and statistical manual of mental disorders (4th ed.). American Psychiatric Association, American Psychiatric Press Inc. Washington, DC.

[4] APA. (2000). DSM IV TR: Diagnostic and statistical manual of mental disorders. American Psychiatric Association, American Psychiatric Press Inc. Washington, DC.

[5] Asukai, N., Tsuruta, N., & Saito, A. (2011). Pilot study of traumatic grief treatment programme for Japanese women bereaved by violent death. *Journal of Traumatic Stress*, 24(4), 470-473.

[6] BBC (2009). Pain of India's 'tiger widows'. Available at: http://news.bbc.co.uk/go/pr/fr/-/1/hi/world/south_asia/8411225.stm

[7] Ball, J.F. (1977). Widow's grief: the impact of age and mode of death. *Omega, Journal of Death & Dying*, 7(4), 307-333.

[8] Banerjee, M. (2008). Man-animal conflicts threaten tiger. Available at: http://bigcatrescue.blogspot.co.uk/2008/03/man-animal-conflict-threatens-tigers.html

[9] Bhabani, S. (2008). Tiger attacks on rise in Indian Sundarbans after cyclone. Available at: http://www.thaindian.com/newsportal/enviornment/tiger-attacks-on-rise-in-indian-sundarbans-after-cyclone_10077600.html

[10] Bhattacharya, S. (2012). The tiger widows of the Sundarban. Available at: http://www.thenational.ae/news/world/south-asia/the-tiger-widows-of-the-sundarbans

[11] Butler, R. W., Mueser, K. T., Sprock, J., & Braff, D. L. (1996). Positive symptoms of psychosis in posttraumatic stress disorder. *Biological Psychiatry*, 30(10), 839-844.

[12] Census of India. (2001). Primary Census Abstract: West Bengal and Orissa. *Office of the Registrar General, Govt. of India, New Delhi.*

[13] Chakrabarti, K. (1986a). Tiger (Panthera tigris tigris) in the mangrove forests of Sundarbans- an ecological study. *Tiger Paper*, 13(2), 8-11.

[14] Chakraborty, K. (1986b). Fish and fish resources in the mangrove swamps of Sundarbans, West Bengal- an indepth study. *The Indian Forester*, 112, 538-542.

[15] Chatterjee, P. (2010). Fishing community issues in the Sundarban Tiger Reserve (STR). Available at: http://www.docstoc.com/docs/30745428/Fishing-community-issues-in-the-Sundarban-Tiger-Reserve-_STR_

[16] Chowdhury, A. N., Chowdhury, S., & Chakraborty, A. (1999). Eco-stress, quality of life and mental health in Sundarban delta of India. *International Medical Journal*, 6, 59-63.

[17] Chowdhury, A. N., Chakraborti, A. K., & Weiss, M. G. (2001). Community mental health and concepts of mental illness in the Sundarban Delta of West Bengal, India. *Anthropology and Medicine*, 8, 109-29.

[18] Chowdhury, A. N., Shasmal, R. K., Ramkrishna, J., & Weiss, M. G. (2001). Eco-stress of human-animal conflicts in the Sundarban delta of West Bengal, India. *Eastern Anthropologist*, 54, 35-50.

[19] Chowdhury, A. N., Sanya,l, D., Dutta, S. K., & Weiss, M. G. (2003). Deliberate self-harm by ingestion of poisons on Sagar island in the Sundarban Delta, India. *International Medical Journal*, 10, 85-91.

[20] Chowdhury, A. N., & Weiss, M. G. (2004). Eco-stress and Mental health in Sundarban Delta, India. In, The Dying Earth: People's action and Nature's reaction, Eds. M Desai and MK Raha, acb Publications with Netaji Institute for Asian Studies, Kokata, 108-119, 8-18750-021-2.

[21] Chowdhury, A. N., Banerjee, S., Chakraborty, A. K., & Weiss, M. G. (2004). Eco-psychology of deliberate self-harm. *Eastern Journal of Psychiatry*, 8, 22-27.

[22] Chowdhury, A. N., Banerjee, S., Brahma, A., & Weiss, M. G. (2007). Pesticide practices and suicide among farmers of Sundarban region. *Food and Nutrition Bulletin*, 28(2), S381-391.

[23] Chowdhury, A. N., Sarkar, P., Das, S., Maity, T., Brahma, A., & Banerjee, S. (2008a). An ethnographic study of health system at Maisani island: Role of HCPs. *Journal of Indian Anthropological Society*, 42, 165-176.

[24] Chowdhury, A. N., Mondal, R., Brahma, A., & Biswas, M. K. (2008b). Eco-psychiatry and Environmental Conservation: Study from Sundarban Delta, India. *Environmental Health Insights*, 2, 61-76.

[25] Chowdhury, A. N., Brahma, A., Banerjee, S., & Biswas, M. K. (2009). Deliberate self-harm prevention in the Sundarban region needs immediate public health attention. *Journal of Indian Medical Association*, 107, 88-93.

[26] Chowdhury, A. N., & Jadav, S. (2012). Ecopsychiatry: Culture, mental health and ecology with special reference to India. *In, Textbook on Community Psychiatry in India, Eds. BS Chavan, N Gupta, P Arun, AK Sidana, S Jadhav, Jaypeebrothers, New Delhi*, 521-541, 978-9-35025-805-7.

[27] Das, C. S. (2012). Tiger straying incidents in Indian Sundarban: statistical analysis of case studies as well as depredation caused by conflict. *European Journal of Wildlife Research*, 58(1), 205-214.

[28] Datta, D., Chattopadhyay, R. N., & Deb, S. (2011). Prospective livelihood opportunities from the mangroves of the Sunderbans, India. *Research Journal of Environmental Sciences*, 5, 536-543.

[29] Decan, Herald. (2010). Sundarbans tigers frequently straying to nearby villages. Available at: http://www.deccanherald.com/content/71444/sunderbans-tigers-frequently-straying-nearby.html

[30] De Jong, J.T.V.M. (2007). Traumascape: an ecological-cultural-historical model for extreme stress. In, Textbook of Cultural Psychiatry, Eds. D Bugra, K Bhui, Cambridge University Press, 347-363, 100521173388.

[31] Distefano, E. (2005). Human-Wildlife Conflict Worldwide: A collection of case studies, analysis of management strategies and good practices. SARD Initiative Report, FAO, Rome. Available at: http://www.fao.org/SARD/common/ecg/1357/en/HWC_final.pdf

[32] DSA, Department of Sundarban Affairs (2008). Government of West Bengal. Available at: http://www.sadepartmentwb.org/Socio_Econimic_1.htm

[33] Falsetti, S. A., Resick, P. A., & Davis, J. L. (2003). Changes in religious beliefs following trauma. *Journal of Traumatic Stress*, 16(4), 391-398.

[34] Floros, G. D., Charatsidou, I., & Lavrentiadis, G. (2008). A case of PTSD presenting with psychotic symptomatology: a case report. *Case Journal*, 1, 352, 10.1186/1757-1626-1-352.

[35] Frank, R. S., Mahabir, R. C., Magi, E., Lindsay, R. L., & Haas, W. D. (2006). Bear maulings treated in Calgary, Alberta: Their management and sequelae. *Canadian Journal of Plastic Surgery*, 14(3), 158-162.

[36] Fortuna, L. R., Porche, M. V., & Alegria, M. (2009). A qualitative study of clinicians' use of the cultural formulation model in assessing posttraumatic stress disorder. *Transcultural Psychiatry*, 46, 429-450.

[37] Gangopadhyay, S., Das, B., Ghosal, G., Das, T., Ghosh, T., Ganguly, R., & Samanto, K. (2008). The prevalence of musculoskeletal disorders among prawn seed collectors of Sundarban. *Journal of Human Argology*, 37(2), 83-90.

[38] Hinton, D.E. (2009). Introduction to the special section: Nightmares of trauma victims- cross-cultural perspectives. *Culture, Medicine and Psychiatry*, 33(2), 216-218.

[39] Hussain, A., Weisaeth, L., & Heir, L. (2011). Changes in religious beliefs and the relation of religiosity to posttraumatic stress and life satisfaction after a natural disaster. *Social Psychiatry & Psychiatric Epidemiology*, 46(10), 1027-1032.

[40] Jain, S., & Sastry, A. (1983). *Botany of Some Tiger Habitats in India.*, Botanical Survey of India, Howrah., 40-44, Pub ID 102520101.

[41] Jalais, A. (2008). Bonobibi: Bridging worlds. *Indian Folklore Serial*, 28, 6-8.

[42] Ji, L., Xiaowei, Z., Chuanlin, W., & Wei, L. (2010). Investigation of posttraumatic stress disorder in children after animal-induced injury in China. *Pediatrics*, 126(2), e320-324.

[43] Johannesson, K. B., Lundin, T., Hultman, C. M., Froid, T., & Michel, P. O. (2011). Prolonged grief among traumatically bereaved relatives exposed and not exposed to a tsunami. *Journal of Traumatic Stress*, 24(4), 456-464.

[44] Kalayjian, A., Kanazi, R. L., Aberson, C. L., & Feygn, L. (2002). A cross-cultural study of the psychological and spiritual impact of natural disaster. *International Journal of Group Tensions*, 31(2), 175-186.

[45] Kanjilal, B., Mazumder, P. G., Mukherjee, M., Mondal, S., Barman, D., Singh, S., & Mandal, A. (2010). Healthcare in the Sundarbans (India): Challenges and plan for a better future. Future Health Systems Research Programme, IHMR, India. Available at: http://www.dfid.gov.uk/r4d/PDF/Outputs/FutureHealth_RPC/sundarbans.pdf

[46] Kazim, H. (2011). Bangladesh's tiger widows fight exclusion. Available at: http://www.spiegel.de/international/world/0,1518,744594,00.html

[47] Kilpatrick, D. G., Resnick, H. S., Freedy, J. R., Pelcovitz, D., Resick, P. A., Roth, S., et al. (1998). Posttraumatic stress disorder field trial: Evaluation of the PTSD construct-criteria A through E. In, DSM-IV Sourcebook, Eds. TA Widiger, AJ Frances, HA Pincus, R Ross, MB First, W Davis, M. Kline, 4th ed., American Psychiatric Press, Washington DC., 803-844.

[48] Krieger, N. (2001). Theories for social epidemiology in the 21st century: an ecosocial perspective. *International Journal of Epidemiology*, 30, 668-677.

[49] Loucks, C., Meyer, S. B., Hossain, A. A., Barlow, A., & Chowdhury, R. M. (2010). Sea level rise and tigers: predicted impacts to Bangladesh's Sundarban mangroves. *Climate Change*, 98, 291-298.

[50] Mallick, J.K. (2011). Status of the mammal fauna in Sundarban tiger reserve, West Bengal, India. *Taprobanica*, 3(2), 52-68, 0180-0427X.

[51] Marsella, A.J. (2010). Ethnocultural aspects of PTSD: An overview of concepts, issues and treatments. *Traumatology*, 16(4), 17-26.

[52] Mc Laren, L., & Hawe, P. (2005). Ecological perspectives in health research. *Journal of Epidemiology and Community Health*, 59, 4-14.

[53] Mitra, P., & Chakraborty, M. (2008). Tiger walks into the kitchen. Available at: http://articles.timesofindia.indiatimes.com/2008-06-10/kolkata/27750976_1_bengal-tiger-niraj-singhal-gosaba

[54] Mishra, A. (2007). No let up in human-animal conflicts in Bhitarkanika National Park. Available at: http://www.downtoearth.org.in/node/5883?quicktabs_1=0

[55] Molla, M. A. G., Islam, M. R., Islam, S., & Salam, M. A. (2009). Socioeconomic status of crab collectors and fatteners in the southwest region of Bangladesh. *Journal of Bangladesh Agricultural University*, 7(2), 411-419.

[56] Mukherjee, S. (2003). Tiger human conflicts in Sundarban Tiger reserve, West Bengal, India. *Tiger Paper*, 30(2), 3-6.

[57] Nandi, N. C., & Pramanik, S. K. (1994). *Crabs and crab fisheries in Sundarban.*, Hindusthan Publishing Corporation, Delhi., 8-17075-034-2.

[58] Neria, Y., Nandi, A., & Galea, S. (2008). Post-traumatic stress disorder following disasters: a systematic review. *Psychological Medicine*, 38, 467-480, S0033291707001353.

[59] Niyogi, T. (2009). Tiger cult of the Sundarvans. *Anthropological Survey of India, No 95 of Memoir*, Ministry of Human Resource Development, Dept. of Culture, Govt. of India, 8-18557-937-7.

[60] Ojha, S., & Chakraborty, M. (2009). Living in the Tiger's shadow. Available at: http://articles.timesofindia.indiatimes.com/2009-12-07/kolkata/28077584_1_tiger-attack-royal-bengal-tiger-sunderbans

[61] Oneindia (2008). Woman saved from jaws of crocodile in Sundarbans. Available at: http://news.oneindia.in/2008/10/29/woman-saved-from-jaws-of-crocodile-in-sundarbans-1225285507.html

[62] Peters, V., Sottiaux, M., Appelboom, J., & Kahn, A. (2004). Posttraumatic stress disorder after dog bites in children. *The Journal of Pediatrics*, 144(1), 121-122.

[63] Pradhan, K. (2010). India: Rising number of "Tiger Widows". Available at: http://www.allvoices.com/contributed-news/6172520-india-rising-number-of-tiger-widows

[64] Rooyen, K. V., & Nqweni, Z. C. (2012). Culture and posttraumatic stress disorder (PTSD): a proposed conceptual framework. *South African Journal of Psychology*, 42(1), 51-60.

[65] Sarkar, S. (2008). Woman chewed up by crocodile in Sundarbans. Available at: http://www.merinews.com/article/woman-chewed-up-by-crocodile-in-sunderbans/shtml

[66] SBR (2006). Sundarban Biosphere Reserve. Available at: http://www. Sundarbanbiosphere.org/html_fi les/man_animal_confl ict.htm

[67] Shelby, J., Mazure, C., & Prigerson, H. (2000). Diagnostic criteria for traumatic grief. *Death Studies*, 24, 185-199.

[68] Shear, K. (2007). Managing grief after disaster. Available at: http://www.ptsd.va.gov/professional/pages/managing-grief-after-disaster.asp

[69] Singh, S.S. (2009). In Sundarbans, crocodile devours tiger. Available at: http://www.expressindia.com/latest-news/in-sunderbans-crocodile-devours-tiger/829699/

[70] The Hindu (2009). Frequent tiger, crocodile attacks in Sundarban villages. Available at: http://www.thehindu.com/news/states/other-states/article39317.ece

[71] TOI (Times of India) (2009a). Crab collector lifted by tiger. Available at: http://articles.timesofindia.indiatimes.com/2009-09-08/flora-fauna/28077664_1_crabs-tiger-sundarbans

[72] TOI (Times of India) (2009b). Straying tiger trapped in Gosaba. Available at: http://articles.timesofindia.indiatimes.com/2009-11-01/kolkata/28081954_1_pug-marks-gosaba-forest-officials

[73] TOI (Times of India) (2009c). Sundarbans proving black hole for men searching livelihood. Available at: http://articles.timesofindia.indiatimes.com/2009-08-16/flora-fauna/28163458_1_sheba-mridha-jamespur-and-annpur-villages-sundarbans

[74] TOI (Times of India) (2010). Tiger strays into village. Available at: http://articles.timesofindia.indiatimes.com/2010-12-31/kolkata/28269038_1_tiger-strays-big-cat-forest-officials

[75] Udomratn, P. (2008). Mental health and the psychosocial consequences of natural disasters in Asia. *International Review of Psychiatry, Abingdon England*, 20(5), 441-444.

[76] Wilson, J. P. (2008). Culture, trauma, and the treatment of posttraumatic syndromes: A global perspective. *In, Ethnocultural perspectives on disaster and trauma: Foundations, issues, and Applications*, Eds A J Marsella, J Johnson, P Watson, J Gryczynski, Springer SBM: New York, 351-378, 101441925163.

[77] Wilson, J. P. (2010). The lens of culture: Theoretical and conceptual perspectives in the assessment of psychological traumas and PTSD. *In, Cross-Cultural Assessment of Psychological Trauma and PTSD*, Eds. JP Wilson, CS Tang, Springer SBM, New York., 3-30, 139781441943705.

[78] WHO. (1992). The ICD-10 Classification of Mental and Behavioural Disorders. 9th Edition. *World Health Organization, Geneva.*, 9-24154-422-8.

[79] Wittmann, L., Schredl, M., & Kramer, M. (2007). Dreaming in posttraumatic stress disorder: A critical review of phenomenology, psychophysiology and treatment. *Psychotherapy and Psychosomatics*, 76, 25-39.

Chapter 16

Attention – Deficit Hyperactivity Disorder (ADHD) in Psychiatry and Psychoanalysis

Crístia Rosineiri Gonçalves Lopes Corrêa

Additional information is available at the end of the chapter

1. Introduction

In this article, we will be talking about the symptoms of lack of attention and hyperactivity, mainly on the fields of learning process

1.1. Attention – Deficit Hyperactivity Disorder (ADHD) in psychiatry

It is possible to find attention - deficit hyperactivity disorder (ADHD) in reference [1], a psychiatric manual which points out its identification based in a group of symptoms referred to carelessness, hyperactivity and also referred to impulsivity. Regarding carelessness, it can be identified by a frequent hard time on paying attention on details; on making mistakes on simple school written activities; on having problems on paying attention on playful activities; on permanent refusal to follow instructions and on finishing school works; do not accept house keeping or professional duties; they have a large difficulty to organize tasks and activities, avoiding or showing aversion and reluctance on getting involved on tasks that require constant mental effort such as: school tasks or home work; frequent loss of their school objects need to perform the same tasks and exercises, it all connect to the fact that they are distracted by any stimulus not concerned with their daily activities.

Hyperactivity, thus, shows a permanent state of "high speed", or as if the person was always on "full battery charge"; the frequently speak non stopping; they keep on moving their feet and hands or are always moving around when are sat still. When they are in the classroom they keep on leaving their desks and do the same in some other situations when they are expected to seat and being easy; they are frequently running around even when they are not supposed to do so; do not stop to play or get quietly involved on playing activities. There are also the impulsivity symptoms that are marked by precipitate answers given even before the question are fully done; they show a very hard time to wait for their turn to do things; and always interrupt or get involved on issues that are not of their business.

It is very important to say that [1] point out as a min item for a ADHD diagnosis just if there is a persistence for, "at least, 6 months, on bad adaptive degree and being inconsistent with the development levels" (p.71)[1], if six or more of the listed symptoms related to attention deficit or, yet, if six or more of the already mentioned symptoms of hyperactivity are shown.

However, despite of the mentioned psychiatric catalog on ADHD, a certain polemic debate referred as to it be or not a mental disturbance, takes place nowadays. [2] well known researchers on the ADHD theme, argue that critics concerning the validity of ADHD as a mental disturbance come from a large variety of academic areas, such as: social critics which turns the question to the teachers and parents intolerance with exuberant children [2], smaller political-religious groups and some non specialized professionals that state out the agreement between the mental health care community and the pharmacy industry [3]. Even though there are variations on the place where the problem would really lay on, under those critics point of view, we can see that the core of this criticism is the belief that ADHD is not more than a myth. These critics look forward to bring up to the surface their claims to state the argument that normal children, full of energy, have been designated as "mentally disturbed" because they end up being under a hyperactivity or ADHD diagnosis – based on an academic logic in which teachers, moored on this supposed disturbance get rid off their responsibility regarding their intolerant and deficient practices, also putting aside the anxiety related to the education levels expected to these children.

But, according to [2] there are, actually, in these critics, not just one, but two arguments that can apparently state the same thing, as known, that ADHD is a myth and that it is not a mental disturbance, in a sense that the problem can be real and not necessarily be characterized as a valid mental disturbance. As concerning its feasibility, regarding these researchers, as an evidence, in the opposite way of calling this concept a myth, among other things, we can point out easily found "important cognitive, behavioral or social differences among children with or without ADHD designations" (p. 105[2]). Besides that, it is possible to show "numerous differences among children with or without ADHD designations" (p. 105[3]). But as it was already said, its validity, concerning the construction or not of a mental disturbance is not automatically done by its feasibility. In accordance to the referred authors it is ultimate to ask about the criteria used to define what a mental disturbance is in order to determine, with these criteria, the ADHD validity as a category as such.

Regarding these criteria, it is possible to underline a lecture under this pretense suffering way of these children in school moored on an "organicist" position by stating the ignited configuration by the symptoms presented as shown on the ADHD characteristics in a biological dimension – requiring, thus, in hard way the use of medication to the shown problems in school for those "hyperactive" children. It is seen on the technical literature, on this

1 Translated from the Portuguese edition.

2 Translated from the Portuguese.

3 Translated from the Portuguese.

particular issue, that such biological dimension has two paths. The first one establishes, as the etiology of this "disturbance", a specific neurological damage that creates a correlation, not scientifically proved yet, to the pre frontal functions of the Central Neural System.

On the other hand [2] do not state the validity of this configuration as a legitimate psychiatric syndrome based on a supposed bad brain work. The contribution taken by [2]. to this determination comes from [5]. [5] developed the Boorsian[4], approach [6–8] providing a biological account on the concept of disorder based on an evolutionary theory. Wakefield promotes natural function as a scientific concept that can not be reduced to values. Dysfunction is considered a demarcation criterion to separate natural processes once called disorder from those known as not. According to Wakefield, the former condition disrupts a natural function.

For Wakefield, a specific condition only constitutes disorder if it involves functional breakdown of an internal mechanism. Both physical and mental disorder must be accounted within the biological sciences, which provides scientific basis to the physical medicine as well as to psychological medicine. Wakefield classifies accounts of disorders on evolutionary fields in three types:

1. [11][5], [12][6], and [6-8] defined the criteria to establish disease conditions as: lowered survival or lowered reproductive fitness.
2. Organism disorder takes place when some mental mechanism (such as perception) does not perform as it is expected to (e.g. to convey information about the environment, it was designed to perform by evolution).

4 References [6-8] established the distinction between illness and disease. According to Boorse's argument whereas disease is defined in factual terms and refers to theoretical concepts in technical contexts, illness is a value-term derived from disease used in non-technical contexts. For Boorse, illness is a value-term, which refers to most serious diseases, namely those who have incapacitating effects [6]. "A disease is an illness only if it is serious enough to be incapacitating and therefore it is (i) undesirable for its bearers; (ii) a title to special treatment; and (iii) a valid excuse for normally "criticisable" behavior" ([6], p.61). Health and disease are purely descriptive terms, which refer to organism function. The central functions of this disease account are survival and reproduction. Therefore, Boorse understands the concept of disease in terms of functionalism, which is a theory in which disease is described in terms of specific functions that are typically found in members of a given species [9]. Thus, Boorse endorses the account given by [10] on normality, which is defined as a function in accordance with its design, claiming that the main idea of this statement is that "normal" means "natural". Boorse assumes the idea of a natural design and claims that the crucial element in it is the notion of a natural function. He defines disease in terms of dysfunction and it turns to be defined as the disturbance physical (in case of physical disease) and mental (in case of mental disease) functions of the species. Disease is defined as a deviation from the natural functional organization of the species. The core of Boorse argument is that health within medical theory is value-free, that it is descriptively definable. Consequentially disease also is descriptively definable – disease is value-free. Illness in opposite comprises negatively evaluated connotations derived from disease diagnosis. One of the main implications of it is that one may have a disease (Boorse gives homosexuality as an example) without being said to be ill. Wakefield, in the other hand, attempts to escape from the charge of an abusive classification regarding homosexuality, advocating the addition of a harm requirement to the failure of the reproductive function. According to Wakefield, the equation between lowered fertility and longevity with harm fails to account for cases in which reduced fertility does not cause real harm and cases constituted by many harmful conditions that are clear cases of disorder without implying reduced fertility or longevity for the person affected by the disorder.

5 [11] reviews the notion of disease defined only from abnormality (defining characteristic) and argues that the presence of disturbance per si cannot be regarded as disease. Rather, in physical terms, disease refers to the quantitative rather than qualitative aspect of the disturbance. Disease is characterized by the former. Scadding suggests that it is crucial to observe whether or not the investigated abnormality placed the individual at a 'biological disadvantage' to establish disease diagnosis. However, Scadding does not provide a clear definition of 'biological disadvantage', what exactly it means.

3. The account claimed by him as correct, consists in combining the second account with a value component. As a result, one is only said to be disordered when some mechanism fails to perform the specific function it was designed to and when the failure of the mechanism causes real harm for the person affected.

Then, dysfunction is conceptualized as the failure of the physical and mental mechanisms to perform their natural functions – what they were designed to perform. Phobia for example consists in the failure of the fear response function, which exists to help a person to avoid danger ([5], p. 383). Phobia therefore constitutes a disorder on this field.

Starting by [2] approach, it is possible to state that, although these researchers do not claim the existence of a specific neural damage that can justify the ADHD under a fundamentalist biological base, they place an argument that constitutes the second path of the already mentioned biological matrix, keeping the medication dimension to the problems shown by "Hyperactive" children in school. The question could be solved regarding ADHD's biological basis if it would not be possible to verify in a study done by MTA Cooperative Group, taken off the "Archivos Generales de Psiquiatria" from 1999, number 56 2.10831086 that was also published by the American Academy of Pediatrics (AAP) – specifically by a sub committee set to investigate attention deficit and hyperactivity, that researchers have shown that in 38% of the cases drugs were not effective (apud [13]).

But, right at this point, analyzing statistic numbers, once it is possible to see a considerable percentage of people that have used medication with no efficient results, it brings up the need of a new question: "regarding this particular disturbance, what can other fields, which do not regard the biological basis of ADHD, bring as a contribution to the pertinent treatment for this complaint"? It is once more ultimate to say that regarding the large number of alternatives, the present article target means to analyze the possible contributions of the psychoanalysis field related to the subject in place.

To start, as argued by [14], studies on attention - deficit hyperactivity disorder (ADHD) "have been showing that children with this syndrome present an increased risk to develop other psychiatric disturbances during childhood, or in their adolescence or even at adult age" (p. 7[7]). Thus, Psychoanalysis literature does not question the legitimacy of the real configurations on diagnosis about attention deficit/hyperactivity frames treated on clinics that actually show the real and serious difficulty of these children regarding attention and soon difficulties involving memory, acknowledgement, and, because of that, also with intelligence. "Phenomenology is real: there are children with memory, attention, learning, language and psychomotor problems" ([13], p.5[8]). Regarding attention, and, consequently

6 [12] concerned with the validity of mental illnesss argues that Scadding defines illness not aetiologically - in causal terms - but by its consequences since that 'biological disadvantage' is the effect rather than the cause of the abnormality. Then Kendell endorses the concept of 'biological disadvantage' of Scadding and argues that although Scadding avoided elaborating on what he meant by biological disadvantage, presumably it applied to mental illness, it must embrace both increased mortality and reduced fertility. Kendell claims it on the grounds that fertility is very important biologically speaking and death is the most important consequence of the disease. And supported by great number of researches whose findings suggest that reduction in the fertility and an increased risk of death are features shared by at least some of the conditions commonly thought of as mental illnesses, including for example schizophrenia

7 Translated from the Portuguese.

memory: children who "forget" too much, who are extremely distracted, unorganized, with unstable thinking, impatient, who do not stand a question with no answer and neither can shortly support a question made to them. Children who are insistent, but this insistence is deeply articulated with the great difficulty they have on being annoyed, because regarding persistence, it does not take place on children who come to the specialized professional with a attention disorder and hyperactivity diagnosis. Those are children who are too aggressive, who heat their classmates, kick chairs and tables, and have a very hard time to follow the rules and stand the established limits of the school polices they are in, precluding their living in this particular situation because of their lack of social interaction.

In terms of "knowledge" and, consequently, "intelligence", it is not deniable how often children under hyperactivity diagnosis show up facing ups and downs, a real suffering time because of "organization and practices issues as well as because of their lack of learning at school or even because of their miss comprehension on how to deal or set their interpersonal relation with people and objects" ([13], p.4[9]). Even though, as stated by [13], it is possible to argue against the extreme and exclusive rational-logic dimension that modernity has placed on "intelligence", and claim the psychoanalytic version "that intelligence includes logic without being reduced to it" ([13], p.4[10]), it is not deniable the ups and downs as well as the suffering that these ADHD diagnosis children who come to the professionals face during their learning activities. These children experience such ups and downs and suffering in relation to the competences moored on the rational-logic operations and thoughts, presenting, thus, a deep difficulty on learning language and math.

But, if in one hand, psychoanalysis does not deny this sad reality, on the other one, we will to underline, in this article, that in accordance to what was stated by [13], we can find the phenomenology described above in "children who 'supposedly' fit to what researchers call 'lack of social interaction'" (p.5[11]). Along with this author, we want to place the following question: "would it be the lack of social interaction a consequence of the syndrome itself or would this lack of social interaction just a signal of the main point in this etiology that happened to these children?" (p.5[12]).

2. What can psychoanalysis say and contribute on the symptoms of inattention and hyperactivity approach?

Aiming to answer the question brought up in the end of the last section: "would it be the lack of social interaction a consequence of the syndrome itself or would this lack of social interaction just a signal of the main point in this etiology that happened to these children?"

8 Translated from the Portuguese.

9 Translated from the Portuguese.

10 Translated from the Portuguese.

11 Translated from the Portuguese.

12 Translated from the Portuguese.

([13], p.5[13]), we argument that, even though the phenomenology concerning this frame of diagnosis on Attention - Deficit Hyperactivity Disorder is true, as mentioned a while ago, is true, it is possible to find, in the psychoanalytic theory, a good contribution to the theme, in the sense that such theory puts its mark on the cause and not on the manifestations of the phenomenon placed on the symptom's dimension, in our case, on the area of symptoms regarding inattention and hyperactivity, not antedating, and not being allow to antedate this last dimension (a symptomatic dimension regarding phenomenology).

But, another question resulting directly from the one before, becomes relevant: the question, based on a psychoanalytic point of view, about the mentioned cause, regarding Attention - Deficit Hyperactivity Disorder. To answer such a question, the path chosen starts at the sign of a aforesaid requirement, done by Freud, on privileging the etiology and not the symptomatology to construct a diagnosis, and, thereafter, the direction of the treatment. It was also a lacanian request: "impel the diagnosis effort away beyond the phenomenon classification of a symptomatology" ([15], p.64), moving the question about symptomatic manifestation towards, according to the individual's position in his or hers fantasies. Why pointing it here? It is relevant to say that to psychoanalysis, fantasy comes, structurally, to rediscover the puzzle of the desire of the "Other "[14], the point that is missing on this Other, that touches the inconsistency of his knowledge which the child has to face in order to be grabbed out of the endless and evil circuit of a demand between the individual and the maternal Other, where the Other is raised in a place of omnipotence.

However, such meeting always traumatic[15], but structural, and, therefore, necessary, between the child and the aforesaid puzzle of the desire of the Other which intervenes, by the operational entre of the father, in the relation between mother and offspring, put on the place of the imaginary phallus, can fail. It can fail even in a non radical way, as in cases like psychotic structures, but in the sense of cases, as for example, cases which configure ADHD, of the mentioned phantasmatic coverage of the enigmatic character show by the desire of the Other, causing in this palming operation of the hiatus in his knowledge, an excessive idealization of such knowledge.

Palming takes place once the traumatic alluded meeting between child and the inconsistent Other, even though, is structural and necessary, it is also unbearable and, as said, a source of extreme anguish. Taking this direction, the axiomatic consistency of fantasy by covering the unbearable "unknown", presents itself as a safe place, even being source of mistake and, paradoxically, of suffering. And the dimension of an excessively idealized father, which paradigm is the father of Hamlet, in Shakespeare's tragedy: a father "all love and comprehension", who, even though, does not know "everything", because "everything" is structurally impossible, knows a lot, introduces consequences inside the dimension of the desirable act of the infant, which includes the act of learning, that, somehow, requires attention, mem-

13 Translated from the Portuguese.

14 Other: a symbolic place to which the subject directly drives its questions and where he/she search answers and guarantees. The notion of Other will be brought up in details, and, because of that, more explicit information will be given along the text.

15 Just as a fast comment, this is the meaning of trauma in Freud's Psychoanalysis with Lacan.

ory, discipline and other categories shown along the present article. In these configurations, it is frequently seen, an unstopping curiosity, although, paradoxically, it does not occur, in the learning process.

In acoordance with [16] and [17], such excessive and insistent child's questions look forward to argue about the issue on the desire of the Other which, even though, it lays on a structural place filled by the mother, the father, the teacher, the psychiatrist, the psychoanalyst, etc., it is the Other of the language: "He tells me this, but what is it that he wants?" ([16], p.203). The aforesaid paradox of the unstopping curiosity happens exactly because does not exist, in these frames, the break that slows down this curiosity, whose the first matrix is the curiosity that takes the place early in early childhood. It happens during the endless "why's" time, when the sexual themes are highlighted, even if such curiosities are not restricted to it. [18] underlined the importance of the structural sexual inhibition in terms of a break to slow down the unstopping infant sexual curiosity in order to access cognitive development, in the sense of turning these sexual interests, that in early ages are in the top of the list, into the interest to learn. From this point on, when it happens in a "normal" way, it was not out of the blue that reading and writing start at the incidences of latency period, in which a certain "calm" captures the place of the unstopping sexual curiosity. By reading Freud, it is visible that such breaks over the intense sexual curiosity, expressed by endless "Why's" from infants, is caused by the crash between the child and the structural impossible "knowledge" introduced by the enigma's dimension, during the infant investigations.

But if Freud talks about "Why's", restricting them to the dimension of sexual curiosity, [16] says that the endless "Why's" regards to a curiosity that touches the incomprehensible, so, the inconsistency on the Other's knowledge, which sex and death, but not just these two, by excellence, are witnesses. Based on Freud and Lacan psychoanalytic approach, it is the question of the puzzle of the desire of the Other, introduced by the traumatic meeting with the point that is missing on his knowledge, that can be seen in children's unstopping sexual curiosity that Freud discusses. Thus, according to a psychoanalytic literature, the child, facing the impossible knowledge that touches the incomprehensible, therefore, the real[16]of the castration, does not goes on with his/hers endless "why's". Children's efforts end up in a certain retreat when they face their investigations that, at this point, are, mainly, sexual. Such retreating is necessary to canalize the individual's interests to other things and give them access to the cognitive development.

According to [19], the impossible of the knowledge regarding the missing point on the knowledge of the Other introduces the inconsistency on the Other: the Other does not know everything. This inconsistency is introduced by sustaining the puzzle, by keeping the questions instead of supplying the answers to the child's "why's". Such approach, which has a

16 Real, in Freud's and Lacan's psychoanalysis means a distinct notion of reality. Real points toward to what makes no sense; toward what resists and escapes to all and any attempt of symbolization, toward the inconsistency (in the logical sense of the term: here the reference is the Gödel theorem) on the Other's knowledge, to the missing object between the significant and the significance, to the puzzle of the desire of the Other, that the subject veils with fantasy. This puzzle of the desire of the Other happens by the incidence of the father function: the incidence of the father operating a distance between the mother and the offspring. Enlightened by psychoanalysis, it is possible to state that to face the dimension of real is the way out to the act of desire. It must be included in this dimension: the act of learning.

Freudian matrix, which introduces the fundamental dimensions of the inconsistency on the Other's knowledge, in the access to learning, suggests to us the need of a precision over the knowledge of the Other, given that on the one hand, it is notorious and largely accepted that the transference, namely the supposition of the knowledge in the Other, it is a condition to the learning process to take place.

According to [19], [20], in one side, institutes the Other as a place of supposition of knowledge. But, in the other side, he places the missing point of the knowledge of the Other, a point that touches the impossible of the real and once supported at the act, opens possibilities, included the possibility of learning, the main interests of this discussion. So, it is possible to figure that the Other is structurally the place of supposition of knowledge, based on the paradigm of supposition of knowledge in Socrates by Alcibiades in the Plato's *Banquet* [21]. But the knowledge is not all, because the Other of knowledge is castrated. The Other does not know everything. The Other's castration concerns to an opaque spot in his knowledge. The missing point on the knowledge of the Other introduces the subject's always traumatic meeting with the puzzle of desire of the Other that launches the separation operation which is one of the two operations of the subject's constitution in the fields of the Other [16] and [17]. But such approach overpasses the limit of the current article. The missing point found in the Other appears in gaps, inside blanks on the Other's discourse. Those blanks are resistant to the glue effect: *what would be the reason that the adult Other tells me that?* [16]. The desire of the Other is beyond or above what the Other says just as what the child understands as a meaning.

At this point, it is important to say that, according to [22], the question does not consists on not supplying the child with the explanations that he/she is investigating and that is required by the unstopping curiosity. The problem is that the educator's trammel ends up in some positions that obstruct the invention of a missing knowledge coming from the redial "not-known". Such positions move from one extreme to the other, or totally denying any explanation to the child, somehow, treating the sexual issue as a taboo, leaving the child in a complete state of emptiness, or giving excessive explanations, leaving to the child the chance to get to know too much, without the possibility of keeping the missing point of knowledge which would stimulate a kind of "going ahead" that, regarding the cognitive level, manifests itself in the act of learning. In this idealizing educating position regarding to want to explain "everything", it is not considered that, as already said, even when there is a real wish for this "everything", it is structurally impossible, once no exposition will be clarifying enough. But, even though, as already pointed out as well, the "knowing too much" does not ends up unpunished.

[19] argues that although knowledge and knowing are not the same thing. so, here, what really matters is to privilege that there is no any possibility to get out of the excess of embarrassment got from the demand of material to be learn if there is an excess of embarrassment caused by the missing point on the knowledge of the Other regarding to the truth that the educator Other does not know everything. It is important to say that the knowledge Lacan talks about, is an unconscious one. So, the possibility of appeasing the excess of embarrassment felt by the infant that faces the puzzle of the desire of the Other - a puzzle quite fre-

quently found on the frames of ADHD - and the following possibility of the learning act and of the joy feeling that comes from the learning process, only takes place by the missing meeting with the inconsistency on the Other [20] which is introduced by his enigmatic desire.

Still, moored at [19], it is a good time to point out something that was already mentioned, namely, the aforesaid structural inhibition of the sexual curiosity on children can be read on the always traumatic meeting between the child and the hiatus on the knowledge of the Other. As a corollary, it is found as a legitimate possibility of this approach: the possibility to read the relation of structural sexual inhibition and the access to the cognitive development based on the relation between the missing meeting with the inconsistent knowledge in the Other and the learning act. Such approach is a legitimate possibility, in the sense that the sustainability, before the hiding of the missing point on the knowledge of the Other[17], causes the repositioning of the subject facing the Ideal. Ideal that, according to [23] and [24], as already said, hides the hiatus on the knowledge of the Other. Such repositioning of the child facing the Other extremely idealized, holds a subversive relation of child and knowledge on the learning process. Such subversion provides an open space to the learning process avoiding the individual's tiring of modeling regarding to an idealizing dimension that can be found on the educational fields, giving the possibility to the subject to put something of his/hers own, inside what they have gotten from the Other.

After this analysis, it is possible to go back to the question based on a psychoanalytic view, regarding the cause of Attention - Deficit Hyperactivity Disorder, and to argue that the cause of these symptoms (inattention and hyperactivity) is paradoxically the cause of the desire of the Other[18] hided, imaginatively covered because the extreme anguish launched by the object of desire of the Other. About this point, the following sentence: "He tells me that, but what is it that he wants?", is paradigmatic. This is just one more way of saying that in regard to the cause of the symptoms of inattention and hyperactivity which obstructs the act of learning and the joy feeling that comes from the learning process, we can, frequently, verify an excessive embarrassment of the subject that suffers from these symptoms with the opacity point on the knowledge of the Other closely connected to his enigmatic desire.

So, the question: "would it be the lack of social interaction a consequence of the syndrome itself or would this lack of social interaction just a signal of the main point in this etiology that happened to these children?" ([13], p.5[19]), that is taken as a starting point to present what psychoanalysis could say and contribute to the approaches on symptoms on inattention and hyperactivity, gives the possibility to argue against the organicit literature that ends up unaware of the possibilities, proof by psychoanalytic treatment on children, that the symptoms on these same children[20], "can represent the truth of the family couple" ([25], p. 369[21]). Somehow, Lacan, once placing this statement, means that "what can be seen as symp-

17 The hiding operation of the hiatus of knowledge of the Other, is what we can see, frequently, on ADHD frames.

18 It is important to point out that the mentioned cause of the enigmatic desire of the Other comes from an object that is missing, as an specific object. So, it is unbearable and a source of extreme anguish, and, because of that, this cause regards to the register of real, a register of the impossible of knowing. In addition, this cause is hided and imaginatively covered. In other words, the subject, in its fantasy, gives an imaginary consistency to this object.

19 Translated from the Portuguese.

tomatic in these children depends on questions that devastate the couple or the mother. These are unconscious questions, which refer to what they do not know about themselves" ([26][22]). But, even if the symptoms are kept this way, the children do not receive peacefully the difficulties of the family couple. Actually, children have their own fault in the symptoms, in a sense that the symptoms take place by "the way they capture what was transmitted and how they invest on their own symptoms, all the gains they get from it and it will constitute the resistance in which they will grab on their illness" ([27] apud [26][23]).

Regarding the investments a subject does on the symptom and the gains that he/she gets from this symptomatic dimension, we can say that this point reaches the question referred to the subject's responsibility over the symptom which he/she suffers and complains about. And, according to this point, even though the present section is concerned with the psychoanalytic view of symptoms on inattention and hyperactivity, regarding a logical rhythm which is privileged in this article and not a chronological one, again, it is impossible to stay away from doing an insertion in the psychiatric scenario to present a psychoanalytic counterpoint, aiming to walk forward on this theme.

Inside psychiatry, [28-31], determined to demonstrate the legitimacy of the medical concept of mental illness and to find a criteria of diagnosis, effective enough to avoid mean practices and abusive mistakes on the psychiatric practices that anti-psychiatrists had the merit of denouncing, introduces an approach of mental illness in which the demarcation criterion to distinguish the latter from other conditions is based in a medical and philosophic interface. Fulford argues that the mentioned demarcation criterion is the failure of intentions and actions, and, because of that, a breakdown of rationality is seen. "He claims that one who is mentally ill fails to act harmoniously with his intention and suffers from that" ([32], p.397): "I did not want to have done it, I do not know why I did it".

Fulford's arguments, that have found large acceptance on the british psychiatric and philosophical fields, extracts direct consequences from delicate and polemic questions that belong to mental health, as for example, the exemption of the responsibility over the mental illness which reaches what we are talking about. According to his argument, exemption of responsibility is a logical consequence and an ethical practice on the mental illness once the subject that suffers from mental illness presents a disturbance on the harmony between intention and action. After Fulford, the debate about exemption of responsibility by psychiatry and philosophy got fresh air, because he got the ward of introducing an intermediate approach inside the rusted and foreseeable debate between orthodox psychiatrists and anti-psychiatrists, welcoming the criticisms from the anti-psychiatrists, but sustaining the legitimacy of the medical concept of mental illness. The question would be answered if we agree with the approach developed by Fulford on intention restricted by the imaginary dimension, that is

20 In accordance to psychoanalytic approach on ADD, lack of attention and hyperactivity are symptoms presented by the children.

21 Translated from the Portuguese.

22 Translated from the Portuguese.

23 Translated from the Portuguese.

conscious, apprehensible, cognitive and transparent in itself. However, the question gets even more complicated, once psychoanalysis has a lot more to say about the intentional acts and the responsibility.

Freud's literature left us a great legacy about intention. [33], [34] and [35] are texts in which Freud, in a rigorous and beautiful way, shows the core of the intention in the unconscious registers. Not in the registers of a transparent knowledge to itself which is the conscious knowledge, but of an unconscious knowledge that does not aware of itself. Even though it is not aware of itself, the subject suffers from its effects. Since the beginning of his clinical experiences, Freud sustained an ethical position regarding unconscious intention and responsibility of his hysterical patients' psychopathologies. Freud strongly remarks this point when he says, for example, at the end of Elizabeth's case [36] that the psychopathology depends much less on personal and volunteer factors than we could think of. With the Freud's subversive cuts on all and any of literature about an alleged rationality of actions based on a conscious intention, and, because of that, about a psychopathology based on a breakdown of racionality, and, consequently, on a failure of this intention [32], "we can effectively call the argument given by Fulford, namely, the failure of intention in mental illness, into question since Freud's argument implies the presence of an unconscious intention" ([32], p.401). Freud's ethical position regarding this issue becomes radical when he tells that *the ego is no longer the master in its own house.*

However, it is important to restrict the elements of intention and responsibility in this discussion, to the symptoms of inattention and hyperactivity. In this sense, it is a good time to say that, based on Psychoanalysis, a possibility is opened to the "inattentive", "hyperactive" and, consequently, "failed" subject, regarding the categories involved with the act of learning and the joy of the learning process by the time when these subjects are taken to a psychoanalytic treatment and can be heard. Being heard does not mean been taken as a "victim", because it is also part of Freud's legacy, the ethical warning of not exempting the subject who claims suffering of any kind from his personal responsibility. Listening to the "inattentive", "hyperactive" subject means put him/her to work, in the sense that they must question themselves by the jouissance[24] dimension related to this "failure". Questioning the "failed" subject about his/hers responsibility over their complains about things that do not work out well, even if the "failed" subject claims that the causes of symptoms on inattention and hyperactivity show something that is beyond his intention, a fail of the conscious intention which ends up pointing toward, even if implicitly, a pure psychic determinism, as suggested by Fulford's approach.

According to [37], something new on Psychoanalysis was, actually, indicating that at the exact point in which the individual seems tight to a certain determinism, being forced to act by a natural force, it is recognizable the dimension of an agreement that points toward the range of the subject's responsibility over the complains and his/hers wish to place themselves as the "victim". By the "failure", jouissance is put into question, moving the individu-

24 Jouissance: psychoanalytic notion closely articulated to the problematic satisfactions as, for example, satisfaction on an act that would cause contempt (being a "failed" at school), or still feel nausea for an act that would bring pleasure)

al towards an extraction of satisfaction in this dissatisfaction. And, actually, because of that, "different from a real determination, in which the individual cannot be blamed by its acts, the jouissance is what allows the talk about a responsible individual" ([37], p.37[25]).

Thus, questioning the range of "inattentive" and "hyperactive" subject's responsibility, even though there can be the claim possibility related to objective conditions which would exempt him from his personal responsibility, it means questioning the satisfaction issue extracted by this subject in the referred position of "inattentive", "hyperactive" and, consequently, "failed" and "victim". Talking about the subject's range of responsibility over the "failure", it means that the cause of the "failure", differently from the cause in place at the game played at the fields of natural sciences, is a cause under an agreement [37]. Even if the psychoanalytic approach does not eliminate the psychic determinism dimension on the structural submission of the subject's desire to the desire of the Other [16] and[17], there is a possibility of questioning, in a certain level, this submission, in a sense that there can be a range of freedom introduced by the desire in its separating function, and not just a pure psychic determinism ([16] and [17]).

Such range of freedom introduced by the desire in its separating function gives the possibility to the subject to put something of his/hers own, inside what they have gotten from the Other. As in Goethe: "what you have inherited from your parents, conquer it, to make it yours", this idea is just possible by making holes in the axiomatic consistency of the fantasy and the trimming of the Ideal, once they are structural and, thus, can not the eliminated. Thus, questioning the subject's range of responsibility on its symptoms of inattention and hyperactivity means working over their position by facing the hiatus of knowledge in the Other, walking towards changing the subject's position when facing the opacity point in the knowledge of the Other, in a way that the subject is not deceived by fantasy and can question this Ideal dimension, when excessive, submitting to it minimally and sustaining his/hers differences.

Also, this article aims to say that to privilege during the treatment of inattention and hyperactivity symptoms the subject's position does not imply, in any ways, by psychoanalysis, the disregards of the ethical accomplishment of people, places and entities able to occupy the Ideal's place. If it would be the case, once the subject under psychoanalytic treatment, inevitably, puts the psychoanalyst in this place, for the psychoanalyst it would not be any interest to not respond from this place of the Ideal, assuming that what really matters is the subject's position facing the Ideal. The psychoanalyst would believes that he or she have nothing to do with it. Actually, it's the opposite, the psychoanalyst must not respond from this place of the Ideal. He must hear the subject inside its difference, sustaining the questioning about what he or she desires, instead of guide a kind of orthopedic and modeling practice, supported by a "a priori" knowledge that assesses and says what is the "best" for the patient. The psychoanalyst must question about the range of responsibility over what the subject apparently does not have: "I did not want to be inattentive, but there is something stronger that goes beyond my intention and makes me failed". He must support a non totalizing di-

25 Translated from the Portuguese.

mension of knowledge in the Other facing the demand of an knowledge that was idealized in this psychoanalyst, by the subject.

3. Final considerations

After placing this short psychoanalytic approach on symptoms in general terms, we will argue that in relation to the symptoms of lack of attention and hyperactivity, it is possible to see, quite often, on these frames, a regular fail on the father function that operates a necessary distance between mother and offspring. According to [38] apud [26][26]), the agitation comes to be put in the spot of this missing distance, on these frames, between the offspring and the mother. "Such distance searchs a way to refuse the maternal demands that are made to them" ([38] apud [26][27]). As soon as this distance is missed, the puzzle of the desire of the maternal "Other" can be the source of the extrem anguish, introducing symptomatic effects in many different dimensions, including in attention, which is the main interest of this article.

Taking this direction, it is important to say that, as stated by [13], "this syndrome enlightened by neurosis is not a mystery, not even a recent discovery" (p. 6[28]). It suggests the problematic dimension given by the "new symptoms", because when these called "new symptoms" are analyzed closely, they do not look as new. Such problematic dimension seems based in a logical thought that intends to privilege the reference given by Frege in his text: *On the sense and the reference*.

[39] in this classic article, states the need of the construction of a relation, in equal terms, between two names that refer to the same thing – even if they have a different sense, it means, different presentation ways. To picture it, the famous example given by Frege: "Morning Star" and "Evening Star" would be names which would place an equal relation, in the sense that even being a different sign with a different sense, they refer to the same thing, as be pointed out, *Venus*. Thus, equality concerns to reference. So, even if Frege is stuck in this article with the logical equality, it shows the difference concerned with the dimension of "something else" in the place of the "same thing". This logical indication of the difference as concerning not to a difference in the sense, but to the reference, is actually what seems to be in place in the logic of the natural sciences, which have the intension to be always launching a "something else" to be called a radical new precept that seems to be moored on the reference empire.

This logical writing about difference also interests psychoanalysis. However, as argues [40], [41] gives more contributions to this logical reference issue. He goes one step ahead in this particular question saying that the reference is always phallic[29], once this dimension of "the same thing" or "the something else" assigned by Frege veils another dimension, namely the

26 Translated from the Portuguese.

27 Translated from the Portuguese.

28 Translated from the Portuguese

dimension of real[30] of the structure. Therefore, as by this new step given by Lacan, it became possible to think that the "other thing" regarding the logical approach by Frege is a mask of the real, an apparent difference, even if this same difference, that can be veiled, points toward to the real, in the sense that the phallus is the "presence of the missing real object" ([42], p.45[31]). Therefore, from this precise and rigorous contribution of Lacan, it is legitimate to question this new radical precept on contemporary symptoms, such as, our object of analyses in this article: Attention Deficit Disorder / Hyperactivity.

That is exactly why, in psychoanalysis, Attention - Deficit Hyperactivity Disorder (ADHD), cannot be taken as a diagnosis. However, it does not exclude, as argued, the psychoanalysis contribution on this symptomatic configuration, but not restricted to the new presentation ways assumed by this question, but facing the real of the structure veiled and pointing at the same time by the reference, namely, the excessive idealization of the father's knowledge in the place of the Other, and, because of that, a fail in the incidence of the father function that operates a necessary distance between the mother and the offspring.

Author details

Crístia Rosineiri Gonçalves Lopes Corrêa[1,2*]

Address all correspondence to: crlopes2001@yahoo.com.br

1 University of Warwick, UK

2 Universidade Federal de Juiz de Fora, Brasil

References

[1] American Psychiatric Association – Referência Rápida aos Critérios Diagnósticos do DSM-IV-TR. Porto Alegre: Artmed; 2003.

[2] Barkley, R. (org.). Transtorno de Déficit de Atenção/Hiperatividade: Manual para Diagnóstico e Tratamento. Porto Alegre: Artmed; 2008.

[3] Kohn, A. (1989 november) Suffer the restless children. Atlantic Monthly 1989; November 90-100

29 Phallus, in psychoanalyses, is the support of something that is missing. Therefore, the phallic reference, in psychoanalyses, covers the radical missing of the object between the significant and the significance. But, even veiling it, it also points toward to the real of the missing object, in the sense that the phallus is the "presence of the missing real object" ([42], p. 45, translated from the Portuguese).

30 See footnote number 16.

31 Translated from the Portuguese.

[4] Timimi, S. A critique of the international consensus statement on ADHD. Clinical Child and Family Psychology Review 2004;7 59-63.

[5] Wakefield, J. The Concept of Mental Disorder: On the Boundary Between Biological Facts and Social Values. American Psychologist 1992;47(3) 373-88.

[6] Boorse, C. On the Distinction Between Disease and Illness. Philosophy and Public Affairs 1975;5(Fall): 49-68.

[7] Boorse, C. Wright on Functions. The Philosophical Review 1976; 85(1) 70-86.

[8] Boorse, C. (1982). What a Theory of Mental Health Should be. In: Psychiatry and Ethics, ed. Edwards, R. B. (Buffalo: Prometheus Books).

[9] Sadler, J. Z. & Agich, G. J. Disease, Functions, Values and Psychiatric Classification. Philosophy, Psychiatry and Psychology 1996;2(3) 219-31.

[10] King, C. D. 1945. The Meaning of Normal. Journal of Biology and Medicine 1945;17 493-94.

[11] Scadding, J. G. 1967. Diagnosis: The Clinician and the Computer. Lancet 1967; (ii) 877-82.

[12] Kendell, R. E. 1975. The Concept of Disease and its Implication for Psychiatry. British Journal of Psychiatry 1975;127 305-15.

[13] Jerusalinsky, A. 2006 Diagnóstico de Déficit de Atenção e Hiperatividade, o que Pode Dizer a Psicanálise? http://www.appoa.com.br/noticia_detalhe.php?noticiaid=35&PHPSESSID=bbea8b84cbb064f37445c2e5eac26344. (Accessed 2011)

[14] Rohde, L. A. et. al. Transtorno de Déficit de Atenção/Hiperatividade. Revista Brasileira de Psiquiatria 2000;22(II) 7-11.

[15] Leguil, F. (1989). Mais-além dos fenômenos. In: Lacan, J. et. al. A querela dos diagnósticos. Rio de janeiro: Jorge Zahar Editor, p.60-69.

[16] Lacan, J. O Seminário, livro 11: Os quatro conceitos fundamentais da psicanálise. Rio de Janeiro: Jorge Zahar editora; 1964.

[17] Lacan, J. Posição do inconsciente. In: Escritos. Rio de Janeiro: Jorge Zahar editora; 1964.

[18] Freud, S. (1905) Três Ensaios sobre a Teoria da Sexualidade. In S. Freud, Edição standard brasileira das obras psicológicas completas de Sigmund Freud. Rio de Janeiro: Imago; 1905. p. 118-229 .

[19] Corrêa, C.R.G.L. A Inauguração da Interlocução entre a Educação e a Psicanálise no Brasil: Arthur Ramos, Transferência Ideal e Autoridade. Revista Psicologia USP (USP) 2011;22 (4) 789-811.

[20] Lacan, J. O Seminário, livro 20: Mais, ainda. Rio de Janeiro: Jorge Zahar editora; 1972-73.

[21] Platão. O banquete. Rio de Janeiro: Bertrand Brasil; 1995.

[22] Corrêa, C.R.G.L. & Pinheiro, G. S.. Período de latência e tempo para compreender nas aprendizagens. Revista Psicologia em Estudo (Maringá), forthcoming.

[23] Lacan, J. O Seminário, livro 10: A angústia. Rio de Janeiro: Jorge Zahar editora; 1962-63.

[24] Lacan, J. Proposição sobre o analista da escola. In: Escritos. Rio de Janeiro: Jorge Zahar editora; 1967.

[25] Lacan, J. Nota sobre a Criança. In: Outros Escritos. Rio de Janeiro: Jorge Zahar editora; 1969.

[26] Bonfim, F. Hiperatividade e Psicanálise. Available at: http://flaviabonfim.blogspot.com.br/2011/03/hiperatividade.html (accessed 2011)

[27] Lamy, M Resistência e desejo do analista: quem trabalha na psicanálise com crianças. In: Ford-Da, nº 4/5, Rio de Janeiro: Revinter; 1998.

[28] Fulford, K. W. M. Moral theory and medical practice. Cambridge: Cambridge University Press; 1989.

[29] Fulford, K. W. M. Psychiatry, compulsory treatment and the value based model of mental illness. In: Almond. B. (ed.). Introducing Applied Ethics. Oxford: Blackwell; 1995.

[30] Fulford, K. W. M. Chapter 9. In: Bloch, S.; Chodoff, P.;Green, S. (orgs.). Psychiatric ethics. Oxford: Oxford University Press; 1999.

[31] Fulford, K. W. M. & Dickenson, D. In two minds: A casebook of psychiatric ethics. Oxford: Oxford University Press; 2001.

[32] Corrêa, C.R.G.L. Suicide in Anti-Psychiatry and in Pychoanalysis. Revista Latinoamericana de Psicopatologia Fundamental 2008;11(3) 392-404.

[33] Freud, S. The interpretation of dreams. Hertfordshire: Wordsworth Editions; 1900.

[34] Freud, S. The psychopathology of everyday life. The Standard Edition of the complete psychological works of Sigmund Freud., Vol.6. Vintage The Hogarth Press; 1901.

[35] Freud, S. (1905). The joke and its relation to the unconscious. London: Penguin Books.

[36] Freud, S. (1893-95). Caso Elisabeth Von R. In S. Freud, Edição standard brasileira das obras psicológicas completas de Sigmund Freud. Rio de Janeiro: Imago; 1893-95. p. 118-229.

[37] Freire, A.B. & Lustoza, A.Z. (2005). A psicanálise entre a razão e a causa. Pulsional Revista de Psicanálise, 2005 XVIII(184), 28-39.

[38] Roy, M. ROY, M. "Tiens-toi tranquille!" In: "La petite girafe" Paris, Ed. Agalma, revue de la Diagonale francophone du Cereda 2003; 18.

[39] Frege, G. Sobre o Sentido e a Referência. In Lógica e Filosofia da Linguagem. São Paulo: Cultrix; 1892.

[40] Corrêa, C.R.G.L. Transmissão e Castração. Revista Cadernos de Psicanálise (SPCRJ) 2011;27(30) 233-261.

[41] Lacan, J. O Seminário, livro 18: De um Discurso que não Fosse Semblante. Rio de Janeiro: Jorge Zahar editora; 1971.

[42] Becker, P. A Economia do Gozo. Rio de Janeiro: Garamond; 2010.

Chapter 17

Quality in Delivery of Mental Health Services

Mary Ditton

Additional information is available at the end of the chapter

1. Introduction

Quality in health care is an important contemporary topic because of rising consumer expectations of health care amidst constrained health care budgets. Historically mental health services have been the poor cousin of health care services generally, and acute health care services specifically. At this time when quality in health care is occupying more space in the health care literature, it is opportune to review what inroads have been made as far as quality in delivery of mental health services.

This chapter will examine the movement towards quality management in health care and explore the divide between quality in general health care and quality in mental health care. After this, what is considered quality in delivery of mental health services is discussed and finally the challenges to quality in delivery of mental health services and methods to overcome these challenges are analysed.

2. The significance of mental illness and the costs of mental health services

The Australian national survey of mental health and wellbeing [1] estimated that 45% of Australians aged between 16-85 years, that is, approximately seven million people, experienced a mental disorder over the course of their lifetimes, while 20% experienced symptoms of a mental disorder over the the twelve months prior to the survey. Anxiety, affective and substance disorders were experienced by fourteen per cent, six per cent and five per cent of the population respectively [2].

Mental disorders are ranked third after cancer and cardiovascular in the major morbidity and mortality disease burden groupings and mental disorders account for thirteen per cent of the total disease burden in Australia [3]. Generally the disease burden for mental illness is non-fatal with only 718 deaths in 2008, excluding suicide and dementia, due to mental illness as a result of substance abuse involving alcohol and heroin [4]. The most mental illness burden is attributable to anxiety, depression, alcohol abuse and personality disorders.

Mental health services are complex and the Australian government has divided them into groupings based on point of contact for treatment [5]. Mental health services consist of mental health-related care in general practice, in emergency departments, community mental health-related care and hospital outpatient services, ambulatory equivalent mental health-related admitted patient care, Medicare–subsidised psychiatrist and allied health services, admitted patient mental health-related care, residential mental health care, mental health-related supported accommodation assitance program services, support services for people with a psychiatric disability, and specialised mental health care facilities. These groupings are arranged from simple to more highly specialised treatment and accommodation arrangements and usually reflect the increasing seriousness of the impact of the mental health-related problem on the individual, family and society.

Australia spent $5.8 billion on mental health-related services during 2008-2009 [6] and this equated to an avergae annual increase of 4.8% on expenditures over the previous four years. The total health care expenditure in the same peiod was $112.8 billion with health taking up 9.0% of Australia's Gross Domestic Product (GDP). If mental disease accounts for thirteen per cent of the burden of disease [3], then it is clear that mental health services are not getting a proportional allocation of Australian government health funds.

The United States spends far more proportionally on health care than most Western countries, spending 16 % of GDP in 2008-2009 amounting to $2.5 trillion [7]. Mental health care costs contribute to about 100million in 2003 which amounted to 6.2% to these health care costs [8]. Apart from these direct costs the indirect costs of mental illness are incurred through reduced labour supply, public income support payments, reduced educational attainment and costs associated with other consequences such as incarceration or homelessness. In fact serious mental illness is associated with the annual loss of earnings totally $193.2 billion [9].

In 2007-2009, an average annual 3.2 million or 8.6% of young adults aged 18-26years had some health ecpenses for mental disorders. Direct medical spending to treat mental health disorders in young adults totally $6.5 billion as a average annual cost [10]. According to the latest US Agency for Healthcare Research and Quality [11] treating America's youth for mental disorders is the most expensive children's medical condition, costing almost 9 billion dollars in 2006.

Mental ill health is the largest single cause of disability in the UK accounting for 23% of the overal burden of disease, compared to 16% each for cancer and cardiovascular disease [12]. In 2010-2011, The United Kingdom spent £118.58billion on health care which was approximately 8.7% of GDP [13], whereas the cost to the NHS for mental health problems and social care costs was over £21 billion a year. The economic and social costs of mental health problems is estimated at £102.5 billion in 2009-2010 [12]. However the majority of the impact of mental illness falls on patients and their families and amounts to costing about £53.6 billion a year. Mental health conditions tend to affect people early in life with 50% of cases occuring before 14 years.

3. Movement towards quality management in health care

Much of the work on quality in health services rests on the influential framework of Donabedian [14] which focused on three components: the structure of the services, the process of provider-client intervention, and the outcomes of the care. This is a comprehensive framework including public services and resources, providers, and consumers. However the movement towards quality management in health care only got traction some time after Donabedian's framework because of the public concern about the apalling low level of quality of health care.

Patient safety started in 1999, when the Institute of Medicine, an agency of the US Government, issued the report, called *To Err is Human*, [15] which stated the following:

- Between 44,000 and 98,000 Americans die each year from preventable medical errors in hospitals alone. That does not account for those who die from medical errors outside the hospital.
- It is the equivalent to the number of people who would die if a jumbo jet crashed every day, and all its passengers died.
- Medical errors cause more deaths than motor vehicle accidents, breast cancer or AIDS.

The report highlighted the reasons the reported deaths happened, calling for a shift from placing blame, to finding the reasons and fixing them. It further outlined a series of proactive recommendations for doing just that. The recommendations [15] from *To Err is human* were:

1. Establishing a national focus to create leadership research tools and protocols to enhance the knowledge base about safety.
2. Identifying and learning from errors through immediate and strong mandatory reporting efforts as well as the encouragement of voluntary efforts both with the aims of making sure the system continues to be made safer for patients
3. Raising standards and expectations for improvements in safety through the action of oversight organisations group purchasers and professional groups.
4. Creating safety systems inside health care organisations through the implementation of safe practices at the delivery level. This level is the ultimate target of all recommendations.

The health care system is complex and Australia has developed a National Health Performance Framework that has been modified since its inception in 1999. The safety of the health care system has been defined by the National Health Performance Framework as the avoidance or reduction to acceptable limits of actual or potential harm from health care management or the environment in which health care is delivered. Similar definitions are in wide use in Australia. For instance, the former Australian Council for Safety and Quality in Health Care, replaced by the Australian Commission for Safety and Quality in Health Care, defined safety as the degree to which potential risk and unintended results are avoided or minimised. The WHO [16] developed a Conceptual Framework for the International Classification of Patient Safety in 2009 so that all health systems are talking the same language about patient safety.

Quality is a multi-faceted concept which can be defined in different ways. At a broad level, quality reflects the extent to which health care service or product produces a desired outcome [17]. At a more detailed level, the National Health Performance Framework views quality as a guiding principle in assessing how well the health system is performing in its mission to improve the health of Australians. The Framework's dimensions for the assessment of health system performance include effective, responsive, continuous, sustainable, efficiency, accessible and safety, all considered relevant to the quality of health care services. In its report Charting the Safety and Quality of Healthcare in Australia [18], the former Australian Council for Safety and Quality in Health Care presented information relating to the dimensions of effectiveness, appropriateness, accessibility and responsiveness as relevant to the quality of health care in Australia. Complementing the information on those dimensions was information on safety, and also on equity, or the degree to which all Australians could benefit equally from health care service provision.

Improvements in quality and safety in health care are important because of rising cost of health care and an increasing concern of poor value for money. In spite of the money and effort spent on health care, poor quality and variations in practice, medical errors, injuries and lack of accountability abound [19]. It is a dilemma to know where to begin because performance of health systems and quality of health care are often used interchangeably although there are differences. Nolte [20] differentiates between quality and performance by referring to the definition of 'quality' proposed by the US Institute of Medicine which is the 'degree to which health services for individuals and populations increase the likelihood of desired health outcomes and are consistent with current professional knowledge' (1992) and definition of 'performance' suggested by Girard and Minvielle [21] as a broader, multidimensional concept that also includes dimensions of equity and efficiency.

In Australia there are National Standards for Mental Health Services [22] designed for implementation in public, private and NGO mental health services. The Australian Council of Healthcare Standards [23] is an independent not-for profit organisation. The Council reviews health care organisations and mental health services for perfomance, assessment and accreditation. It aims to provide a framework through the Evaluation and Quality Improvement Program (EQuIP) to deliver consumer centered services focussing on the continuum of care by providing systematic external peer review. The Council reviews mental health services against the National Standards for Mental Health Services and EQuIP.

The Standards within the National Standards for Mental Health Services [22] are:

1. Rights and Responsibilities
2. Safety
3. Consumer and Carer participation
4. Diversity Responsiveness
5. Promotion and Prevention
6. Consumers
7. Carers
8. Governance Leaderships and Management
9. Integration
10. Delivery of Care

Accreditation by meeting standards is a minimum requirement for mental healath services and healthcare generally. Accreditation is a static achievement that needs to be renewed every few years. In Australia 93% of public (that is 637 hospitals) and private hospitals (that is, 543 hospitals) are accreditated with either the Australian Council of Healthcare Standards, Business Excellence Australia, Quality Improvement Council or the certification of the International Organisaiton for Standardisation's 9000 quality family [24]. Funding sources demand that health care facilities are accreditated. Being an accrediated hospital has not stopped significant problems in patient care.

The drive towards improvements in health care is faced with many challenges, such as countless providers and patients, institutions and communities, and incremental policies driven by experience and evidence rather than theory and ideology. Health system performance measurement and reporting are part of a global move for accountability and transparency in health services and consumer engagement and contribute to the continuous quality improvement cycle [25]. Quality improvements can occur without measurements, for example clinical guidelines, peer review, videoing consultations, and patient interviews, however, measurement is important to quality improvement.

Kohn, Corrigan, and Donaldson [26] consider health care to be a highly complex and tightly coupled system which are the types of systems that are more prone to accidents. In complex systems one component of the system may interact with multiple of the components of the system in sometimes unexpected and invisible ways. Complex systems are both specialised and interdependent. Coupling is a dynamic term that means there is no slack or buffer between two items. Large systems that are tightly coupled have more time dependent processes and sequences that are more fixed. Tight coupling contributes to more accidents because things unravel quickly and prevent errors from being intercepted or prevent speedy recovery from an event.

Latent errors or system failures, according to [26] pose the greatest threat to safety in a complex system because they lead to operator errors. They are failures built into the system and present long before the active error. Latent errors are difficult for people working in the system to see because they may be hidden in computers or layers of management and people become accustomed to working around the problems.

Such is the difficulty of getting health care right, [17] regard health care as characterised by islands of excellence in a sea of mediocrity. So there has been a steady increase in emphasis on continuous improvement of health care rather than leaving safety and quality to a static achievement of accreditation once every three or four years.

The approach to improvement in quality has been systemic and systematic, with the consumer perspective. Runciman, Merry, and Walton [17] have seven dimensions of quality in health care that involve:

1. Access
2. Efficacy and effectiveness
3. Efficiency
4. Safety
5. Timeliness
6. Acceptability
7. Appropriateness

These 7 dimensions operate at world international; state/national; organisational; team; clinicians; and patient levels.

Within health care there has been changes about safety and quality and managing problems that arise. Vincent [27] summarised these in a table:.

Past	Future
Fear of reprisal common	Generally blame free reporting
Individual scapegoat	Individuals held to account where justified
Disparate Adverse Errors databases	All database coordinated
Staff do not always hear the outcome of investigation	Regular feedback to frontline staff
Individual training dominant	Team based training more common
Attention focuses on individual error	Systems approach to hazards and prevention
Short term Fixing of problems	Emphasis on sustained risk management
Many Adverse Drug Events (ADE) regarded as one offs	Potential for replication of similar ADE recognised
Lessons from adverse events seen as primarily for the team concerned	Recognition that lessons may be relevant to others
Individual learning	Team based learning and developing of non-technical skills

Table 1. Changes in Approach to Safety and Quality in Healthcare

Indicators are explicitly defined and measurable items referrring to structures processes and outcomes of care [28]. Developing and applying quality indicators is not easy. There are three types of indicators. Activity indicators measure how frequently an event happens. Quality indicators infer a judgement about the quality of care provided. Performance indicators are statistical devices for monitoring performance without any necessary inference about quality. Indicators do not provide answers but they are indicative of problems or may indicate good quality care.

Continuous improvement is a planned way of improving care for patients and carers step by step over time. The reflective cycle for continuous improvement follows the Plan-Do-Study-Act model of improvement of Langley, Nolan and Nolan [29]. Ferlie and Shortell [30] in discussing quality improvement in healthcare in the UK and the US, said that there are four essential core properties that must operate at individual, group/team, organisational and larger system level. These four essential core properties are: 1) leadership at all levels; 2) a pervasive culture that supports learning throughout the care process; 3) an emphasis on effective teams; and 4) greater use of information technologies for both continuous improvement work and external accountability.

3.1. Consumers and health care

Consumers' expectations of health care are certainly different from those of health care providers. As far as quality in health care is concerned [31] study found that consumers described quality in health care in terms of access to care, having competent and skilled providers, and recieving the proper treatment. From nurses consumers in the same study wanted caring behaviour, competence and skill, good communication and discussion about their condition.

Engagement with consumers in health care can occur at three levels [32]. Informed choice is the role that is most actively promoted for consumers and within that sphere shared decision making is promoted to a lesser extent. The two other levels of engagement are less often encouraged and supported. These levels deal with consumers as active participants in their care (co-producer role) and consumers evaluating the care they recieve (evaluator role).

Although speaking of health care reform in the United States, [33] take the importance of consumer engagement further and state that 'engaging consumers is an essential component to health care reform'. Consumers of higher education, higher incomes, no health insurance and good self reported health have higher levels of engagement with their health care. Interestingly, people with depression have lower levels of consumer engagement in thie health care. Hibbard and Cunningham's research shows that consumers that are more involved in their health care have lower levels of unmet needs and recieve greater support from health care providers.

The value of consumers to the drive for quality in health care is part of incorporating the end user into the design and delivery of health services. Health services however are not like industrial complexes. [34] compares the quality improvement strategies in reshaping Toyota with quality attempts in health care. The problems for health care lie in providers not being able to anticipate that quality improvements will result in higher prices, increased volume or decreased costs.

[35] take the point about consumer involvement in quality in health care further and delineate five principles to improve the effectiveness and impact of public reporting in health care quality. These principles are:

1. Consumers must be convinced that health care quality problems are real that they have serious consequences and that quality can and should be improved.
2. Quality reporting must be standardised and universal
3. Consumers are given quality information that is relevnt and easy to use
4. Dissemination of quality information is improved
5. Purchasers reward quality improvements and providers create the information and organisational infrastructure to achieve them

Certainly, [36] were cautious about consumer led quality improvements in health care. These authors stressed that greater clarity has to be obtained about what consumer satisfaction with the health system (not just health treatments) is all about.

The UK has moved forward with consumer engagment in healthcare with the Care Quality Commission forming in 2009 as the independent regulator of health and adult social care in England. It replaced the Healthcare Commission, Commission of Social Care and the Mental Health Act Commission. Every year the Commission conducts patient surveys on the NHS Trusts throughout England. The survey is based on the Picker Patient Experience Questionnaire that has been validated across five countries in, Germany, Sweden, Switzerland and, Germany as well as the UK [37]. The dimensions of patients' experience in the Picker adult in-patient questionnaire are:

- Information and education
- Coordination of care
- Physical comfort
- Emotional support
- Respect fro patient preference
- Involvement of family and friends
- Continuity and transition
- Overall impression

The commission's patients survey compares the responses with previous years results and these reports are given back to the specific Trusts with comparison data from other Trusts. Trusts are expected to improve their performace because the Commission is the regulator and has a Judgement Framework and an Enforcement Policy.

Consumer input to improving mental health services has been recognised in the US with the development of the Consumer-Orientated Mental Health Report Card which is organised around prevention, access, appropriateness, and outcomes with consumer satisfaction included under each area and each of these areas is associated with indicators. The Mental Health Statistics Improvement Program [38] has taken the Consumer Orientated Mental Health Report Card and it has been adapted for use with inpatients, youths and families and translated into French and Spanish.

In an era when there is sustained political rhetoric in favour of consumers involvement in health care [39] the media's interest in critical contributions is limited, preferring to sensationalise issues as part of the production of news [40]. However the media does have a legitimate role to play in health policy and health services within democratic societies.

The media is significant in the relationship between health decision makers and patients, providing a communication channel influencing the demand and supply of medical treatments sometimes reagardless of evidence of effectivenss, providing a voice for whistleblowers and a platform for patient safety disasters to be exposed. In reporting medical errors the media often takes the simple approach of blaming those doctors who fail to live up to some imaged medical paragon [41], and missing the failures of the poorly developed and managed health systems that allow these mistakes to occur.

There have been situations in which the media has been involved in the ongoing exposure of major health system failures such as Dr Jayant Patel in Queensland [42], Sydney Morning Herald's coverage of the Cambelltown and Camden hospitals problems in 2004 [43], and The Guardian's report of Professor Bolsin's account of events at the Bristol Royal Infirmary in the 1990s [44]. Even the power of the press however, finds it hard to make much of an impression against the medical fraternity which is backed by the government. Most system failures take years to pass through the process of breakdown in patient safety, whistleblower, public exposure with the press, public inquiry and recommendations, to implementation of changes within the health system and system improvements to prevent the same problems occuring again. Not only does this process take years there are many casualities on the way as patients suffer and whistleblowers lose their jobs and their reputation's suffer as was the case with Professor Bolsin.

In 2002 the World Health Assembly urged the WHO and Member states to pay the closest possible attention to patient safety and in 2004 launched the WHO patient safety program with Sir Liam Donaldson as the WHO envoy for patient safety. The WHO definition of patient safety is simply: the absence of preventable harm to a patient during the process of healthcare. WHO patient safety has initiated two patient safety campaigns involving hand washing and a safety checklist to improve compliance with surgey standards and decrese complications.

One initiative of the WHO Patient Safety is Patients For Patient Safety (PFPS) [45]. Patient For Patient Safety (PFPS) is a collective voice of patients and consumers concerned about patient safety issues. This active process involves patients and consumers as partners in healthcare and operates in countries and globally.

4. The global burden of mental disorders

The global burden of mental disorders is considerable. The [46] reports that as many as 450 million people suffer from a mental or behavioural disorder, nearly 1 million people commit suicide every year, four of the six leading causes of years lived with disability are due to neuropsychiatric disorders (depression, alcohol-use disorders, schizophrenia,and bipolar disorder) and those suffering from a mental illness are also victims of human rights violations, stigma and discrimination both inside and outside public institutions. The gap between the need for treatment for mental disorders and resources available is greater in developing countries than in developed countries. In developed countries between 44% and 70% of patients with mental disorders do not recieve treatment, whereas in developing countries the treatment gap is close to 90%.

Disadvantages are accumulative in health and mental functioning is fundamentally connected to physical and social functioning and health outcomes. Depression is often associated with chronic physical illness and requires comprehensive treatment to achieve the best physical outcomes. The family bears the burden of a family member with mental illness but the extent of this burden is hard to quantify. Sometimes the stigma associated with mental illness extends to the family and causes isolation and discrimination.

Reputable sources such as the [46] report situations of mental patients being chained as a form of treatment. The New York Times in 2009 reported examples of abuse during psychatric treatment in Kings County Hospital [47]. The political abuse of psychiatry which is the misuse of psychiatric diagnoses and treatment to obstruct the human rights of individuals is well documented in a recent review by [48].

The huge treatment gap in mental health in developing countries requires innovative thinking rather than repeating the clinic or hospital based patient management by specialist mental health professionals as occurs in Western countries. Vikram Patel [49], a psychiatrist from the London School of Hygiene and Tropical Medicine, said that mental health care in developing countries needs to shift treatment to appropriately trained and supervised lay people. The precise model of care for mental health in developing countries depends greatly on the local health system factors and in particular the state of the general health system and the political commitment to public health [50]. A great deal has to be done about mental health advocacy and raising the priority of mental health with donor agencies.

There is a complex interaction between poverty and mental disorders. Mental disoders are costly in terms of treatment and loss of productivity. Other factors such as low educational levels, poor housing and malnutrition contribute to common mental disorders. Povery contributes to mental disoders and mental disorders contribute to poverty. Similarly, work education, violence and trauma are linked in a vicious cycle to mental disorders [46].

Traditionally underserved groups include those who are geographically remote, those of disadvantaged socioeconomically minorities, people with disabilities, women and indigenous people, lesbian gay and bisexual people and the aged. Developing mental health services to meet the needs of these diverse and underserved groups has recieved increasing attention both globally with the Nations for Mental Health [51] final report (2002) and nationally.

The important issue about meeting the mental health needs of traditionally underserved groups is that no one approach is going to satisfy the needs of these widely diverse populations. However as research is acculmulating about health needs for these populations then strategies can be developed to promote mental health, prevent mental illness and provide treatments for early recovery and prevention of long term disability.

5. Quality in delivery of mental health services

Health services that deal with mental illness have not be subjected to the same scrutiny as have health services that deal with physical illness. There are many reasons for this, not the least of which is the social stigma associated with mental illness. Patients in general health services who experience poor care have avenues to complain and have their complaints dealt with so that services can be improved. Patients in mental hospitals have the burden of social stigma to negotiate before complaining about poor care. Also, many general health services struggle to provide culturally competent services. For sufferers of mental illness the cultural differences between providers and mental health consumers can be a barrier to treatment and recovery.

In 2002 President Bush in the United States set up the New Freedom Commission on Mental Health because the health system should treat people with mental illness with the same urgecny as a physical illness. Bush identified three barriers to excelelnt care for those with mental illness: the stigma attached to mental illness, unfair limits that stems from inadequate health insurance, and a fragmented system for delivering services. The Commission [52] produced its report and tied its 19 recommendations to six goals: building greater understanding among Americans that mental health is essential to overall health; mental health care is consumer and family driven; eliminating disparities in the delivery of mental health services; early mental health screening assessment and referral to services is common practice; excellent mental health care is delivered and research is accellerated; and technology is used to access mental helth care and information.

Goal 1

Building greater understanding among Americans that mental health is essential to overall health;

Recommendations

1. Advance and implement a national campaign to reduce the stigma of seeking care and a national strategy for suicide prevention
2. Address mental heatlh with the same urgency as physical health

Goal 2

Mental health care is consumer and family driven;

Recommendations

1. Develop an individualised plan of care for every adult with the sersious mental illness and for every child with a serious emotional disturbance
2. Involve consumers and families fully in orienting the mental health system towards recovery
3. Align relevant federal programs to improve access and accountability for mental health services
4. Create a comprehensive state mental health plan
5. Protect and enhance the rights of people with mental illnesses

Goal 3

Eliminating disparities in the delivery of mental health services;

Recommendations

1. Improve access to high-quality care that is culturally competent
2. Imporve access to high-quality care in rural and geographically remote areas

Goal 4

Early mental health screening assessment and referral to sesrvices is common practice;

Recommendations

1. Promote the mental health of young children
2. Improve and expand school mental health programs
3. Screen for co-existing mental and substance use disorders and link with integrated treatment strategies
4. Screen for mental disorders in primary health care, across the life span, and connect to treatment and supports

Goal 5

Excellent mental health care is delivered and research is accellerated;

Recommendations

1. Accelerate research to promote recovery and resilience and ultimately to cure and prevent mental illness
2. Advance evidence based practices using dissemination and demonstration projects and create public-private partnerships to guide implementation

3. Improve and expand the workforce providing evidence-based mental health services
4. Develop the knowledge base in four understudied areas: disparities in mental health care; long term effects of medication, trauma and acute care

Goal 6

Technology is used to access mental helth care and information

Recommendations

1. Use health and information technology to improve access to and coordination of mental health care, especially in remote areas and underserved populations
2. Develop and implement integrated electronic health record and personal health information systems

The recommendations of the Commision may not have been fully implemented [53]. It has been, however, a line drawn in the sand stating that the system to provide services to treat mental illness was a shambles and that the mental health maze had to be transformed starting from community perceptions of mental health and eradicating stigma associated with mental illness treatment. The stigma of mental illness is pervasive. It limits people seeking care, influences the provider-client realtionship and impacts public funding of mental heatlh services.

Simpson and House [54] conducted a systematic review about involving users in the delivery and evaluation of mental health services. They found that the few comparative studies of users' involvement that have been published indicate that involving users as employees, trainers, or researchers has no negative effect on services and may be of benefit.

The priority towards a limited biomedical model of medical training rather than an expanded bio-psycho-social model greatly impedes recognition of mental illness in primary health care. The biomedical model of medical education is reflective of the philosophy of medicine [55] and is reflective also of the dominance of physical acute health care in public funding of health services and health research.

In spite of the dominance of acute physical health care there have been some inroads made with mental health services as an area of academic interest. Although there are many journals that deal with mental health issues a smaller number deal specifically with mental health services. In 2006 the journal Mental Health Services Research combined with the journal of Administration and Policy in Mental Health under the editorship of Leonard Bickman to form Springer's Administration and Policy in Mental Health and Mental Health Services Research journal. Another Springer journal dealing with mental health services is the Journal of Behavioural Health Services and Research (JBHS&R).

6. Challenges to quality in delivery of mental health services and methods to overcome them

There is an argument that the escalating cost of mental health services reflects the need for these services. There is also the argument that the cost of mental health services reflects an imbalance in budgetary allocation between treatment services and mental health promotion and mental illlness prevention programmes. Knapp McDaid and Parsonage [56] presented an imposing economic argument for mental health prevention programs having a beneficial impact on the economic burden of mental illness over the long term. Fifteen interventions were modelled. These were a range of health interventions across the life span that had evidence of their effectiveness. Some of these interventions were: health visiting to reduce post natal depression, school based interventions to reduce bullying, school based social and emotional programmes to prevent conduct problems in childhood, early detection of psychosis, workplace screening for depression, population-level suicide awareness training and intervention, and tackling medically unexplained symptoms. The estimated economic payoffs per £ of expenditure from each of the models varied, with the sector involved such as the NHS, other public sector bodies and non- public sector impacts and the timeline considered such as short term (in the first year) through to long term (year 6 and beyond). Early intervention for conduct disorders had a 7.89 return on inventment per £1 expenditure, suicide training course provided to all GPs had a 43.99 return and workplace health promotion programmes had a 9.69 return on investment.

Preventive mental health strategies targeting families, schools, and workplaces could be developed to promote healthy child development, resilience, personal achievement, healthy relationships, career satisfaction, work-life balance and healthy ageing. Secondary specialist care in mental health services is urban and needs to be expanded to meet the needs of traditionally underserviced consumers.

The major challenge to quality in delivery of mental health services is the adequate diagnosis and treatment of mental illness in the primary care sector of health care services. After analysing the results of the US National Comorbidity Survey Replication study, [57] found that most people with mental disorders in the United States remained either untreated or poorly treated. They recommended that interventions were needed that enhanced treatment initiation and quality.

The internet as a menal health intervention and prevention tool is being explored more as adults and youth integrate the internet into their daily lives. Obviously the use of the internet can eliminate the stigma associated with accessing a real world facility and therapist. Emental health service is defined as including 'all forms of electronic mental health services delivered over the internet, ranging from informational and educational products to direct services offered by professionals' [58].

Ybarra and Easton [59] provide an assessment of internet-based mental health interventions and were generally cautious but positive about their effectiveness. Transferring face to face mental health interventions to the internet presents challenges that have to be addressed. The health literacy level of the traditionally underserved populations which is usually lower than advantaged populations is an important issue that needs consideration, the marketing and presentation of mental health interventions will be in competition with the glitz of abundant websites, and the training of mental health professionals will have to change to encompass a different skill base that will be necessary for operating on the internet.

7. Conclusion

Mental health services lag behind general health services as far as seeking to develop a quality management approach to the delivery of mental health services. The global burden of mental illness on individuals, families, communities and the public purse is enormous and is beginning to be recognised. Funding for mental health services is not proportional to the impact of mental illness. The disconnenct between the need for mental health services and the services available is related to the prioritisation of physical acute health over mental health. This prioritisation relfects cultural attitudes towards mental illness which generally encompass various forms of stigmatisation of mental illness and ostrasizing the people and sometimes the families of those who suffer mental illness.

There are some signs globally and nationally that reducing the stigma of mental illness will lessen the burden of mental illness. As part of a social justice approach, there are movements to be more inclusive towards the mental health needs of the traditionally underserved populations. Prevention programs may have a beneficial impact on the economic burden of mental illness. The integration of the internet into the lives of so many people means that it may provide an opportunity for greater accessibility of more people to innovative mental health interventions.

Author details

Mary Ditton

University of New England, Australia

References

[1] Australian Bureau of Statistics (ABS). National survey of mental health and wellbeing: summary of results, Australia, 2007. ABS cat. No. 4326.0. Canberra: ABS. 2008.

[2] Department of Health and Ageing (DoHA). The mental health of Australians 2: Report on the 2007 national survey of mental health and wellbeing. Canberra: DoHA. 2009.

[3] Begg, S., Vos, T., Barker, B., Stevenson, C., Stanley, L. & Lopez. A. The burden of disease and injury in Australia, 2003. AIHW cat. No. PHE 82. Canberra: Australian Institute of Health and Welfare. 2007.

[4] Australian Bureau of Statistics (ABS). Causes of death, Australia, 2008. ABS cat. No. 4102.0. Canberra: ABS. 2010.

[5] Australian Institute of Health and Welfare (AIHW). Mental Health Services in Australia, Key Concepts. 2010. Available from http://www.mhsa.aihw.gov.au/key-concepts/ (accessed 30 June 2012).

[6] Australian Institute of Health and Welfare (AIHW). (2010). Health expenditure Australia 2008-2009. 2010. Health and welfare expenditure series no. 42. Cat. No. HWE 51. Canberra: AIHW.

[7] US Government Spending. Spending. 2012. Available from http://www.usgovernmentspending.com/year_spending_2003Usbn_13bsln_10 (accessed 1 July 2012).

[8] Mark TL, Levit KR, Coffey RM, McKusick DR, Harwood HJ, King EC, Bouchery E, Genuardi JS, Vandivort-Warren, R, Buck JA, Ryan K: National Expenditures for Mental Health Services and Substance Abuse Treatment, 1993–2003: SAMHSA Publication SMA 07-4227. Rockville, Md, Substance Abuse and Mental Health Services Administration, 2007.

[9] Insel, TR. Assessing economic costs of serious mental illness. American J of Psychiatry 2008; 165(6) 663-665.

[10] Medical Expenditure Panel Survey (MEPS). Statistical Brief #358. 2012. Available from: http://www.meps.ahrq/mepsweb/data_stats/PubResults_Details_jsp?pt=Statistical Brief&opt=2&id=1041 (accessed 14 June 2012).

[11] Agency for Healthcare Research and Quality (AHRQ) (2009). Mental Disorders are the Most Expensive Children's Medical Conditions. 2009. Available from: http://www.healthcare411.ahrq.gov/featureAudio.aspx?id=956 (accessed 20 July 2012).

[12] Centre for Mental Health. Promotion, prevention and early intervention dramatically cut the costs of mental ill health, says government-sponsored report. 2011. Available from http://www.centreformentalhealth.org.uk/news/2011_promotion_prevention_cut_costs.aspx (accessed 24 June 2012).

[13] HM Treatury. Public Expenditure Statistical Analyses 2010. Available from http://www.hm-treasury.gov.uk/pespub_economic_functional_analysis.html (accessed on 5 July 2012).

[14] Donabedian, A. The Quality of Care: How can it be assessed? JAMA 1988; 260(12) 1743-1748.

[15] Institute of Medicine (IOM). Medicare: A strategy for quality assurance. Vol 2. Washington, DC: National Academy Press. 1990.

[16] WHO. "More than words: Conceptual Framework for the International Classification of Patient Safety Version 1.1 Technical Report January 2009." Available from http://www.who.int/patientsafety/implementation/taxonomy/icps_technical_report_en.pdf (accessed 7 July 2012).

[17] Runciman, B., Merry, A., Walton, M. Safety and Ethics in healthcare: A guide to getting it right. Aldershot: Ashgate. 2007

[18] Health Policy Analysis. Charting the Safety and Quality of Healthcare in Australia 2004. Report for the former Australian Council for Safety and Quality in Health Care, 29 july 2004.

[19] Kelly, E., Hurst, J. Health Care Quality Indicators Project - Conceptual Framework. Working Paper No 23 (March 2006). Paris: OECD. Available from : www.oecd.org/els/health/workingpapers (accessed 29 September 2010).

[20] Nolte, E. International benchmarking of health care quality: A review of the literature. A Rand publication and London School of Hygiene and Tropical Medicine. 2010.

[21] Girard, JF., Minvielle, E. Summary and Conclusions. In: Smith P. (ed.) Measuring up: Improving Health System performance in OECD countries Paris: OECD Publishing; 2002. p337-350.

[22] National Standards for Mental Health Services (NSMHS) 2010. Available from http://www.health.gov.au/internet/main/publishing.nsf/content/mental-pubs-n-servst10 (accessed 24 June 2012).

[23] Australian Council of Healthcare Standards (ACHS). EQuIP. 2012. Available from http://www.achs.org.au/equip5/ (accessed 10 July 2012).

[24] Australian Institute of Health and Welfare (AIHW). Hospital performance Accreditation. 2012. Available from http://www.aihw.gov.au/haag09-10hospital-performance-accreditation/ (accessed 30 June 2012).

[25] Hurst, J. Performance measurement and improvement in OECD health systems: Overview of issues and challenges. In: Smith P. (ed.) Measuring Up: Improving health system performance in OECD countries. Paris: OECD Publishing; 2002. p35-54.

[26] Kohn, LT. Corrigan, JM. Donaldson, M.S. To err is Human: building a safer health care system. Washington: National Academy Press; 2000.

[27] Vincent, C., editor. Patient Safety. Chichester: BMJ Books; 2010.

[28] McGlynn, EA. Asch, SM. Developing a clinical performance measure. Am J of Prev Med. 1998; 14 14-21.

[29] Langley, GJ., Nolan, KM., Nolan, TW. The Foundation of Improvement. Silver Spring: API publishing; 1992.

[30] Ferlie, EB. Shortell, SM. Improving the quality of health care in the United Kingdom and the United States: A framework for change. Milbank Quaterly 2001; 79(2) 281-315.

[31] Oermann, MH. Consumers' Descriptions of Quality health Care. Nursing Care Quality 1999; 14(1): 47-55.

[32] Hibbard, JH. Engaging Health Care Comsumers in Quality of Care. Medical Care 2003; 41(1) Supplement, 161-171.

[33] Hibbard, JH., Cunningham, P.J. How engaged are Consumers in their Health and Health Care and Why does it matter. Research Briefs 2008; Oct. No. 8 1-10.

[34] Coyle, MJ. No Toyotas in health care: why medical care has not evolved to meet patients' needs. Health Affairs 2001; Nov-Dec; 20(6) 44-56.

[35] Shaller, D., Sofaer, S., Findlay, SD., Hibbard, JH., Lanksy, D., Delbanco, S. Consumers and Quality-Driven Health Care: A Call to Action. Health Affairs 2003; 22(2) 95-101.

[36] Bleich, SN., Özaltin, E., Murray, CJL. How does satisfaction with health care system relate to patient experience? Bulletin of World Health Organisation 2009; 87 271-278.

[37] Jenkinson, C., Coulter, A., Ruster, S. The Picker Patient Experience Questionnaire: development and validation using data from in-patient surveys in five countries. International Journal for Quality in Healthcare 2002; 14(5) 353-358.

[38] Mental Health Statistics Improvement Program (MHSIP). MHSIPon line 2012. Available from http://www.mhsip.org/toolkit/index.html (accessed 30 June 2012).

[39] Milewa, T. Valentine, J. and Calnan, M. Managerialism and Active Citizenship in Britain's Reformed Health Service: Power and Community in the Era of Decentralisation. Social Sciencce and Medicine 1998; 47(4) 507-517.

[40] Benelli, E. The role of the media in steering public opinion on healthcare issues. Health Policy 2003; 63 179-186.

[41] Jackson, T. How the media reports medical errrors. BMJ 2001; 322(7285) 562.

[42] Dunbar, J. Reddy, P. May, S. Deadly healthcare. Brisbane: Australian Academic Press; 2011.

[43] Sydney Morning Herald. System Failure. 2004 Available from http://www.smh.com.au/specials/hospitals/index.html (accessed on 15 July 2012).

[44] Guardian. Whistle-blower accuses NHS. 2001 Available from http://www.guardian.co.uk/society/2001/jul/18/1 (accessed on 18 July 2012).

[45] WHO. Patient Safety. 2012. Available from http://www.who.int/patientsafety/patients_for_patient/en/ (accessed on 15 July 2012).

[46] WHO. Investing in mental health. 2003 Geneva. Available from http://www/who.int/mental_health/media/investing_mnh.pdf (accessed on 30 June 2012).

[47] New York Times (2009) Abuse is found at Psychaitric Unit run by the City. 2009 Available from http://www.nytimes.com/2009/02/06/myregion/06kings.html (accessed 2 June 2012).

[48] Van Voren, R. Political Abuse of Psychaitry. Schizophrenia Bulletin 2010; 36(1) 33-35.

[49] Patel, V. Mental Health in the Developing World: Time for innovative thinking. Science and Development network. 2008 Available from http://www.scidev.net/en/opinions/mental-health-in-the-developing-world-time-for-inn.html (accessed 18 July 2012).

[50] Patel, V. And Cohen A. Mental health services in primary care in developing countries. World Psychiatry 2003; 2(3) 163-164.

[51] WHO 2002. Nations for Mental Health Final report. 2002 Available from http://www.who.int/mental_health/media/en/400.pdf (accessed 15 June 2012).

[52] New Freedom Commision on Mental Health. Achieving the Promise: Transforming Mental Health Care in America. 2003. Available from http://www.nami.org/Content/NavigationMenu/inform_yourself/About_Public_Policy/New_Freedom_Commission/Default1169.htm (accessed 28 June 2012).

[53] Iglehart, JK. The Mental Health Maze and the Call for Transformation. New England Journal of Medicine 2004; 350(5) 507-514.

[54] Simpson, EL., House, AO. Involving users in the delivery and evaluation of mental health services: systematic review. BMJ 2002; 325, 30 November 1-5.

[55] Marcum, JA. An Introductory Philosophy of Medicine: Humanising Modern Medicine, US: Springer; 2008.

[56] Knapp, M. Mc Daid, D. & Parsonage, M. (2011). Mental health promotion and mental illness prevention: The economic case. London: Department of Health. Retrieved from: http://www.centreformentalhealth.org.uk/pdfs/Economic_case_for_promotion_and_prevention.pdf

[57] Wang PS., Lane, M., Olfson, M., Pincus, HA., Wells, KB., & Kessler, RC. Twelve-Month use of Mental Health Services in the United States. Arch Gen Psychiatry 2005; 62 629-640.

[58] Lambousis, E. Politis, A., Markidis, M. and Christodoulou, GN. Development and use of online mental health services in Greece. Journal of Telemedicine and Telecare, 2002; 8 51-52.

[59] Ybarra, ML. And Easton, WW. Internet-based mental health nterventions. Mental Health Services Research 2005; 7(2) 75-87.

Permissions

The contributors of this book come from diverse backgrounds, making this book a truly international effort. This book will bring forth new frontiers with its revolutionizing research information and detailed analysis of the nascent developments around the world.

We would like to thank Prof. Robert Woolfolk and Lesley Allen, for lending their expertise to make the book truly unique. They have played a crucial role in the development of this book. Without their invaluable contribution this book wouldn't have been possible. They have made vital efforts to compile up to date information on the varied aspects of this subject to make this book a valuable addition to the collection of many professionals and students.

This book was conceptualized with the vision of imparting up-to-date information and advanced data in this field. To ensure the same, a matchless editorial board was set up. Every individual on the board went through rigorous rounds of assessment to prove their worth. After which they invested a large part of their time researching and compiling the most relevant data for our readers. Conferences and sessions were held from time to time between the editorial board and the contributing authors to present the data in the most comprehensible form. The editorial team has worked tirelessly to provide valuable and valid information to help people across the globe.

Every chapter published in this book has been scrutinized by our experts. Their significance has been extensively debated. The topics covered herein carry significant findings which will fuel the growth of the discipline. They may even be implemented as practical applications or may be referred to as a beginning point for another development. Chapters in this book were first published by InTech; hereby published with permission under the Creative Commons Attribution License or equivalent.

The editorial board has been involved in producing this book since its inception. They have spent rigorous hours researching and exploring the diverse topics which have resulted in the successful publishing of this book. They have passed on their knowledge of decades through this book. To expedite this challenging task, the publisher supported the team at every step. A small team of assistant editors was also appointed to further simplify the editing procedure and attain best results for the readers.

Our editorial team has been hand-picked from every corner of the world. Their multi-ethnicity adds dynamic inputs to the discussions which result in innovative outcomes. These outcomes are then further discussed with the researchers and contributors who give their valuable feedback and opinion regarding the same. The feedback is then collaborated with the researches and they are edited in a comprehensive manner to aid the understanding of the subject.

Apart from the editorial board, the designing team has also invested a significant amount of their time in understanding the subject and creating the most relevant covers. They scrutinized every image to scout for the most suitable representation of the subject and create an appropriate cover for the book.

The publishing team has been involved in this book since its early stages. They were actively engaged in every process, be it collecting the data, connecting with the contributors or procuring relevant information. The team has been an ardent support to the editorial, designing and production team. Their endless efforts to recruit the best for this project, has resulted in the accomplishment of this book. They are a veteran in the field of academics and their pool of knowledge is as vast as their experience in printing. Their expertise and guidance has proved useful at every step. Their uncompromising quality standards have made this book an exceptional effort. Their encouragement from time to time has been an inspiration for everyone.

The publisher and the editorial board hope that this book will prove to be a valuable piece of knowledge for researchers, students, practitioners and scholars across the globe.

List of Contributors

John D. Matthews
Harvard Medical School, USA

Afusat Olanike Busari
University of Ibadan, Ibadan, Nigeria

Mohamed Dammak
Sfax, Tunisia

Maja Rus-Makovec
University Psychiatric Hospital Ljubljana & School of Medicine, University Ljubljana, Slovenia

Karin Sernec
University Psychiatric Hospital Ljubljana, Slovenia

Velko S. Rus
Department of Psychology, Faculty of Arts, University Ljubljana, Slovenia

Narong Maneeton and Benchalak Maneeton
Department of Psychiatry, Faculty of Medicine, Chiang Mai University, Thailand

Gregory Patrick Garvey
Quinnipiac University, Hamden, USA

Apu Chakraborty, Lance Patrick and Maria Lambri
University College London, UK

Lesley A. Allen and Robert L. Woolfolk
Department of Psychology, Princeton University, Princeton, NJ, USA

Sharon Lawn
Flinders Human Behaviour and Health Research Unit, Flinders University, Australia
Mental Health Carer, Adelaide, Australia

Jeannette Walsh, Margaret Springgay and Patricia Sutton
Mental Health Carer, Adelaide, Australia

Anne Barbara
Mental Health Carer, Adelaide, Australia
Central Adelaide Mental Health Directorate, Adelaide, Australia

Lawrence T. Lam
The School of Medicine Sydney, The University of Notre Dame, Sydney, Australia
Discipline of Paediatrics and Child Health, Sydney Medical School, The University of Sydney, Australia

Gatta Michela, Dal Zotto Lara and Battistella Pier Antonio
Woman and Child Department-University of Padua, Italy

Testa C. Paolo, Del Col Lara
Neuropsychiatric Unit of Child and Adolescent - ULSS Padua, Italy

Spoto Andrea
Department of General Psychology- University of Padua, Italy

De Sauma Maxim
Brent Centre For Young People, London, UK

Ashok Kumar Jainer and Bettahalasoor Somashekar
Coventry & Warwickshire Partnership NHS Trust, Coventry, UK

Rajkumar Kamatchi and Marek Marzanski
Coventry & Warwickshire Partnership NHS Trust, Coventry, UK
Warwick Medical School, Coventry, UK

Adeyi A. Adoga and Taiwo J. Obindo
Ewa Wojtyna and Agnieszka Wiszniewicz
Institute of Psychology, University of Silesia, Katowice, Poland

Arabinda N. Chowdhury
Northamptonshire Healthcare NHS Foundation Trust, Stuart Road Resource Centre, Corby, Institute of Psychiatry, Kolkata, India

Ranajit Mondal, Mrinal K Biswas and Arabinda Brahma
U. K. & Research Assistant, Institute of Psychiatry, Kolkata, India

Crístia Rosineiri Gonçalves Lopes Corrêa
University of Warwick, UK
Universidade Federal de Juiz de Fora, Brasil

Mary Ditton
University of New England, Australia